Manual of Surgical Infections

Manual of Surgical Infections

Sherwood L. Gorbach, M.D.

Professor of Medicine and Microbiology, Tufts University School of Medicine; Chief, Infectious Diseases Division, New England Medical Center Hospital, Boston

John G. Bartlett, M.D.

Professor of Medicine, Johns Hopkins University School of Medicine; Chief, Division of Infectious Diseases, Johns Hopkins Hospital, Baltimore

Ronald Lee Nichols, M.D.

Henderson Professor and Vice-Chairman, Department of Surgery, and Professor of Microbiology and Immunology, Tulane University School of Medicine; Attending Surgeon, Tulane University Hospital and Ambulatory Care Facility, and Charity Hospital of Louisiana, New Orleans

Little, Brown and Company
Boston/Toronto

First Edition

Library of Congress Catalog Card No. 83-82836

ISBN 0-316-32070-6

Printed in the United States of America

HAL

To our students, house officers, and colleagues who showed us what we know and what we don't know; and to our wives—Judy, Jean, and Elsa—who gave us the inspiration to write it down

Contents

Preface

If a surgeon from the last century were to be transported by a time warp to a modern operating room, he would no doubt be lost in the panoply of surgical instruments and electronic monitoring equipment. However, on venturing into the surgical wards this transplanted surgeon would be familiar with the clinical conditions of many of the patients, especially those with wound suppuration and sepsis. These infectious processes have an eternal character, spanning the centuries, overriding the advances in surgical technique. Since the sixteenth century when Ambroise Paré introduced revolutionary concepts of local care of gunshot injuries—by stopping the practice of pouring boiling oil into the wound—each advance has been accompanied by the hope, always unfulfilled, of eliminating surgical infections. Every development—the listerian principles, the advent of vaccines and immunizations, and most recently, the era of antimicrobial wonder drugs—has improved the outlook for surgical infection, but none has caused the problem to disappear. Indeed, the rates of infection and the outlook for survival with some conditions have not changed substantially in the past half-century. Infection remains a leading cause of morbidity and mortality in surgical patients.

This manual represents an effort to restate the traditional approaches to surgical infections, at the same time applying the latest developments in diagnosis, surgical management, and antimicrobial therapy. It is intended to be practical, readable, and, above all, helpful—what was called in ancient times a *vade mecum* (literally, go with me), to accompany the surgeon on rounds or in the office.

We have relied heavily on the recorded literature of surgical infection, but we have also added a measure of our own experience by evaluating the conventional wisdom and by stating our opinions in controversial areas. Above all, we emphasize that neither the surgical blade nor the antimicrobial drug can, in isolation, produce good results in surgical infection. The first principle is diagnosis, followed by an intelligent treatment plan that combines judicious surgical intervention with appropriate antimicrobial agents and physiologic support measures.

We are grateful to the many colleagues who read portions of the manuscript, contributing their sage advice and encouragement: Michael Barza, M.D., Allan W. Hackford, M.D., John M. Kellum, M.D., Edwin M. Meares, Jr., M.D., and Francis P. Tally, M.D. To David R. Snydman, M.D., we owe a special debt for reviewing the epidemiology sections and contributing the hepatitis section. We are also grateful to the many people who helped in the preparation of the manuscript, including Luci Aran, Allie Broadway, Mary Calderazzo, Joan Donoghue, Florence Hagins, Louise Kelly, Virginia Lindsey, and Jeffrey Smith. Our thanks also go to Tracy Scannell-Keating, who played an important role in putting the manuscript into its final form. The editors of Little, Brown showed great patience during the gestation period and helped us in many ways: Cynthia Baron and Jim Krosschell. While many people have contributed their talents to this endeavor, the authors accept the ultimate responsibility for its veracity.

S. L. G.
J. G. B.
R. L. N.

Manual of Surgical Infections

Notice. The indications and dosages of all drugs in this book have been recommended in the medical literature and conform to the practices of the general medical community. The medications described do not necessarily have specific approval by the Food and Drug Administration for use in the diseases and dosages for which they are recommended. The package insert for each drug should be consulted for use and dosage as approved by the FDA. Because standards for usage change, it is advisable to keep abreast of revised recommendations, particularly those concerning new drugs.

1 Initial Antimicrobial Therapy of Bacterial Infections

I. **General principles.** In the initial evaluation of a patient with suspected sepsis, three fundamental questions should be posed:

A. Is infection actually present? It must be remembered that noninfectious processes, such as collagen diseases and disseminated neoplasms, can simulate the clinical features of infection.

B. If infection is present, what is the likely type of pathogen—viral, bacterial, fungal, or protozoal?

C. If **bacterial** infection is suspected, what is the most appropriate antimicrobial agent(s)?

Viruses probably are responsible for the majority of mild infections. Of the potentially treatable infections, however, bacteria are the major pathogens.

II. **Guidelines for selecting antimicrobial drugs.** The selection of antimicrobial agents is obviously simplified when a specific pathogen and its susceptibility pattern are known (Table 1-1). In practice, however, immediate decision-making may be required before laboratory analyses are available, or it may be impossible to obtain reliable specimens for culture. For example, patients with diverticulitis must be treated without cultures, since the infected site cannot be sampled unless a laparotomy is performed.

When presumptive therapy is necessary, a rational selection of drugs can be made on the basis of **the most likely pathogen associated with a specific clinical setting.** In Table 1-2, likely causative agents according to site of infection are specified, in order of frequency, along with the antimicrobial recommendation for them. Several alternative regimens are listed, since certain variables can modify the initial selection of drugs, i.e., the Gram's stain findings, severity of the illness, concomitant infections at other sites, renal or hepatic insufficiency, a history of adverse reactions to antimicrobial drugs, and previous therapy. Although antimicrobial therapy is emphasized here, the need for additional forms of treatment such as surgical drainage and supportive measures should also be considered.

Finally, the limitations of this empiric format must be emphasized. Table 1-2 is simply a guide to the initial therapy of infections in which the causative agent has not been determined. This initial therapy should be supplemented by careful culture and Gram's stain of specimens. Changes must be made in the drug regimen on the basis of subsequent cultures and susceptibility reports, other diagnostic studies, or an inadequate clinical response. (More information is contained in the chapters dealing with each clinical entity. Specific drugs in each class and their dosages are found in Chap. 12.)

Specific Infections

I. Intraabdominal infections

A. **Intraabdominal sepsis** is caused by a variety of microorganisms that are determined by the organ involved and the source of the infecting inoculum. Bacteria derived from the bowel flora can be cultured in cases of intraabdominal abscess, diverticulitis, appendicitis, peritonitis, and infections associated with colonic surgery or penetrating trauma. Several bacterial species are found in the same

Table 1-1. Drugs of choice for specified bacterial agents

Organisms	Preferred agents (based on predictable susceptibility patterns)
Gram-Positive Cocci	
Pneumococcus	**Penicillin,** cephalosporin, erythromycin, clindamycin, chloramphenicol
Staphylococcus aureus	
Penicillinase-producing	**Penicillinase-resistant penicillin,** cephalosporin, clindamycin, vancomycin
Nonpenicillinase-producing	**Penicillin,** cephalosporin, clindamycin, vancomycin
Methicillin-resistant	**Vancomycin,** aminoglycoside
Staph. epidermidis	Cephalosporin, penicillinase-resistant penicillin, vancomycin
Streptococci	
Streptococcus pneumoniae	**Penicillin,** cephalosporin, erythromycin, clindamycin, chloramphenicol
Strep. pyogenes	**Penicillin,** erythromycin, cephalosporin, clindamycin
Anaerobic *Streptococcus*	**Penicillin,** ampicillin, clindamycin, cephalosporin, chloramphenicol
Enterococci	**Penicillin + aminoglycoside,** ampicillin, vancomycin, chloramphenicol
Strep. viridans	**Penicillin,** cephalosporin, vancomycin
Gram-Positive Bacilli	
Actinomyces	**Penicillin,** cephalosporin, tetracycline, clindamycin, chloramphenicol, erythromycin
Bacillus anthracis (anthrax)	**Penicillin,** erythromycin, tetracycline
Clostridium perfringens	**Penicillin,** clindamycin, cefoxitin, cephalosporin
Clostridium (other)	**Penicillin,** clindamycin, cefoxitin
Corynebacterium acnes	**Penicillin,** tetracycline, clindamycin, erythromycin
C. diphtheriae	**Penicillin,** erythromycin
Listeria monocytogenes	**Penicillin or ampicillin plus aminoglycoside,** tetracycline, erythromycin, chloramphenicol
Gram-Negative Cocci	
Gonococci	**Penicillin,** ampicillin, tetracycline, cefoxitin, spectinomycin
Meningococci	**Penicillin,** ampicillin, chloramphenicol, tetracycline, erythromycin
Gram-Negative Bacilli	
Achromobacter	Aminoglycoside, ampicillin, tetracycline, chloramphenicol
Bacteroides fragilis	Clindamycin, cefoxitin, metronidazole
Bacteroides (other)	Penicillin, clindamycin, cefoxitin, metronidazole
Bordetella pertussis	Erythromycin, ampicillin, tetracycline
Brucella	**Tetracycline,** chloramphenicol, tetracycline, or chloramphenicol plus streptomycin
Citrobacter	**Aminoglycoside**
Enterobacter	Aminoglycoside, ticarcillin, cefamandole
Escherichia coli	Ampicillin, cephalosporin, aminoglycoside
Fusobacterium	**Penicillin,** clindamycin, cefoxitin, metronidazole
Hemophilus influenzae	Ampicillin, chloramphenicol, tetracycline, penicillin plus aminoglycoside, sulfamethoxazole/trimethoprim, cefamandole
H. ducreyi (chancroid)	**Tetracycline,** sulfonamide
Klebsiella	**Cephalosporin,** aminoglycoside

Table 1-1 (continued)

Organisms	Preferred agents (based on predictable susceptibility patterns)
Legionella pneumophila	**Erythromycin,** rifampin
Pasteurella multocida	**Penicillin,** tetracycline, chloramphenicol
Pasteurella pestis (bubonic plague)	Streptomycin plus tetracycline, or chloramphenicol
Pasteurella tularensis (tularemia)	Streptomycin plus tetracycline, or chloramphenicol
Proteus mirabilis	**Ampicillin,** aminoglycoside, cephalosporin
Pr. vulgaris, morganii, or rettgeri	Ticarcillin, aminoglycoside
Providencia	Ticarcillin, aminoglycoside
Pseudomonas aeruginosa	**Aminoglycoside,** ticarcillin
Ps. pseudomallei (meliodiosis)	**Tetracycline,** tetracycline plus chloramphenicol
Salmonella typhi	**Chloramphenicol,** ampicillin, sulfamethoxazole/trimethoprim
Salmonella (other)	Ampicillin, amoxicillin, chloramphenicol, sulfamethoxazole/trimethoprim
Serratia marcescens	Aminoglycoside, ticarcillin, chloramphenicol, cefoxitin
Shigella	Ampicillin, chloramphenicol, sulfamethoxazole/trimethoprim
Vibrio cholerae	**Tetracycline,** chloramphenicol

Note: 1. "Aminoglycoside" refers to gentamicin, tobramycin, or amikacin. These are considered equally efficacious for infections involving susceptible bacteria.
2. Amoxicillin is considered equivalent to ampicillin for oral therapy of infections other than shigellosis.
3. Ticarcillin is equivalent to carbenicillin.

culture, including anaerobes (especially *Bacteroides fragilis*) and enteric gram-negative rods such as *Escherichia coli*. Antibiotic decisions must take into account the complex bacteriology; for this reason a combination of antibiotics often is required.

B. Biliary tract infections, including cholecystitis and ascending cholangitis, follow a somewhat different set of rules. The infecting flora is relatively simple. The most frequent pathogens are *E. coli* and streptococci; less commonly, *Klebsiella* and *Clostridium* are encountered. Elderly patients (older than 70 years) and those with obstruction of the common duct are apt to have anaerobes such as *Bacteroides*. A cephalosporin or a combination of ampicillin and an aminoglycoside can be used in most cases. When anaerobes are suspected, one of the following should be included in the regimen: cefoxitin, clindamycin, chloramphenicol, or metronidazole.

C. Diarrheal disorders are caused by a diverse group of pathogens. A distinction should be made between small-bowel and large-bowel diarrhea. Small-bowel diarrhea is associated with epigastric pain and large volumes of watery, fecal material that does not contain blood or mucus. The etiologic agents are viruses (rotavirus in children, and the Norwalk agent in all ages) or enterotoxin-producing bacteria such as *E. coli*. Food-poisoning organisms such as *Staphylococcus aureus, Clostridium perfringens,* and *Bacillus cereus* act in a similar fashion. Antibiotics are seldom required, since these diseases are self-limited. The main therapeutic consideration is fluid and electrolyte replacement.
Diarrhea originating from the large bowel tends to be associated with a smaller fecal volume, lower abdominal pain, and tenesmus. Some patients pass gross

Table 1-2. Antimicrobial recommendations for initial therapy of bacterial infections

Type of infection	Likely pathogens	Systemic antimicrobial therapy
Intraabdominal		
Peritonitis Appendicitis Diverticulitis Intraabdominal abscess	*Bacteroides fragilis* *Peptostreptococcus* *Clostridium* Coliforms	Clindamycin, chloramphenicol, or metronidazole, + aminoglycoside; or, cefoxitin ± aminoglycoside
Spontaneous peritonitis in cirrhosis	Coliforms *Streptococcus pneumoniae* *Streptococcus*	Cephalosporin or ampicillin, + aminoglycoside
Liver abscess	*Peptostreptococcus* *Bacteroides/Fusobacterium* Coliforms	Clindamycin, chloramphenicol, or metronidazole, + aminoglycoside Cefoxitin ± aminoglycoside
	Entamoeba histolytica	Metronidazole
Biliary tract	*Escherichia coli* *Klebsiella* *Enterococci* *Clostridium*	Cephalosporin or ampicillin, + aminoglycoside
Diarrheal disorders		
Small bowel	Viral *E. coli*	None
Food poisoning	*Staphylococcus aureus* *Clostridium perfringens* *Bacillus cereus*	None
Large bowel (dysentery)	*Shigella*	Trimethoprim/sulfamethoxazole, or ampicillin
	Campylobacter	Erythromycin
Salmonella		None
Genitourinary		
Pyelonephritis and cystitis		
First episode	*E. coli*	Sulfonamide Trimethoprim/sulfamethoxazole Nitrofurantoin Ampicillin
Recurrent; previous antibiotics, association with catheter or instrumentation	*Enterobacteriaceae* *Pseudomonas*	Cephalosporin Aminoglycoside
Urethritis	*Neisseria gonorrhoeae* *Enterobacteriaceae* *Chlamydia* *Ureaplasma*	Penicillin (gonorrhea) Trimethoprim/sulfamethoxazole Tetracycline
Prostatitis		
Acute	*Enterobacteriaceae* *N. gonorrhoeae*	Ampicillin Trimethoprim/sulfamethoxazole
Abscess	*Enterobacteriaceae* Anaerobic bacteria	Clindamycin + aminoglycoside Cefoxitin

Table 1-2 (continued)

Type of infection	Likely pathogens	Systemic antimicrobial therapy
Female genital tract		
Pelvic abscess Post-gynecologic surgery infection	*Peptostreptococcus* *Bacteroides* *Clostridium* *Enterobacteriaceae*	Clindamycin or metronidazole, + aminoglycoside Cefoxitin
Pelvic inflammatory disease	*N. gonorrhoeae* *Chlamydia* Anaerobic bacteria	Penicillin, tetracycline, or spectinomycin (gonorrhea) Clindamycin or metronidazole + aminoglycoside Cefoxitin
Upper respiratory tract		
Otitis media		
Acute	*Streptococcus pyogenes* *Strep. pneumoniae* *Hemophilus influenzae*	Erythromycin Ampicillin Amoxicillin
Chronic	*Pseudomonas* Anaerobic bacteria *Staph. aureus* *Enterobacteriaceae*	Aminoglycoside Penicillin Clindamycin
Otitis externa	*Pseudomonas* *Staph. aureus* *Strep. pyogenes* *Enterobacteriaceae* *Aspergillus niger* *Candida*	
Sinusitis		
Acute	Viral *H. influenzae* *Strep. pyogenes* *Strep. pneumoniae* *Staph. aureus*	Ampicillin Erythromycin Tetracycline PR-Pen (*Staph. aureus*)
Chronic suppurative	*Strep. pneumoniae* *Staph. aureus* Anaerobic bacteria *H. influenzae*	Erythromycin Tetracycline Ampicillin
Pharyngitis	Viral *Strep. pyogenes* Infectious mononucleosis	Penicillin Erythromycin
Epiglottitis	Viral *H. influenzae*	Ampicillin Tetracycline
Eye		
Sty	*Staph. aureus*	
Blepharitis	*Staph. aureus*	
Conjunctivitis	Viral *Chlamydia* *Staph. aureus* *Strep. pneumoniae* *Hemophilus aegyptius* *H. influenzae* *Strep. pyogenes*	Tetracycline (*Chlamydia*)

Table 1-2 (continued)

Type of infection	Likely pathogens	Systemic antimicrobial therapy
Keratitis	*Herpes* *Moraxella* *Pseudomonas* *Strep. pneumoniae* *Candida* *Alternaria*	
Dental	*B. melaninogenicus* *Fusobacterium* *Peptostreptococcus*	Penicillin Clindamycin
Pulmonary		
Bronchitis		
Acute	Viral	
Exacerbation of chronic bronchitis	*H. influenzae* *Strep. pneumoniae*	Ampicillin Tetracycline Trimethoprim/sulfamethoxazole
Pneumonia		
0–4 yr	Viral *Staph. aureus* *H. influenzae*	Ampicillin ± PR-Pen Trimethoprim/sulfamethoxazole
5–30 yr	Viral *Mycoplasma* *Strep. pneumoniae* *Strep. pyogenes*	Erythromycin Tetracycline Penicillin
Adult (≥ 30 yr)	*Strep. pneumoniae* Viral	Penicillin Erythromycin Clindamycin Cephalosporin
Aspiration	*B. melaninogenicus* *Fusobacterium* *Peptostreptococcus* *Staph. aureus*	Penicillin Clindamycin
	Enterobacteriaceae or Pseudomonas (hospital-acquired)	Clindamycin + aminoglycoside
Immunosuppressed host	*Pseudomonas* *Aspergillus* *Pneumocystis carinii* *Enterobacteriaceae* *Nocardia* *Strep. pneumoniae* *Staph. aureus*	Etiologic diagnosis essential for therapy
Respiratory-induced or tracheostomy	*Enterobacteriaceae* *Pseudomonas* *Staph. aureus*	Carbenicillin, ticarcillin, or piperacillin, + aminoglycoside
Postinfluenzal	*Staph. aureus* *Strep. pneumoniae*	PR-Pen Cephalosporin
Lung abscess	*B. melaninogenicus* *Fusobacterium* *Peptostreptococcus* *Staph. aureus* *Klebsiella*	Penicillin Clindamycin Cefoxitin

Table 1-2 (continued)

Type of infection	Likely pathogens	Systemic antimicrobial therapy
Empyema		
With pulmonary infection	Anaerobic bacteria *Staph. aureus* *Enterobacteriaceae*	Penicillin Clindamycin Cefoxitin
Postthoracotomy	*Staph. aureus* *Enterobacteriaceae* *Pseudomonas*	PR-Pen or cephalosporin, + aminoglycoside
Infant	*Staph. aureus*	PR-Pen Cephalosporin
Central nervous system		
Brain abscess		
Nontraumatic	*Peptostreptococcus* *Bacteroides* *Fusobacterium* *Streptococcus* (facultative) *Enterobacteriaceae*	Metronidazole, or penicillin + chloramphenicol Moxalactam, cefotaxime
Traumatic and postsurgical	*Staph. aureus* *Enterobacteriaceae* *Strep. pneumoniae*	Moxalactam, cefotaxime PR-Pen + aminoglycoside PR-Pen + chloramphenicol
Subdural empyema	*Peptostreptococcus*	Metronidazole + chloramphenicol
	Streptococcus (facultative) *Staph. aureus* *Enterobacteriaceae* *H. influenzae*	Chloramphenicol + PR-Pen Moxalactam, cefotaxime
Meningitis		
Neonatal	*Enterobacteriaceae*	Moxalactam, cefotaxime Aminoglycoside
3 mo–8 yr	*H. influenzae* *Strep. pneumoniae* *Neisseria meningitidis*	Ampicillin Chloramphenicol Erythromycin
Adult	*Strep. pneumoniae* *N. meningitidis*	Penicillin Chloramphenicol Erythromycin
After spinal surgery or spinal anesthesia	*Enterobacteriaceae* *Pseudomonas* *Staph. aureus*	Moxalactam, cefotaxime Aminoglycoside + chloramphenicol Aminoglycoside + PR-Pen
Chronic	Tuberculosis *Cryptococcus* Coccidioidomycosis *Histoplasma*	INH + another 1st-line drug (TB) Amphotericin B + 5 FC (mycotic)
Epidural abscess	*Staph. aureus* Tuberculosis	PR-Pen INH + another 1st-line drug (TB)
Skin and soft tissue		
Pyoderma		
Furunculosis	*Staph. aureus*	PR-R Pen Cephalosporin Clindamycin
Cellulitis	*Strep. pyogenes* *Staph. aureus*	Penicillin + PR-Pen Cephalosporin
Burns	*Staph. aureus* *Streptococcus* *Pseudomonas* *Enterobacteriaceae*	Cephalosporin + aminoglycoside

Table 1-2 (continued)

Type of infection	Likely pathogens	Systemic antimicrobial therapy
Decubitus ulcer	*Enterobacteriaceae* *Bacteroides* sp. *Peptostreptococcus* *Staph. aureus* *Pseudomonas*	If septic: Clindamycin, metronidazole, or cefoxitin, + aminoglycoside
IV catheter site	*Staph. aureus* *Enterobacteriaceae* *Pseudomonas* *Candida*	If septic: Cephalosporin + aminoglycoside Amphotericin B
Bone and joint		
Osteomyelitis		
Child	*Staph. aureus* *Strep. pyogenes*	PR-Pen Cephalosporin
Hemoglobinopathy	*Staph. aureus*	PR-Pen, cephalosporin, or clindamycin
	Salmonella	Ampicillin, trimethoprim/sulfamethoxazole or chloramphenicol
Adult	*Staph. aureus* *Enterobacteriaceae* *Pseudomonas*	PR-Pen, cephalosporin, or clindamycin Ticarcillin or piperacillin ± aminoglycoside
Addict	*Staph. aureus* *Enterobacteriaceae* *Pseudomonas*	PR-Pen, cephalosporin, or clindamycin Ticarcillin or piperacillin, ± aminoglycoside
Joint		
Child	*Staph. aureus* *H. influenzae* *Strep. pyogenes*	PR-Pen, cephalosporin, ampicillin Penicillin
Young adult	*N. gonorrhoeae* *Staph. aureus*	Penicillin Tetracycline PR-Pen (*Staph. aureus*)
Adult (40 years)	*Staph. aureus* *Strep. pneumoniae*	PR-Pen Penicillin
Postoperative infection	*Staph. aureus* *Enterobacteriaceae* *Pseudomonas*	PR-Pen + aminoglycoside Cephalosporin + aminoglycoside
Chronic	Tuberculosis Atypical mycobacteria Mycotic	INH + another 1st-line drug (TB) Amphotericin B
Addict	*Staph. aureus* *Enterobacteriaceae* *Pseudomonas*	PR-Pen, cephalosporin, or clindamycin Ticarcillin or piperacillin, ± aminoglycoside

PR-Pen = penicillinase-resistant penicillin.

blood and mucus. Microscopic examination of the stool reveals sheets of WBCs, and the appellation "bacillary dysentery" is based on these findings. The principal pathogens in this type of diarrhea are *Shigella* and *Campylobacter*. Rare pathogens are *Salmonella, Vibrio parahemolyticus,* penetrating strains of *E. coli,* and *Yersinia*. Most patients with mild symptoms respond to symptomatic therapy. Patients with moderate to severe bacillary dysentery should receive antibiotics. Trimethoprim/sulfamethoxazole or ampicillin is used in shigellosis, and erythromycin in *Campylobacter* infections.

Salmonella infections of the gastrointestinal tract usually are associated with diarrhea. For mild *Salmonella* gastroenteritis, antibiotic therapy is contraindicated. These drugs do not alter the clinical course of this disease, but they may prolong the carrier state and increase public health problems. Bacteremic salmonellosis, typhoid fever, and localized infections (e.g., joint and bone) are indications for antibiotic therapy with chloramphenicol, trimethoprim/sulfamethoxazole, or amoxicillin. There are, however, an increasing number of antibiotic-resistant *Salmonella* strains.

II. Urinary tract Infections. The initial attack of an uncomplicated urinary tract infection usually is caused by *E. coli*. Most cases respond to a variety of oral antimicrobials, including sulfonamides, ampicillin, and tetracycline. The bacteriologic possibilities multiply when the infection is recurrent or is associated with manipulations of the GU tract such as catheterization, cystoscopy, or a surgical procedure. In the uncomplicated case, when symptoms are mild, antimicrobial therapy can be started with an oral agent and modified, if necessary, according to the results of urine culture and sensitivity. If the patient is severely ill, therapy should be initiated empirically on the basis of the worst possibilities; an aminoglycoside is the logical choice in such a case.

III. Female genital tract infections. Many infections of the female genital tract are comparable to intraabdominal infections in that they involve the flora of adjacent mucosal surfaces, in this setting the vagina and cervix. These infections include endomyometritis, salpingitis, pelvic inflammatory disease, pelvic abscess, and wound infection following gynecologic surgery. The infecting flora is complex and includes both aerobic and anaerobic bacteria. Because of the mixed nature of these infections, antibiotic combinations are recommended. Milder forms of pelvic inflammatory disease are caused by gonococci, *Chlamydia,* or mixed vaginal flora.

IV. Upper respiratory tract. The vast majority of upper respiratory tract infections (including pharyngitis, laryngitis, acute sinusitis, and acute bronchitis) are viral in origin, and viruses do not respond to antimicrobial therapy. Group A β-hemolytic streptococcal pharyngitis is suspected when symptoms are severe, fever is high, exudate is present, and lymph nodes are involved. Although these findings suggest bacterial infection, it is difficult for even the most astute physician to make an accurate etiologic diagnosis on clinical grounds, particularly in the case of children. Infectious mononucleosis is an additional possibility in adolescents and young adults; these patients do not respond to antimicrobial therapy, and they may have a severe skin rash to ampicillin. Splenomegaly, peripheral adenopathy, and appropriate laboratory findings (Mono spot test and atypical lymphocytosis) are useful clues to this diagnosis.

Hemophilus influenzae, an important pathogen in children with acute otitis media, epiglottitis, or laryngotracheal bronchitis, is not very frequently pathogenic in adults except in exacerbations of chronic bronchitis and in some cases of sinusitis. *H. influenzae* merits particular emphasis since some strains are highly resistant to ampicillin. Oral drugs of choice for sensitive strains include ampicillin, amoxicillin, and tetracycline, or combinations of penicillin with sulfonamide or streptomycin. Ampicillin-resistant strains usually are sensitive to trimethoprim/sulfamethoxazole, erythromycin, tetracycline, or chloramphenicol.

V. Pulmonary infections

A. Likely pathogens in **pneumonitis** are determined largely by the patient's age and the clinical setting. Among infants and young children the most common agents are viral, such as respiratory syncytial virus and parainfluenza virus. When children over 5 years old and young adults are affected, *Mycoplasma pneumoniae* is an important possibility. Severe infections with this organism generally respond to tetracycline or erythromycin. The therapeutic efficacy of these agents for mild symptoms is not well established. Pneumonitis in adults usually is caused by bacteria, particularly in patients who require hospitalization. The principal pathogen is the pneumococcus, which accounts for more than 90% of community-acquired acute bacterial pneumonias. Other bacterial pathogens, however, are common in specific clinical settings. For example, the association of *Staph. aureus* and influenza is well established.

B. Another special setting is **aspiration pneumonia,** which is caused by bacteria normally colonizing the oropharynx. The principal organisms are anaerobic species, which are generally susceptible to penicillin. *Staph. aureus* and gram-negative rods also may be involved, especially when the aspiration occurs in the hospital. Occasionally, the symptoms of aspiration pneumonia are acute or are complicated by wheezing or hypotension. These symptoms may indicate chemical pneumonitis due to the massive aspiration of gastric acid or other irritants. Respiratory support is the most important facet of therapy in such cases, and the role of antibiotics has not been clearly established.

C. The **immunosuppressed host** requires special consideration, since the responsible pathogen frequently is difficult to determine. Likely possibilities include fungi, parasites, bacteria, and viruses, each requiring a specific therapeutic approach. The pursuit of the diagnosis in this setting should be aggressive, with transtracheal aspiration often followed by a lung biopsy.

D. Pulmonary infections characterized by **cavitation** are seldom, if ever, caused by pneumococci. Anaerobic bacteria are the major pathogens in these cases. *Staph. aureus, Klebsiella,* and *Nocardia* are less frequently involved. A characteristic clinical picture of necrotizing pneumonia may be caused by *Pseudomonas aeruginosa* or other gram-negative rods; this diagnosis is an important consideration in the immunosuppressed patient.

E. Although the pneumococcus was once the principal pathogen in **empyema,** in the chemotherapeutic era this organism is seldom recovered in pleural fluid. More common pathogens in recent studies are anaerobic bacteria, *Staph. aureus,* and gram-negative bacilli. A useful guide to a presumptive diagnosis is a Gram's-stained slide of the infected pleural fluid.

VI. Central nervous system infections. The commonest pyogenic infections of the central nervous system are meningitis, brain abscess, and subdural empyema. The penetrative ability of antibiotics into the central nervous system (blood-brain barrier) is an important consideration. Metronidazole, chloramphenicol, and tetracycline penetrate well, while penicillin penetrates satisfactorily only in the presence of inflammation. Cephalosporins and clindamycin generally are not recommended for CNS infections. The third-generation cephalosporins, moxalactam and cefotaxime, penetrate well into the CSF, and they can be used, especially in gram-negative meningitis. When the pathogen requires aminoglycoside therapy, intrathecal, along with intravenous, administration may be necessary.

Brain abscess usually is related to a suppurative process in contiguous structures, such as the sinuses or middle ear, or to metastatic spread from a pulmonary process. The principal pathogens are anaerobic bacteria, especially *Peptostreptococcus, Bacteroides,* and *Fusobacterium;* facultative streptococci and enteric gram-negative rods are found less frequently. Subdural empyema is usually a sequel to infections of the middle ear or sinuses or may be associated with *H. influenzae* meningitis.

In pyogenic meningitis the range of pathogens is entirely different. The most common pathogens in neonates are gram-negative enteric bacilli, especially *E. coli.* Among children 3 months to 5 years of age the vast majority of cases are caused either by *H. influenzae* (40–50%), *Streptococcus pneumoniae,* or *Neisseria meningitidis.* Acute pyogenic meningitis in older children and adults is almost invariably caused by one of the latter two organisms. Infection related to spinal surgery or spinal anesthesia may be caused by other pathogens, especially enteric bacteria; in these cases a toxic, "aseptic" meningeal reaction related to irritants in the spinal anesthetic is an important consideration. *Listeria* and unusual gram-negative rods are important pathogens in the immunosuppressed patient. In all cases of meningitis, a Gram's stain of the CSF is a valuable aid in the initial selection of drugs.

VII. **Skin and soft tissue infections.** The specific pathogen in infections of the skin and soft tissues can be suspected from the nature of the lesion and the clinical setting. Furunculosis and pyoderma generally are caused by *Staph. aureus,* whereas cellulitis associated with lymphagitis is highly suggestive of *Strep. pyogenes.* In cellulitis, however, these two pathogens can be mixed, and it is difficult to identify them from clinical findings. Thus, therapy for both *Staph. aureus* and *Strep. pyogenes* is indicated in severe cases of cellulitis. Hyperalimentation lines and intravenous catheters are important portals of entry for opportunistic infections, especially staphylococci and fungi. Their presence may be difficult to determine, since chemical phlebitis can simulate infection. The most important factor in therapy is removal of the catheter. Should fever and toxicity persist, specific chemotherapy is required. Surgical removal of the vein is rarely indicated.

2 Abdominal Infections

I. Anatomic landmarks in the abdominal cavity. The peritoneal cavity is divided into several compartments by natural anatomic barriers:

A. The transverse colon and mesocolon form the division between the **supracolonic area,** which lies above, and the **infracolonic area,** which lies below.

B. The **vertebral column** divides the peritoneal cavity into right and left segments.

C. The **sacral promontory** and **psoas muscle** demarcate the **pelvis** from the abdominal cavity.

II. Spaces in the abdominal cavity

A. Supracolic (superior to the transverse colon and mesocolon). The supracolic space is divided into **right** and **left subdiaphragmatic spaces** by the falciform suspensory ligament.

1. **Right subphrenic space** (limited posteriorly by the coronary ligament). Often divided into **anterior** and **posterior** compartments by pyogenic membranes.
2. **Right subhepatic space**
   a. **Anteroinferior**
   b. **Posterosuperior** (Morison's pouch)
3. **Left subphrenic space** (limited inferiorly by left lobe of liver, stomach, and spleen; limited posteriorly by coronary and triangular ligament)
4. **Left subhepatic space**
   a. **Anterior** (limited posteriorly by lesser omentum and stomach)
   b. **Posterior** ("lesser sac;" limited anteriorly by stomach)

B. Infracolic (below the transverse mesocolon)

1. Internal paracolic region—right and left
2. External paracolic gutter—right and left

C. Pelvic space

III. Spread of sepsis within the peritoneal cavity. Contaminated or irritating substances can be disseminated widely throughout the peritoneal cavity. This movement is controlled by

A. Anatomic landmarks and natural compartments

B. Intraperitoneal pressure gradients, i.e., diaphragmatic movements causing cephalad spread of pelvic infection

C. The position of the patient with relation to gravitational flow

D. The site of introduction of contaminated or irritating substances

IV. Anatomic Determinants. Fluid introduced into the abdomen can traverse the paracolic gutters in both directions and can move from the pelvis to the supracolic spaces. There are, however, certain favored directions of flow based on anatomic relationships.

A. The right external paracolic gutter communicates between the upper and lower abdominal compartments. Infected material from the ileocecal region flows freely into the right subhepatic space, especially in the posterior area (Morison's pouch). The infection may later spread to the right subphrenic space. Gastric or duodenal perforations can present with initial symptoms in the right lower quadrant of the abdomen, simulating acute appendicitis because of these same anatomic relationships ("Valentino appendicitis").

B. The left infracolic space communicates directly with the pelvis downwardly and with the left subphrenic and subhepatic spaces upwardly. Thus, infections or irritating material arising from the left of the root of the mesentery can pass directly into the pelvis; such collections on the right of the mesentery collect in the right paracolic gutter.

C. Left upper quadrant abscesses are rare in peritonitis, since the flow is stopped by the phrenicocolic ligament.

D. Collections in the pelvis can extend to the supracolic area, usually on the left side, probably as a result of negative pressure created by diaphragmatic movement.

Peritonitis

I. General principles. The peritoneum, covering the abdominal and pelvic cavities, has a surface area approximately equal to that of the skin, about 25,000 cm^2. When exposed to injury, this massive surface can exude vast quantities of fluid and electrolytes within the peritoneal cavity. Thus, the initial 12 hours of peritoneal infection are associated with 5–10 liters of fluid loss. This accounts for the hypovolemia, shock, and renal insufficiency often accompanying acute peritonitis. In addition, peritoneal irritation leads to paralytic ileus, which causes further fluid loss into the lumen of the bowel. Vomiting and diarrhea accentuate the loss of fluid and electrolytes.

Reduction in the circulating volume due to loss of fluid into the peritoneal cavity or the lumen of the bowel results in reduced venous return and compromised tissue perfusion. If this is not corrected by fluid replacement, glomerular filtration diminishes and renal insufficiency develops.

The outcome of acute peritonitis is highly dependent on early diagnosis and institution of adequate treatment. Hence, it is urgent to recognize an acute inflammatory process of the peritoneum. Much of the symptomatology is related to exudation of fluid and electrolytes into the peritoneal cavity and the bowel lumen. Penetration of bacteria and the production of endotoxin are contributing factors.

II. Signs and symptoms. Fever, vomiting, and abdominal pain are the earliest signs of peritoneal irritation. The patient usually develops shaking chills, a high spiking temperature, and a rapid pulse rate. Physical examination displays distention, generalized abdominal tenderness, muscle rigidity, and rebound tenderness. Absent bowel sounds are an early sign.

III. Classification of peritonitis. Peritonitis caused by infection can be defined by the **route of entry** (hematogenous vs. direct extension) and the **type of infecting microorganism.**

A. Hematogenous peritonitis ("primary")—monomicrobial infection. *Pneumococcus* and *Streptococcus* infections are seen in cirrhosis, in nephrotic syndrome, and occasionally in young, healthy girls. This condition has an acute onset and is associated with high mortality, if not treated early. In most cases a portal of entry is not apparent, i.e., chest x-ray is negative and there are no signs of sinusitis or otitis media. Abdominal findings may be minimal, but most patients have a high fever and leukocytosis.

1. Diagnosis. The diagnosis of pneumococcal and streptococcal infection of the peritoneum is established by paracentesis. Direct examination of the fluid reveals sheets of PMNs; Gram's stain demonstrates the specific morphology of these gram-positive cocci. Pneumococci are grouped in pairs with the ends slightly sharpened in a "lancet" appearance; diplococci may be arranged in long chains, usually with fewer than five or six sets of pairs. When the light of the microscope is decreased, the pneumococci show distinct capsules. Streptococci are in chains without a disposition to form paired structures, and their chains often consist of 10 or more individual cells.

2. Treatment. The treatment of choice is penicillin G. This drug freely passes the peritoneal surface in the presence of inflammation. Aqueous penicillin G, 3 million units, is given IV q4h.

There is no need for direct instillation of antibiotics into the peritoneal cavity, since these bacteria are exquisitely sensitive to penicillin, and the bloodstream can deliver large concentrations of the drug to the peritoneum. Operative intervention is not indicated, although it is important to be sure that there is no evidence of ruptured viscus.

B. Spontaneous peritonitis in cirrhosis. Coliforms, principally *Escherichia coli* and *Klebsiella,* are the infecting organisms in 70% of the cases. Streptococci and pneumococci account for 25%, and a variety of other bacterial types are seen in the remaining 5%. About 50% of patients have positive blood cultures. The infection is usually caused by a single organism, but in occasional cases, two or even three different bacteria are encountered. The setting is a patient with cirrhosis, either Laennec's or postnecrotic, who has chronic ascites. Such patients are subjected to frequent episodes of bacteremia because of their liver disease; it is probable that the ascitic fluid becomes infected by the hematogenous route. Evidence of intestinal perforation is not found in such cases.

1. Diagnosis. The major diagnostic problem is differentiating primary from secondary peritonitis due to a ruptured viscus, which requires surgical intervention. The diagnosis of primary peritonitis is established by paracentesis and examination of ascitic fluid. This disease may have an insidious onset and be present for several weeks in the patient with cirrhosis without showing specific signs. Many patients are diagnosed at postmortem following an indolent course. Hence, any patient with cirrhosis who complains of abdominal pain, develops a low-grade fever, or has a change in his clinical status, should undergo paracentesis.

Under the microscope, the ascitic fluid usually displays many PMNs. In most instances the infecting organism can be identified by microscopic examination. Gram-negative bacilli, particularly *E. coli* and *Klebsiella*, should be searched for. The laboratory will verify the culture, but the initial Gram's-stain appearance is often a reliable clue. The cell count is variable, usually over 1,000 WBC/mm^3, mostly PMNs. There are cases, however, in which the cellular response is sparse, 200–300 WBC/mm^3. Curiously, the protein content of this fluid is often in the range of a transudate, i.e., 1.0–2.5 gm/100 ml.

2. Treatment. Treatment is based on identification of the organism. Gram-negative bacilli, such as *E. coli* and *Klebsiella,* can be treated with a cephalosporin. Gram-positive cocci, such as streptococci and pneumococci, should be treated with penicillin (see **A.2.**). When the final identification and antibiotic sensitivities are available, changes in antibiotics are appropriate, e.g., ampicillin might be used for *E. coli.* The Gram's stain may fail to show any organisms, and such patients should receive broad-spectrum coverage such as ampicillin and an aminoglycoside.

C. Tuberculosis. TB peritonitis is usually an indolent infection, often presenting without signs of tuberculosis in other organs. Indeed, the chest x-ray may be negative. The abdomen is said to have a "doughy" feel on palpation, and there is often diffuse abdominal pain. However, the signs and symptoms are extremely variable. The tuberculin skin test is negative in approximately 50% of cases, possibly because of anergy.

1. Diagnosis

a. The diagnosis of tuberculous peritonitis is best established by biopsy of the peritoneum in order to demonstrate **granuloma formation** with central caseation. The tubercle bacillus can be gown from peritoneal fluid in only a small percentage of cases. Uncommonly, appropriate staining identifies acid-fast bacilli in peritoneal fluid or within a granuloma. Efforts should be made to culture the urine, sputum, and gastric contents in order to recover the organism, since the peritoneal cultures may prove negative. A positive culture is important to establish the antimicrobial sensitivity of the particular strain of mycobacterium.

b. Peritoneal fluid in tuberculous peritonitis is usually classified as an **exudate,** i.e., the protein content is greater than 3.5 gm/100 ml and the cell count is greater than 1,000/mm^3 with a predominance of lymphocytes and mononuclear cells. The sugar content may be reduced below that of the serum. It must be strongly emphasized that exceptions have been noted to each of these findings. In some cases, tuberculous peritonitis presents with a transudate; in other cases the findings are mixed, such as a normal protein content but an increased concentration of cells. Because of the variable nature of this disease, patients should undergo biopsy and/or laparoscopy whenever the diagnosis is suspected.

2. **Treatment.** Because the disease is hematogenous, the patient should be treated aggressively for 12–18 months with antimicrobial drugs. Initial chemotherapy is as follows:

Isoniazid (INH)	300 mg/day PO in one dose
Ethambutol	15 mg/kg/day PO in one dose
Rifampin	600 mg/day PO in one dose

This regimen may have to be altered when antimicrobial susceptibility results are available.

D. Peritonitis due to contiguous spread ("secondary")—polymicrobial. The commonest form of peritonitis is that caused by **injury to the bowel,** resulting in perforation and leakage of intraabdominal contents. The GI flora invades the peritoneal cavity and its surrounding tissues. A variety of clinical settings are associated with injury to the small bowel or large bowel, or both. Regardless of the type of injury, the end result is an inoculum of fecal microorganisms that includes both aerobic and anaerobic bacteria. **Pelvic organs** can be primarily involved with septic processes that can subsequently spread to the peritoneal cavity. Infections of the **liver, biliary tract, pancreas, kidney,** and **pleural space** can also extend into the peritoneal cavity, resulting in either localized or generalized suppuration.

1. **Diagnosis**

   a. The diagnosis is suspected in the first instance from a **history** of nausea, vomiting, abdominal pain and distention, chills, and spiking fever. The **physical findings** usually are confirmatory of the suspected diagnosis; abdominal tenderness, rebound tenderness, muscle spasm, rigidity, and decreased or absent bowel sounds. In some patients the infection may be localized so that the generalized findings are not apparent. A rectal examination or pelvic examination may be helpful and should always be done. Classic signs of peritonitis may be absent in the very young and the very old patient. Corticosteroids, antibiotics, and potent pain medication may disguise an acute inflammatory response.

   b. **Paracentesis** of peritoneal fluid, by a low, midline tap, is a useful adjunct to diagnosis. Care should be taken to avoid perforation of the bowel. A "four-quadrant tap" can be used to diagnose localized collections of exudate. When only a small amount of peritoneal fluid is present, a specimen can be obtained by placing the patient on hands and knees and inserting a needle in the most dependent area, just above the umbilicus. Peritoneal fluid should be examined in the following manner:

      (1) Gram's staining for microorganisms; acid-fast stains, if tuberculous peritonitis is suspected

      (2) Aerobic and anerobic culture; tuberculous and fungal cultures, when indicated

      (3) Total protein, sugar, amylase, and pH

      (4) Total cell count (WBC and RBC) and WBC differential count

   c. **Abdominal x-rays** show a hazy, glassy appearance, with loss of normal markings such as the psoas shadows and the perirenal fat pad. The bowel is diffusely distended, with gas distributed throughout the small and large intestine.

2. **Bacteriology.** Injury to the bowel produces contamination of the peritoneum and surrounding tissues by the normal flora. Although the intestinal flora comprises many bacterial species, perhaps up to 500 different types, a relatively select group has pathogenic potential and actually is involved in intraabdominal sepsis. Two general principles can be applied:

   a. Cultures of peritoneal fluid in such cases yield a mixture of aerobic and

Table 2-1. Bacteriology of intraabdominal infections

	Frequency of isolation (%)
Aerobes	
E. coli	65
Proteus	25
Klebsiella	20
Pseudomonas	15
Enterococcus	15
Streptococcus (other than groups A or D)	10
Anaerobes	
Bacteroides fragilis	80
Bacteroides (other)	30
Clostridium	65
*Peptostreptococcus**	25
*Peptococcus**	15
Fusobacterium	20

*Sometimes grouped under "anaerobic Gram-positive cocci."

anaerobic bacteria (Table 2-1). It is uncommon to encounter only aerobes (e.g., *E. coli*) or only anaerobes following perforation of the bowel.

b. The average number of different bacterial species in an intraabdominal infection is five, generally consisting of two aerobes and three anaerobes.

3. Therapy

a. Treatment of polymicrobial peritonitis, particularly when related to intestinal injury, requires an aggressive operative approach, appropriate use of antibiotics, and general support measures. Modern surgical opinion favors **operative treatment** of peritonitis after physiologic parameters have been stabilized. At laparotomy there should be a careful search for the source of contamination, particularly perforation of the gastrointestinal tract. At this time, decisions concerning repair, colostomy, exteriorization, or bypass procedures can be made.

b. Lavage of the peritoneal cavity with normal saline solution is recommended to remove gross contamination, blood, necrotic tissue, and foreign bodies. However, experimental studies have shown that it is impossible to completely "wash out" contaminating bacteria.

The question of **antibiotic-contaminating lavage fluid** is controversial. The most effective means of delivering antimicrobial agents to the peritoneum is via the bloodstream. Antibiotic lavage affects only those organisms in the peritoneal fluid or on the immediate surface of the peritoneum. A high serum level of antibiotics delivers the drugs to both the tissues and the peritoneal fluid, since antibiotics are readily transferred across the peritoneal surface in the presence of inflammation.

If the decision is made to use antibiotics in the lavage fluid, the following regimen has been recommended: 500 mg of kanamycin dissolved in 500 ml of saline.

The addition of 50,000 units of bacitracin to this solution is recommended. A potential danger with the use of kanamycin is sudden respiratory arrest or prolonged apnea due to the curare-like action of this drug.

c. It is our view that **continuous instillation and drainage** of antibiotic-containing fluids during the postoperative period offers little benefit and may predispose the patient to superinfection by providing a portal of entry.

4. **Antibiotic therapy.** Successful treatment of intraabdominal sepsis involves judicious surgical resection, debridement, and drainage in addition to the selection of appropriate antibiotics. Operative intervention is surely the most crucial modality, but it should be emphasized that surgery alone may be inadequate. Intraabdominal infections can continue to simmer, with intermittent seticemia and even insidious extension of the process, unless appropriate antibiotics are employed.

   At present, there is no single antibiotic that can be expected to encompass within its spectrum of activity the full range of potential pathogens. Not only is the list of invasive organisms awesomely complex, but the choice of antibiotic therapy must be made before results of bacteriologic culture are available. A combination of antibiotics, active against both aerobes and anaerobes, is recommended in cases of intraabdominal sepsis in which the bacteriology has not been fully defined. When the pathogens have been identified, appropriate changes in therapy can be made.

   Broader-spectrum cephalosporins have become available which may provide sufficient coverage for single-drug therapy. Cefoxitin has proved useful in this manner. The third-generation cephalosporins are other potential candidates, expecially moxalactam. At the time of this writing, however, comparative trials are not available to establish the efficacy of the third-generation cephalosporins in intraabdominal sepsis.

   a. For the aerobes, an aminoglycoside giving wide coverage should be used:

   Gentamicin
   Tobramycin
   Amikacin

   b. For the anaerobes, the major consideration is therapy directed against **Bacteroides fragilis,** for two reasons:

   (1) It is the most virulent anaerobe in abdominal infections, as witnessed by its frequency of isolation in soft tissues and blood cultures.

   (2) It has unique antibiotic sensitivities, being the only anaerobe that is often resistant to penicillins or cephalosporins.

   The only drugs currently available for parenteral therapy which have consistent activity against *B. fragilis* are

   Clindamycin
   Chloramphenicol
   Cefoxitin
   Metronidazole

   c. A regimen composed of **two** drugs—one for aerobes and one for anaerobes—has proved effective in treating intraabdominal sepsis when therapy must be initiated on empirical grounds.

For anaerobes (select one)	**For aerobes (select one)**
Clindamycin 600 mg q6h IM or IV	Gentamicin* 1.5 mg/kg q8h
Chloramphenicol 750–1,000 mg q6h IV	Tobramycin* 1.5 mg/kg q8h
Cefoxitin 2 gm q6h IV	Amikacin* 500 mg/kg q8h
Metronidazole 500–750 mg q8h IV (or PO, if possible)	

   Cefoxitin has broad coverage against coliforms as well as anaerobes, but it is not active against *Pseudomonas, Enterobacter,* and certain strains of

*Dose is adjusted according to renal function. See p. 254.

Serratia and *Klebsiella*. This drug can be used as a **single agent** in acute cases of peritonitis and bowel perforation. Cefoxitin should be combined with an aminoglycoside when antibiotic-resistant bacteria are likely to be encountered: (1) Previous use of antibiotics, within past 30 days. (2) Reoperation, recurrence of infection, or chronic intraabdominal abscess. (3) Long hospitalization preoperatively. When the aminoglycoside is added, subsequent cultures should be examined, since it is possible to discontinue this drug, continuing cefoxitin alone, in the event that all isolates are sensitive.

We do not advocate specific treatment of the enterococcus, for example by adding ampicillin. The regimens listed previously have proved effective in treating intraabdominal infections, without problems related to superinfections or relapses due to enterococci.

Antibiotic treatment of acute peritonitis should be continued until the acute phase has passed and the patient has defervesced (approximately 4–7 days). The drugs should then be stopped in order to witness any localization of fluid or subsequent abscess formation. Long-term maintenance of antibiotic therapy is to be discouraged, as it may obscure the presence of an abscess, thereby delaying appropriate intervention. The main role of antibiotics in acute peritonitis is to control the initial septicemia and to prevent metastatic spread of infection to other sites.

For the same reasons, patients with proved or suspected intraabdominal sepsis should not be discharged with oral antibiotics. It is better to stop parenteral drug treatment before discharge, and then observe the patient for a few days in the hospital. A long course of oral antibiotics may engender a false sense of security while suppressing an area of undrained pus. If the patient has had adequate surgical drainage with removal of purulent material and necrotic tissue, the wound should granulate without prolonged antibiotic treatment. Again, it is better to know of the existence of undrained pus at an early stage, when the patient is in better nutritional status, than to allow a suppurative collection to persist within the abdominal cavity.

Patients who have remained in the hospital for an extended period of time with open wounds may become superinfected by resistant bacteria from the hospital environment. *Pseudomonas, Proteus, Serratia,* and *Providencia* can become significant pathogens during the subsequent course. Superinfection requires alterations in antibiotic therapy based on sensitivity testing.

IV. General Support Measures. The initial physiologic derangements in intraabdominal sepsis are related to massive shifts of fluid and electrolytes into the peritoneal cavity and the bowel lumen. In addition, bacterial products such as endotoxin are released into the circulation and produce hypovolemia and decreased peripheral vascular resistance. These physiologic derangements may be corrected by employing the following general support measures.

- **A.** Circulating blood volume should be restored with appropriate plasma and colloid; fluid and electrolytes should be adjusted to maintain equilibrium. A central venous pressure line should be inserted to ensure that the circulation is not overloaded. Hypotension should be carefully monitored by blood pressure readings and measurement of hourly urine output.
- **B.** Oral intake should be withheld; an intestinal tube with a weighted end should be used for suctioning and decompressing the intestinal tract.
- **C.** The patient should be placed in semi-Fowler's position to localize any potential fluid formation to the pelvis and to ease respiratory movements.
- **D.** Sedation and pain medication should be kept to a minimum, just enough to keep the patient moderately comfortable. Low doses of morphine can be used, although respiratory depression must be avoided.

Intraabdominal Abscess

Intraabdominal abscess is the *bête noire* of surgical infections, often occurring in the wake of an intraabdominal catastrophe. The course is unpredictable to the extent

Table 2-2. Sites of intraabdominal abscess

Site	Percent of total abscesses	
Intraperitoneal		36
Right lower quadrant	16	
Subphrenic	8	
Left lower quadrant	5	
Pelvic	5	
Interloop	1	
Horseshoe	1	
Retroperitoneal		38
Anterior	17	
Posterior	15	
Retrofascial	6	
Visceral		26
Hepatic	13	
Pancreatic	6	
Tuboovarian	5	
Gallbladder and biliary tree	2	

Source: Adapted from W. A. Altemeir et al., Intra-abdominal abscesses. *Am. J. Surg.*, 125:70, 1973.

that the symptoms and localizing signs are cryptic. The eventual outcome in untreated patients, however, is grave.

I. Clinical settings

A. Intraabdominal abscess usually occurs in the setting of contamination from the gastrointestinal tract, biliary tract, GI system, pancreas, or lung; the infection may present as

1. Diffusion peritoneal contamination
2. Localized contamination in which there is no free spillage into the peritoneal cavity

B. Occasional idiopathic cases, without apparent source of contamination, may arise via bacterial spread through the bloodstream or lymphatics.

II. Classification

An anatomic classification divides intraabdominal abscesses into **intraperitoneal, retroperitoneal,** and **visceral** (Table 2-2).

III. Intraperitoneal abscess. The localization of abscesses within the peritoneal cavity corresponds to the natural compartments. In addition to these anatomic spaces, abscesses can arise through formation of purulent membranes, between loops of small and large intestine and their mesenteries; structures such as the omentum and the transverse mesocolon prevent their extension. Multiple abscesses occur in 20% of patients.

An uncommon form of intraperitoneal collection that defies anatomic compartments is the **horseshoe abscess,** an ill-defined, massive collection of pus that occupies a major portion of the intraabdominal cavity in a horseshoe-shaped configuration. Its massive size leads to profound debilitation in the patient. Such a structure is seen in patients whose diagnosis has been delayed.

A. Primary vs. secondary abscesses. An abscess is considered a **primary** event when it is caused by a spontaneous intraabdominal process or trauma, and a **secondary** event when it develops as a complication of an operation or procedure.

B. Predisposing causes. A large number of conditions can produce contamination of the peritoneal cavity (Table 2-3). In clinical practice, the commonest predisposing causes of intraabdominal abscess are **appendicitis; spread from foci in the gastrointestinal, genitourinary, or biliary tract; leakage through an intestinal anastomosis; abdominal trauma; diverticulitis; and perforating tumors of the GI tract.** While perforation of the colon carries a high rate of abscess formation, perforation of a peptic ulcer carries a very low rate.

Table 2-3. Sources of intraabdominal abscess

Source	Percent of total cases
Primary Abscesses (70%)	
Appendicitis	25
Diverticulitis	20
Trauma	15
Colon cancer	10
Inflammatory bowel disease	5
Female pelvic tract	5
Peptic ulcer	5
Pancreatitis	3
Miscellaneous	12
Secondary Abscesses (30%)	
GI surgery	66
Non-GI surgery	14
Endoscopy	10
Biliary surgery	7
Miscellaneous	3

Source: Adapted from S. Saini, et al. Improved localization and survival in patients with intraabdominal abscesses. *Am. J. Surg.* 145:136, 1983.

C. Onset. Intraperitoneal abscess has three clinical presentations:

1. An acute condition that follows in the wake of **diffuse peritonitis** related to intestinal perforation. Septic pockets are loculated during the process of repair and form in the right lower quadrant, pelvis, or beneath the diaphragm.
2. Localization of purulent material that is **contiguous to a septic focus** such as the pancreas, appendix, genitourinary tract, or biliary tract. This situation may be heralded by symptoms relating to the abscess itself rather than to the primary process.
3. An insidious course of fever and sepsis in which there has been **no recognized predisposing event.**

D. Diagnosis

1. **Physical examination, history, and routine laboratory studies** provide enough evidence to institute drainage of an intraabdominal abscess in 40% of patients. However, the localization and operative approach are determined by other diagnostic studies, particularly ultrasound and computed tomographic scan (CT scan). In addition, 20% of patients have multiple abscess, which can only be identified by these techniques prior to a surgical procedure.
2. **X-rays of the abdomen** can identify air bubbles or displaced structures that give a clue to the presence of an abscess.
3. **A CT scan of the abdomen** is the most useful study, with a sensitivity of about 95%, using the newer instruments.
4. **Ultrasound** has a sensitivity of 75%. Although less accurate than the CT scan, ultrasound has the advantages of being inexpensive, easily available, and a bedside technique. It is also used as an adjunct to percutaneous drainage and in pregnant women with suspected abscess. Ultrasound does not add to the accuracy of the CT scan.
5. The **gallium scan** has a 75% sensitivity. Its disadvantages include a 10–20% false-positive rate and a delay of 3–7 days for final report.

Table 2-4. Localization of subphrenic abscess

Location	Percent of total cases		
Unilateral		90	
Bilateral		10	
Multiple (unilateral or bilateral)		15	
Right Side			60
Subphrenic	30		
Subhepatic	15		
Combined	15		
Left Side			30
Subphrenic and subhepatic	27		
Lesser sac	3		

E. Surgical treatment

1. The **transabdominal approach** is required in about 50% of patients. Indications are
   a. Continued leakage from the GI tract
   b. Lesser sac or peripancreatic abscess
   c. Multiple abscesses
   d. Preoperative localization not possible
2. The **extraserous approach** should be used whenever anatomically possible. The advantages are reduced trauma of procedure, no spread of infection to other sites in the peritoneal cavity, and gravitational drainage. The most common routes are
   a. Posterior approach, with or without rib resection
   b. Subcostal approach to a subpleuric or subhepatic abscess
   c. Vaginal cul-de-sac or rectal approach to a pelvic abscess
3. **Percutaneous catheter drainage** is performed with a trocar or pigtail catheter. This technique is especially useful for a single abscess, easily localized by CT scan or ultrasound. It is also employed in the case of high-risk patients who cannot undergo general anesthesia.

F. Medical Therapy

These infections are usually caused by a mixed aerobic-anaerobic flora. The treatment schedules mentioned previously (pp. 18–19) should be used.

G. Mortality

The mortality for intraabdominal abscess before 1975 ranged from 25% to 35%. Since then, the mortality has fallen to 10–15%. This improvement has been ascribed to better preoperative localization due to CT scans and ultrasound and use of antibiotics active against anaerobes and aerobes.

H. Complications

1. **Organ failure** occurs in 10–20% of patients, affecting the heart, kidneys, lungs, or liver. The mortality of such patients is 50–60%. Organ failure accounts for two-thirds of deaths of patients with abscess.
2. **Hemorrhage.**
3. Enterocutaneous, pancreatic or intraabdominal **fistulas.**
4. **Superinfection** by *Candida* or resistant gram-negative bacilli.

IV. Subphrenic Abscesses

A. Anatomic considerations. Subphrenic spaces are divided on the **right** and **left** sides by the falciform ligament. They are further divided on the **right side** by the coronary ligaments into **anterior** and **posterior** compartments; and on the **left side** into **subphrenic** and **subhepatic spaces** (Table 2-4). Any collection of pus that is contiguous to the diaphragm in these anatomic spaces is considered a subphrenic abscess.

B. Pathogenesis of subphrenic abscess. A site of origin can be identified in 90% of cases of subphrenic abscess. Approximately 50% arise as postoperative complications. Spontaneous events such as perforated gastric or duodenal ulcer, abdominal trauma, and acute appendicitis account for the remainder.

Source of subphrenic abscess	Percent of total cases
Stomach	35
Liver and biliary tract	20
Appendix	10
Large bowel	10
Abdominal trauma (multiple injuries)	10
Miscellaneous	15

C. Symptoms and signs. In 90% of cases the onset is **acute or subacute,** occurring within 6 months of the precipitating event, e.g., operation or spontaneous intestinal perforation. Patients usually complain of diffuse **abdominal pain,** but there is poor localization of pain to one side or the other. **Fever,** often associated with chills, is seen in a high percentage of patients. Over 90% of patients complain of **both fever and abdominal pain** at some time during the course of their illness, and these two symptoms, in the setting of a predisposing cause, represent the strongest indications of a subphrenic abscess. **Weight loss** is noted in about two-thirds of patients; about the same number complain of chest pain or some respiratory symptoms.

Signs and symptoms of acute subphrenic abscess	Percent of total cases
Acute (6 mos)	90
Chronic (6 mos)	10
Fever	70–90
Chest findings	70–90
Weight loss	60–70
Abdominal or chest pain	40–70
Abdominal tenderness	40–70
Nausea and vomiting	10–20

Abdominal tenderness can be appreciated in the majority of patients, but the localization may not necessarily correspond to the site of the abscess. The most useful physical findings relate to **abnormalities in the chest,** found in nearly 90% of cases; these are pleural effusion, atelectasis, and an elevated, often immobilized, diaphragm.

Chest X-ray findings in subphrenic abscess	Percent of total cases
Pleural effusion	65*
Elevated diaphragm	50
Immobile diaphragm	30
Atelectasis	25
Pneumonitis	10

An **elevated white blood count** with a shift to the left and a predominance of polymorphonuclear leukocytes is the general rule in subphrenic abscess. Most patients are anemic and show the typical normocytic, normochromic anemia of chronic infection.

Less common signs are intracostal edema or erythema, draining sinus, and, in rare cases, a bulge in the abdominal wall.

The extensive use of antibiotics following surgical procedures has produced a **chronic form** of subphrenic abscess, seen in approximately 10% of cases. The onset is insidious, with few localizing symptoms. Fever, intermittent abdominal

*90% of pleural effusions are on the same side, 10% on the opposite side, and 1% are bilateral.

pain, and weight loss are the commonest complaints. The hiatus between the presumed precipitating event and diagnosis of the abscess can be as long as 10 years. During this period the patient loses weight, becomes anorexic, and appears so feeble as to suggest a diagnosis of carcinoma.

D. Diagnostic clues

1. Fluid introduced into the abdominal cavity has access to the subphrenic spaces on both sides. However, fluid from the right paracolic gutter tends to move upward to the right subhepatic space (Morison's pouch). Fluid from the pelvic space can flow via the left paracolic gutter, but the colon and transverse mesocolon act as barriers to the subphrenic spaces. A ruptured duodenal ulcer favors the right subphrenic spaces, while gastric ulcers favor the left side, usually the anterior spaces.
2. The **right subphrenic space,** when involved with infection, is often associated with an elevated diaphragm, pleural effusion, empyema, and/or pneumonitis in the right lung.
3. The **right subhepatic space (Morison's pouch)** is the watershed of the appendix, duodenum, and biliary tract. It may be contaminated by events following biliary tract or gastroduodenal operation, perforated duodenal ulcer, perforated right colon (appendix or hepatic flexure), or a ruptured gall bladder. The diagnosis often is very difficult. There may be an enlarging, poorly defined, tender mass in the right upper quadrant, which suggests involvement of this space. A flat-plate x-ray of the abdomen may show air bubbles or an air-fluid level. Scanning techniques usually are required to establish the presence of an abscess cavity.
4. The **left subphrenic space** has poorly defined boundaries. The wall of an abscess in this location often is enmeshed in inflammatory tissue and dense vascularized adhesions. This creates operative problems when the abscess arises from pancreatitis, since the wall may bleed profusely, especially in the presence of an operative drain. Other causes of abscess in this area are gastric hemorrhage and splenectomy. There is a tendency for the abscess to form fistulas into the gastrointestinal tract, leading to bleeding and perforated viscus.
5. The **lesser sac** may communicate with an anterior abscess, or it may be involved as an isolated process, usually associated with acute pancreatitis. Scanning techniques are usually required to diagnose an abscess at this site. An upper GI series shows anterior displacement of the stomach and widening of the duodenal loop.
6. When hemorrhage precedes perforation of a gastric or duodenal ulcer, there is a higher risk of subphrenic abscess formation in the postoperative period. The explanation is that blood is an effective buffer of gastric acid, the normal defense mechanism that kills off bacteria from the oropharynx as they are swallowed. Thus, in the presence of blood, the concentration of microorganisms in the stomach and duodenum is extremely high, thereby increasing the risk of infection when perforation of the viscus occurs.

E. Diagnostic procedures

1. **X-rays.** Roentgenographic findings often suggest the diagnosis of subphrenic abscess:

   Pleural effusion
   Elevated and/or fixed diaphragm
   Atelectasis
   Pneumonitis
   Gas bubbles in abscess
   Displacement of adjacent viscus

   In addition to inspiration and expiration chest x-rays, fluoroscopy establishes the immobility of the diaphragm. An upper GI series may show displacement of the stomach, especially when the patient is in the Trendelenburg position. A combined liver-lung scan may be useful to display a space-occupying lesion in the right subphrenic space.

2. **Computerized tomography (CT scan)** is the most successful diagnostic technique currently available. The accuracy in intraabdominal abscesses is over 90%, with a low incidence of false-positives.
3. An **abdominal echogram** is helpful in delineating a mass lesion and in determining whether a structure is fluid-filled or solid.
4. **Gallium scans** have been rewarding in the diagnosis of subphrenic abscess. The isotope is preferentially picked up by white blood cells, and localization can be achieved by this technique when other methods have failed. However, it is important to emphasize that both false-positive and false-negative results have been noted with this technique. Other problems with gallium scanning are uptake by the intestine, localization in recent surgical sites, and the long time (3–5 days) required for a definitive scan.
5. **Percutaneous needle aspiration** of a suspected abscess is disavowed by most surgeons. There are several dangers to this procedure: spreading infection, rupturing into major viscera or blood vessels, and the false security of negative results, since the abscess may be missed by this technique. However, needle aspiration can be used at the time of exploratory laparotomy under direct vision in order to probe a suspected mass for the presence of pus.
6. **Percutaneous drainage** of subphrenic abscesses can be attempted under guidance by **ultrasound or CT scan.** With an 18-gauge needle under CT scan direction, fluid is drawn from the abscess for diagnosis. Drainage can be achieved by guiding a pig-tail catheter into the abscess cavity under ultrasound monitoring.

   Subphrenic abscess may be a cryptic and undiagnosable condition; approximately 10% of cases have been missed during life, the final recognition being made at the autopsy table.

F. **Bacteriology.** Since most subphrenic abscesses are related to contamination by the gastrointestinal tract, their bacteriology is similar to that of other intraabdominal infections, i.e., a mixture of aerobic and anaerobic bacteria (see Table 2-1). **Exceptions** to this general rule include:

1. Septicemia may cause metastatic spread of pathogenic bacteria to the subphrenic space. In this setting a single organism, often *Staphylococcus* or *Streptococcus,* is encountered.
2. Infections following a perforated gastric or duodenal ulcer become contaminated with bacteria derived from the oropharynx. These organisms are contained in saliva and are washed into the stomach with food and drink. *Fusobacterium, Bacteroides melaninogenicus,* and anaerobic streptococci are common pathogens in this setting. *B. fragilis* is less commonly encountered. The implication of these findings is that an abscess caused by oropharyngeal flora can be treated adequately with a penicillin or cephalosporin, whereas an abscess harboring *B. fragilis* requires a specific antibiotic such as clindamycin, chloramphenicol, cefoxitin, or metronidazole.
3. An abscess resulting from biliary tract infection or rupture of an abscess in the liver or spleen can be caused by coliforms such as *E. coli* or *Klebsiella* or by streptococci. The infecting flora is composed of a single or perhaps two pathogens, rather than the complex mixture found in the usual intraabdominal abscess. Anaerobes may be absent.

G. **Treatment.** The cornerstones of treatment are **surgical drainage** and **antimicrobial drugs.** The approach to drainage is based on the anatomic location.

1. **Operative approach**
   a. For a **right subphrenic** abscess (posterosuperior), the extraserous approach by a posterolateral exposure and resection of the 12th rib is recommended by some authorities. A transverse incision through the lumbar fascia and diaphragm at the level of the 1st lumbar spinal process is performed. This exposes the perirenal fascia and the liver. The problem with this technique is the limited area of exposure; other abscesses, often located in the subphrenic space, cannot be easily approached. For this reason, a transperitoneal (subcostal) approach with adequate exposure for inspection and insertion of drains often is the preferred route.

b. A **right subphrenic** abscess, posterior in location, can be drained by a transpleural approach. This procedure is especially useful if there is pleural and/or pulmonary involvement.

c. Subphrenic abscesses that involve the **left side,** either perihepatic or in the lesser sac, are best approached by a transperitoneal route. The extent of suppuration can be appreciated only at operation, and adequate exposure is highly desirable.

2. **Antimicrobial therapy.** Antibiotic treatment of the mixed aerobic-anaerobic abscess is similar to that already listed (pp. 18–19) for other forms of intraabdominal sepsis, i.e., an antianaerobic drug—clindamycin, cefoxitin, metronidazole, or chloramphenicol—in association with an aminoglycoside, such as gentamicin, amikacin, or tobramycin. As noted above, cefoxitin can be used as a single agent when a resistant organism is not present. An abscess with a single pathogen, such as *Staphylococcus* or a coliform, can be treated with the drug appropriate to that pathogen. Usually a cephalosporin such as cefazolin or cephalothin is adequate in this setting.

H. **Dangers of prolonged antibiotic therapy.** A caveat should be inserted regarding the antimicrobial treatment of intraabdominal abscesses. It has become apparent that the presentation of localized purulent collections within the abdomen may be chronic rather than acute. The scenario of a chronic abscess is as follows:

A patient has undergone an intestinal operation or has sustained trauma to the abdomen and developed fever postoperatively that was treated with a long course of antibiotics. The fever relented, and the patient was apparently cured of sepsis. A long hiatus ensues, often months, sometimes years, during which time the patient has intermittent periods of malaise, fever, and abdominal pain, superimposed on a pattern of weight loss and gradual inanition. The diagnosis of chronic intraabdominal abscess is made after a prolonged period, but now the patient is in such poor nutritional status that what should be a relatively simple drainage procedure becomes a high-risk event. Such chronic subphrenic abscesses have an overall mortality of 35%, despite advances in antibiotic therapy and surgical technique.

Chronic intraabdominal abscess is a product of modern antibiotic therapy. In order to avoid such cryptic infections, it is advised that patients not be treated with antibiotics for long periods of time when there is a suspicion of an intraabdominal collection of purulent material. There is an enduring surgical tenet, one that should not be violated by antibiotics: **pus in a closed space must be adequately drained.** Treatment of such infections with injudicious and extended use of antibiotics only suppresses the infection and converts an easily drained purulent collection into a chronic, mysterious septic process. It is better to stop antibiotics and let the infection present itself, rather than attempt to suppress it with drugs.

I. **Complications.** Approximately two-thirds of patients with subphrenic abscess have complications in the abdomen or chest. Sixty percent of these individuals have more than one major complication.

Abdominal complications associated with subphrenic abscess are as follows:

Wound infection
Dehiscence
Impingement on surrounding viscera
Generalized peritonitis and uncontrolled sepsis
Fistula formation
Hemorrhage
Pylephlebitis

The pleuropulmonary complications associated with subphrenic abscess are

Pleural effusions
Pneumonitis
Atelectasis
Empyema

Bronchopleural fistual
Peforation of diaphragm
Lung abscess
Peforation into pericardial sac

A small percentage of patients with subphrenic abscess experience septicemia and even septic shock. This is usually in the setting of the seriously ill patient who cannot undergo adequate surgical drainage.

J. Risk factors. Despite advances in surgical technique and antibiotic therapy, the outcome is unfortunately still guarded for some patients with intraabdominal abscess. In relatively acute cases, the mortality is 10–20%, whereas in more chronic infections, the mortality is 30–40%. Patients treated with antibiotics alone, when a surgical procedure is forestalled or delayed, have a mortality of approximately 50%.

The important determinants of mortality in patients with subphrenic abscess are

1. **Underlying disease.** Patients with carcinoma or severe biliary disease have a poor outlook.
2. **Organ failure.** Cardiac, renal, pulmonary, or hepatic failure portends a poor prognosis.
3. **Location.** Multiple abscesses and those that are intraperitoneal or intravisceral carry a higher fatality.
4. **Chronicity.** Long duration of symptoms has an increased mortality, often related to the poor nutritional status of the patient.
5. **Complications.** Peritonitis, communication with viscera or the GI tract, dehiscence, and perforation into the chest cavity increase the risk.

The relationship between mortality and major complications in subphrenic abscess is as follows:

Complication	Percent mortality
No complications	10–20
Complications	30–40
Wound dehiscence	35
Empyema without bronchopleural fistula	40
Empyema with bronchopleural fistula	60
Organ failure	60
Other intraabdominal abscesses	70
Associated hepatic abscess	75
Perforation into GI tract	80
Generalized peritonitis	90

V. Retroperitoneal abscess. Infection can arise in the potential space existing between the peritoneum and the transversalis fascia. This space has been further divided into an **anterior division,** limited by the peritoneum and the anterior renal fascia; and a posterior **retroperitoneal space,** which can be further divided into the perinephric spaces. The anterior and posterior compartments are involved with septic conditions in approximately equal frequencies. On rare occasions, the **retrofascial space,** behind the transversalis fascia, becomes infected.

A. Predisposing causes. Retroperitoneal spaces account for approximately 40% of intraabdominal abscesses. Common sources of infection are as follows:

Intestinal source 50%
Appendicitis
Diverticulitis
Pancreatitis
Renal source 50%
Pyelonephritis
Intrarenal abscess

Perinephric abscess can arise spontaneously, without a predisposing cause. An intestinal or renal site should be suspected in all retroperitoneal abscesses, but even a conscientious search can yield a negative result.

B. **Symptoms and signs.** The diagnosis is suspected initially from signs of **severe sepsis** with fever and shaking chills, occasionally associated with septic shock. Patients complain of pain in the back, along the psoas muscle, which is referred to the gluteal area, the leg, hip, or thigh. The patient often is restless, thrashing from side to side, finding it impossible to be comfortable. Sometimes a mass can be felt in the abdomen, flank, or back. Tenderness and spasm of the back muscles are related features. A perinephric abscess usually is accompanied by **muscle spasm** and/or **bulging of the flank.**

Appendicitis

I. **Diagnosis.** Acute appendicitis usually presents with a sequence of anorexia, nausea, vomiting, and abdominal pain. The pain is often periumbilical at onset, later moving to the right lower quadrant. There are three pathologic stages of infection that can be recognized at operation: local inflammation, regional inflammation (periappendicitis), and perforation. These stages often have a poor correlation with the clinical signs and symptoms. However, decisions concerning antibiotic therapy and technique of wound closure are based on the intraoperative finding (Table 2-5).
Perforation of the appendix occurs in 30–40% of cases; the incidence is related, in some instances, to delay in diagnosis. Morbidity is associated mostly with perforation and is found in 15–30% of such cases. The major complications are abscess formation and wound infection. The mortality in otherwise healthy individuals is low, less than 1%.
The sites of abdominal abscess following perforated appendix* are

Site	Percent of total abscesses
Right lower quadrant	62
Anterior retroperitoneum	16
Pelvic	13
Subphrenic	7
Interloop	2

II. **Treatment.** Antibiotics are indicated only when local abscess formation or free perforation has occurred. Since the condition of the appendix and its surrounding structures cannot be appreciated until the operation is underway, it is prudent to begin antibiotics (one dose) preoperatively. The decision to continue therapy depends on the operative findings (Table 2-5). If the patient is being observed for evolution of signs of appendicitis, antibiotics (and potent pain medication) should be avoided, since they may obscure the natural course.
The bacteriology of appendicitis is a mixture of aerobic and anaerobic bacteria, similar to those seen with bowel perforation. Thus, antimicrobial therapy is patterned along the same lines, using drugs for aerobes and anaerobes (see pp. 18–19). General support measures, as outlined on p. 19, should be instituted.
Vigorous replacement of fluids and electrolytes, and blood or colloids if necessary, is important in postoperative management. Daily rectal examination by the same surgeon is helpful in the early recognition of a developing pelvic abscess.
Whenever possible, the inflamed appendix should be removed. In cases in which a necrotic appendix is found floating freely in the exudate or in an abscess cavity, drainage alone is indicated. Additional repair may be necessary at a later time, when the inflammation has resolved.
Some surgeons prefer to manage local collections of pus in the paracolic gutter by drainage and delayed primary closure, and they do not employ antibiotics unless there is generalized peritonitis or systemic signs of sepsis. With a perforated appendix, local irrigation is useful for removing debris, necrotic tissue, or exudate.

*Adapted from W. A. Altemeier et al., Intra-abdominal abscesses. *Am. J. Surg.* 125:70, 1973.

Table 2-5. Management of acute appendicitis

Stage	Wound management	Antibiotics
Local inflammation, restricted to appendix	Primary closure; no drains	Only preoperative
Inflammation with periappendicitis; no pus	Primary closure; no drains	Only preoperative
Perforation		
Local abscess	Delayed primary closure; intraperitoneal drain to abscess cavity	Recommended (short-term)
Generalized peritonitis	Delayed primary closure; intraperitoneal drains, if localized collections of exudate are found to be present	Mandatory (full course)

Diverticulitis

I. **General principles.** Diverticula of the colon are extremely common in older individuals who are consuming a standard Western diet. Approximately one-third of patients over age 45 have large-bowel diverticula, usually on the left side of the bowel, with the highest prevalence in the sigmoid colon. These structures are outpouchings or small hernias of the intestinal mucosa through the circular muscular layer at the site of penetration of the terminal branches of the mesenteric artery. About 10% of individuals with diverticulosis experience symptoms at some time in their lives. Such individuals have occasional episodes of colicky, abdominal pain. A small percentage, however, develop severe infection, known as **diverticulitis,** which at times requires surgical intervention.

II. **Pathogenetic mechanisms.** A single diverticulum, or multiple ones in the same area, can become infected, usually due to inflammation and obstruction of the neck of the diverticulum. There is diffuse inflammation (peridiverticulitis) of the bowel wall that can extend through the muscular layer, even to the serosa. Intramural abscesses are formed that can rupture into surrounding tissue, sometimes freely into the peritoneal cavity, or into adjacent structures such as the bladder, a loop of small bowel, or the uterus. Microperforations are seen at the base of the diverticulum. Thus, we see that the septic process is in communication with the intraluminal colonic flora.

III. **Symptoms.** Chronic, relapsing diverticulitis is characterized by crampy, lower abdominal pain with poor localization, which leads to a change in bowel habits—either diarrhea, constipation, or alternating waves of each. This symptom complex is similar to that seen in irritable bowel syndromes.

These symptoms can escalate into an attack of diverticulitis. Fever, malaise, nausea, vomiting, and lower abdominal pain are indicative of an acute episode. A mild attack can be treated at home by "giving the bowel a rest," i.e., advising a semisolid, low-residue diet. The severe attack, however, requires hospitalization and intensive therapy.

IV. **X-rays.** A barium enema demonstrates diverticula in the colon, but this finding only verifies the presence of **diverticulosis,** not necessarily diverticulitis. Since large-bowel diverticula are so common, particularly in older people, a positive x-ray is not useful in a specific individual. More helpful roentgenographic findings of diverticulitis on barium enema include the following.

   A. Persistent spasm and coarse mucosal folds, seen usually in the sigmoid region, the commonest area for diverticulitis.

B. Spicules of barium, occasionally seen to form a fistular tract. A path of barium can sometimes be followed from the diverticulum to an abscess cavity. A caveat should be inserted regarding barium enema examination during a period of acute symptomology. Barium can escape through a ruptured diverticulum, producing a severe case of "barium peritonitis."

C. On a flat plate of the abdomen, small bubbles of gas ("soapsuds bubbles"), outside the bowel, can be seen in an abscess cavity, most often in the left flank, adjacent to the sigmoid area.

V. **Treatment.** Patients hospitalized for diverticulitis should be managed initially with conservative measures:

A. The patient should be allowed nothing by mouth.

B. A nasogastric or intestinal tube should be inserted under intermittent suction to decompress the small intestine.

C. Intravenous fluids and electrolytes should be administered with proper compensation for aspirated fluid and the accumulation within the bowel due to partial obstruction.

D. The use of antispasmodics and narcotics such as meperidine (Demerol) or morphine is controversial; we would recommend that such drugs be withheld, except for unremitting, severe pain.

E. **Antibiotic therapy.** If there is evidence of intestinal obstruction, fever and chills, peritoneal signs, or the presence of a mass suggesting an abscess, it is advisable to initiate antimicrobial treatment. The rational use of antibiotics is predicated on an understanding of the microbiology.

Since the diverticulum communicates with the colonic flora, the resulting infection involves a combination of aerobic and anaerobic bacteria, similar to that in other forms of intraabdominal sepsis (Table 2-1). Large abscesses can occur in this setting, and the purulent contents yield multiple types of enteric bacteria. Bacteremia frequently accompanies severe diverticulitis. The pathogens isolated from the bloodstream are coliforms, *B. fragilis*, and clostridia, in that order of frequency.

On the basis of these pathologic events and the infecting flora, it is recommended that the following antibiotics be used (see pp. 18–19 for details):

1. **For anaerobes:** Clindamycin, cefoxitin, metronidazole, or chloramphenicol.
2. **For aerobes:** Gentamicin, tobramicin, or amikacin.

For patients with a recent onset of symptoms, cefoxitin can be used as a single drug, since resistant bacteria are rarely encountered in this setting.

F. **Indications for operative invention.** When patients fail to respond to conservative measures and antimicrobial therapy, operative intervention is necessary. Indications are

1. Intestinal obstruction, suggested by persistent abdominal distention, increases in abdominal pain, and an x-ray of the abdomen that shows air-fluid levels, dilated loops of bowel, or absence of air in the rectum.
2. Imminent or actual perforation, characterized by increasing peritoneal signs or a sudden change in the clinical course that indicates a catastrophic event.
3. Severe toxicity with chills and fever and unrelenting sepsis, not responding to adequate antibiotics and conventional measures.
4. Demonstration of an abscess, either by palpation of a tender mass, by radiographic appearance of air in the soft tissues, by a barium enema that shows displacement by a cavity, or by evidence of fistula formation with flow of barium into the cavity.
5. Urinary tract symptoms, especially pneumaturia or foul-smelling urine, which suggest a fistula to the bladder.
6. Passage of stool into the vagina.
7. Multiple attacks, despite medical management.

G. Several **operative approaches** have been advocated. The traditional method is a **three-stage procedure** consisting of a diverting transverse colostomy with drainage of the infected area, followed in 3–4 weeks by a resection of the involved bowel with reanastomosis and 2–3 weeks later by a closure of the colostomy. This technique, while giving good results, imposes three operations and long periods of hospitalization.

Most surgeons now attempt a **two-stage procedure:** the diseased segment is excised and drainage performed; the proximal loop is brought out as an end-colostomy, while the distal end is brought out as a mucous fistula, or a Hartmann's pouch is created. The advantage of the Hartmann's pouch is that all the intraperitoneal sigmoid colon can be resected; it can be argued that this is rarely necessary, since ties rarely extend below 25 cm from the anus. Hartmann's turn-in seems to have a higher rate of recurrent abscess than mucous fistula. At the time of the second operation the proximal end-colostomy is refashioned and anastomosed to the opened pouch of distal rectum. An alternative type of two-stage procedure is resection of involved colon with reanastomosis and performance of a diverting proximal colostomy, which is closed at the second operation.

In selected cases, a **primary resection** and anastomosis can be performed, although this invites the possibility of a breakdown of the anastomosis and recurrent suppuration and fistula formation.

H. Several risk factors influence the type of operation and the eventual outcome. The following features are associated with a higher mortality:

1. Chronic disease with multiple recurrences
2. Significant hemorrhage
3. Obstruction
4. Peritonitis
5. Abscess formation
6. Poor nutritional status
7. Advanced age

Drains and Abdominal Wound Irrigation

I. General principles. Drains are usually employed **prophylactically** in cases in which postoperative drainage or bleeding is strongly suspected. In this clinical setting, their presence allows prompt diagnosis of leakage and also prevents intraabdominal or intrathoracic accumulation of fluids.

Drains are also used **therapeutically** to allow the escape of a localized area of accumulation, such as in abdominal or thoracic abscesses.

Drains cannot be used for generalized peritonitis, since the protective mechanisms of the body rapidly wall off the drain from surrounding structures, just as they would isolate a foreign body.

II. Types of drains most frequently used

A. Gauze packing is the simplest type of drain. It functions by capillary action only as long as the fabric can absorb fluid. Once saturated, the gauze must be replaced. It is used only in simple subcutaneous abscesses, mostly for the mechanical debridement that the gauze affords rather than for the initial drainage function.

B. Rubber drains, the most commonly used type, may be either flat strips or hollow (Penrose) tubes (see Table 2-6). The Penrose drain affords excellent passive drainage due to the rubber's capillary action.

C. Plastic drains include both flap-suction catheters and sump drains. Both types act as conduits, with "active" suction delivered to their outer ends. This type of drain is necessary for evacuation against the force of gravity. The sump drain has two lumina; air is accessible to the outer lumen to prevent the vacuum adhesion of the aspirating inner lumen. Newer modifications of the sump-type drainage catheters employ filters at the end of the air conduit, and also disposable collection containers that have microporous filters to retain bacteria, and in addition, have reusable electric suction units that fit into the collection device.

III. Removal

A. All drains should be removed as soon as possible to minimize the possibility of complications.

B. Aseptic technique must be strictly practiced when examining or changing the dressings that overlie the drain site.

Table 2-6. Use of drains in common abdominal operations

Operation	Always use	Occasionally use	Never use	Type of drain
Gastrectomy		X		Sump drain to duodenal stump
Pyeloroplasty			X	
Small-bowel resection			X	
Intraperitoneal colon resection			X	
Extraperitoneal colon resection (low anterior resection)	X			Flap catheter or sump
Cholecystectomy and other biliary procedures		X		Flap catheter or sump
Splenectomy		X		Flap catheter or sump
Pancreatic surgery	X			Sump drain
Drainage of visceral abscess (liver)	X			Combo penrose & sump drains
Drainage of intraperitoneal abscess	X			Combo penrose & sump drains
Large soft-tissue dissections	X			Flap catheter

C. Drains placed **prophylactically** should be removed within the 1st 2 postoperative days if drainage has not occurred. These drains are generally removed completely at one time.

D. Drains placed **therapeutically** are left in place as long as drainage continues. To remove, the drain should be twisted to break off any adhesions and then moved out gradually, a few centimeters each day. This process assures that the drainage tract will fill upward from the deepest portion and prevents the pocketing of suppurative material in the tract.

IV. Complications

A. Drains are a "two-way street": Bacteria from the skin or the environment can easily travel to the depths of the drainage site to cause local or invasive infection. Careful, aseptic dressing of the wound and prompt removal of the drain reduce the possibility of significant exogenous infection.

B. Less pliable plastic drains (sump catheters) left in place for several days may cause pressure erosion of the surrounding tissues. For this reason plastic drains should be fixed away from vital sutures.

C. Drains to intraperitoneal intestinal anastomoses usually are unwarranted and may interfere with the normal process of healing.

IV. Abdominal Wound Irrigation

A. Saline lavage

1. Saline is used widely in the irrigation of the peritoneal cavity and the abdominal wall in contaminated or dirty operations. This technique mechanically dilutes debris, dead cells, bacteria, and gastrointestinal contents, which if retained would increase the sepsis and retard the healing process.
2. In the past a theoretical objection was that saline lavage of the peritoneal cavity in the face of peritonitis would further spread the infecting organisms. Studies have shown, however, that this objection is invalid. A small amount

of colored dye placed in one small area of the peritoneal cavity disperses widely within a few minutes. It must be assumed that bacteria free in the peritoneal cavity act similarly.

3. A greater amount of saline irrigation produces a greater reduction of bacteria. Five to ten liters of saline can be used in cases of generalized peritoneal contamination, unless the signs of cardiac failure are evident. Saline irrigation should be accompanied by a thorough abdominal exploration—including the subphrenic spaces, the pelvis, and any adherent intestinal loops—to discover, open, and drain any pockets of purulence.
4. The subcutaneous space should aslo be vigorously irrigated with saline after peritoneal and fascial closure.

B. Antibiotic lavage of the wound and peritoneal cavity

1. Many antibiotic agents have been used with saline for peritoneal and wound irrigation. Most surgeons who advocate use of antibiotic irrigation recommend it only at the time of operation. Others advocate use of an inlying peritoneal catheter for periodic irrigation in the early postoperative period. When used, this continuous irrigation must include a heparin solution to prevent walling off of the intraperitoneal catheter by fibrinous adhesions.
2. Some studies report a reduction of postoperative wound infection following antibiotic irrigation when compared to saline alone. There is no evidence, however, that antibiotic irrigation is superior to saline irrigation in the prevention of intraabdominal abscesses.
3. Most commonly used peritoneal antibiotic lavages—including kanamycin, neomycin, sulfonamide, ampicillin, and kanamycin/bacitracin—do not suppress the anaerobic gastrointestinal microflora, although they usually retard the growth of aerobic coliforms (see Table 2-7).
4. Complications are reported following antibiotic peritoneal lavage. These complications are usually related to rapid antibiotic absorption by the inflamed peritoneum. Most frequently, prolonged apnea occurs with the use of aminoglycoside agents with curarelike anesthetics. Rarely, there may be hypersensitivity reactions or renal toxicity.

C. Recommendations for wound and peritoneal irrigation

1. Saline lavage of peritoneal cavity and wound should be liberally performed in all patients with evidence of contamination. Peritoneal irrigation **with antibiotics** is controversial.
2. Appropriate parenteral antibiotic agents that are active against both colonic aerobes and anaerobes should be administered immediately preoperatively and continued as indicated postoperatively. (See pp. 18–19.)
3. After facial closure, local wound irrigation with the various safe antibiotics in addition to saline is optional.
4. The once popular use of intraperitoneal irrigation with povidone-iodine solutions is generally discouraged due to reported side effects, which include metabolic acidosis, and to lack of efficacy in experimental models of intraperitoneal sepsis.

Surgical Aspects of Intestinal Amebiasis

I. General principles. Amebiasis is a cosmopolitan disease, respecting neither age nor socioeconomic class. Of the six amebae that may inhabit the human gut, only *Entamoeba histolytica* is a pathogen. The parasite exists in two forms, as a **cyst,** generally measuring 12–20μ in diameter, and in an invasive form, the **trophozoite,** which varies considerably in length, but is usually 10–20μ. The cyst is responsible for transmission by vehicles such as water and food, especially leafy vegetables. The trophozoite is the form seen in tissue sections.

Table 2-7. Qualities of antibiotics commonly employed in peritoneal lavage

Agent	Dose (usually mixed in 500 ml saline)	Suppression of aerobic coliforms	Suppression of anaerobic *Bacteroides*	Complications reported		
				Hypersensitivity	Renal	Prolonged apnea
Ampicillin	1,000 mg	+	–	X		
Kanamycin	500 mg	+	–		X	X
Neomycin	500 mg	+	–		X	X
Kanamycin/ bacitracin	500 mg 50,000 units	+	–		X	X
Sulfonamides	1,000–2,000 mg	+	–	XX		

+ = Effective; – = Not generally effective; XX = Occasionally; X = Rarely.

II. Clinical presentations. The forms of intestinal amebiasis are

Asymptomatic cyst passer
Dysentery (mild to severe)
Chronic amebic colitis
Ameboma
Amebic appendicitis

A. An **asymptomatic cyst passer** is the type of patient most frequently encountered. In the United States approximately 4% of the population have cysts in their stools without experiencing symptoms. Careful studies, however, have revealed mucosal invasion in some individuals, so that this condition may not be totally benign.

B. Most episodes of **acute amebiasis** tend to be subacute in nature, with alternating periods of diarrhea and relative well-being. Symptoms may last for weeks, months, or even years if untreated. While such recurrent cases do exist, it is important to recognize that many patients, even with dysentery, have spontaneous cures.

It has been a custom in the past to label all cryptic diarrheal diseases as "amebiasis," prompting the famous remark of Elsdon-Dew that "amebiasis is the last resort of the diagnostically destitute."

III. Pathology. The most common site of intestinal invasion is the cecum, followed by the sigmoid, rectum, and splenic flexure. The ulcerations tend to be spotty, with normal intervening mucosa. The classic pathologic picture is an initial erosion that leads to a mucosal ulcer that is associated with necrosis of the lamina propria. These events produce a "flask-shaped" ulcer with a small opening on the surface and a large necrotic zone beneath. Typically there is a paucity of inflammatory cells in the necrotic debris, and only a narrow rim of plasma cells, lymphocytes, and eosinophils surrounding the zone of ulceration. Only 50% of mucosal biopsies actually demonstrate the parasite, always seen in its trophozoite form within tissue. Recently, some investigators have reported a diffuse, nonspecific inflammatory reaction in the mucosa. It is claimed that this form of amebiasis cannot be differentiated from other types of inflammatory bowel disease, whether infectious or idiopathic in nature.

IV. Signs and symptoms. Diarrhea occurs in all patients with amebic colitis. Approximately two-thirds of patients have only one attack, while one-third have prolonged diarrhea, from 1 to 8 months in duration. The individual episode of diarrhea lasts 5–10 days, usually with five to eight bowel movements per day, although some individuals experience up to 20 liquid stools in a 24-hour period.

Sign	Incidence in patients with amebic dysentery (%)
Diarrhea	100
Blood in stool	100
Gross blood in stool	60
Crampy abdominal pain	50
Weight loss	50
Fever	40
Tenesmus	30
Nausea and vomiting	15

There is a paucity of physical findings. Weight loss and dehydration are occasionally present. Abdominal tenderness is found in approximately 20% of patients. An enlarged, usually tender liver is encountered in about 25% of patients.

V. Laboratory findings. Routine laboratory studies yield nonspecific results and may be entirely normal in patients with amebic dysentery. Approximately 50% of patients have **mild anemia,** which is usually due to iron deficiency, but it may be a normochromic, normocytic anemia of chronic infection. The **white blood cell count** is elevated in 40% of patients. Eosinophilia is distinctly unusual in amebiasis. As a general rule, protozoan infections do not cause a rise in eosinophils. Such an increase in this cell line would suggest the coexistence of another parasitic infection, such as roundworms or schistosomiasis.

A. Stool examination. The definite diagnosis of amebiasis is based on direct visualization of the parasite in the stool or intestinal mucosa. In most cases of intestinal disease the organism can be identified by collecting three fresh stool specimens, preferably on different days. All such specimens should be examined directly for motile trophozoites. If the stool is loose, semiformed, or frankly bloody, it should also be placed in a fixative such as polyvinyl alcohol (PVA), and the fixed preparation should be examined by a Trichrome stain. Formed stools, in which cysts are more likely to be encountered, should be examined by a concentration method as well as by direct smear. Three careful stool examinations should identify up to 90% of intestinal infections.

Many chemicals and drugs used in treatment or diagnosis can interfere with identification of the parasite in the stool. Such interfering materials include bismuth, kaolin, certain antibiotics such as neomycin and tetracycline, heavy metal compounds, magnesium hydroxide, oils, soaps and irritants used for enemas, and barium sulfate. The preparation for a barium enema x-ray examination invalidates microscopic study of the stool for amebic forms for up to 2 weeks.

B. Amebic serology. The most reliable serologic test for diagnosing amebiasis is the indirect hemagglutination test (IHA). This test measures mostly serum IgG, with some IgM. A diagnostic titer is 1:128 or greater. It is estimated that 3–5% of asymptomatic individuals in the United States have a titer of this level. In invasive intestinal amebiasis, the IHA titer is positive in 95% of proved cases. Other serologic tests have recently become available, but their accuracy has not been as well established as that of the IHA.

C. Sigmoidoscopy and biopsy. If the stool examination is negative, it is advised that sigmoidoscopy, or colonoscopy with a fiberoptic instrument, be performed. By direct vision, ulcerations are seen in the intestinal mucosa of 85% percent of patients with amebiasis. Approximately two-thirds of these have small ulcerations with a background of otherwise normal mucosa, while one-third show edema, hemorrhage, and surrounding inflammation. The ulcers tend to be punched-out, small, and even pinpoint, occasionally only 5 mm in diameter, and they are usually numerous. About 10% of patients show a diffusely hemorrhagic mucosa with no visible ulcers, and the remaining 5% have a normal mucosa, at least as far as the instrument can be passed.

A highly successful method of obtaining motile trophozoites is to sample the base of the ulcer with a spoon or cotton pledget. The material should be examined directly under the microscope, with a small amount of saline. Motile trophozoites, advancing with unidirectional motion, usually with ingested red cells, should be readily apparent. In addition, it is advised that a rectal biopsy be performed below the rectal valves; the tissue should be stained with hematoxylin-eosin as well as with PAS. (The PAS stain allows the pathologist to distinguish trophozoites from macrophages.)

VI. Confusion with inflammatory bowel disease. Careful analysis of history, x-ray findings, and routine laboratory tests cannot always differentiate between **intestinal amebiasis** and **inflammatory bowel disease.** The only positive distinction between these diseases is the presence of the parasite, either in fecal specimens or in intestinal biopsies. In some patients with chronic amebiasis, the parasite cannot be found even by these methods, and a presumptive diagnosis is based on serology (see **V.B**). A response to specific chemotherapy also favors the diagnosis of chronic amebiasis.

VII. Complications. Although most patients with amebiasis experience a self-cure or have relief of symptoms by antiamebic therapy, a small percentage suffer severe complications, as follows:

Perforation of bowel	Stricture
Hemorrhage	Intussusception
Appendicitis	Ameboma
Perianal abscess	Postdysenteric colitis

A. Perforation of the bowel is the common cause of death in patients with intestinal amebiasis. The major site, when it can be identified, is the cecum. The sequelae of perforation are localized inflammatory reaction, either extrinsic to the bowel or intrinsic to the bowel (ameboma); generalized peritonitis; or discrete intraabdominal abscess formation.

Two forms of intestinal perforation are seen in amebiasis, each with distinctive clinical presentation and requiring different forms of surgical management.

1. **Leakage through an extensively diseased bowel wall.** This condition occurs in association with severe amebic dysentery. The presentation is fulminating amebic colitis, much like that of severe ulcerative colitis. Although the bowel may appear grossly intact, it is severely ulcerated, often with a shaggy exudate visible on the serosal surface. The patient is gravely ill, and no specific change in the clinical course signals perforation. Rather, there is a crescendo of abdominal distention and ileus, accompanied by signs of severe toxicity with fever, chills, and hypotension. X-ray of the abdomen may show free air, an important sign of bowel perforation.

   A highly conservative approach is advised whenever possible, since the operative mortality in such cases is prohibitive. The initial treatment could include antiamebic therapy incorporating emetine or intravenous metronidazole, general support measures with fluid and electrolyte supplementation, and antibiotic therapy directed at the contaminated intestinal flora (either cefoxitin, metronidazole, clindamycin, or chloramphenicol, plus an aminoglycoside). At operation, the intestine is extremely friable, hemorrhagic, and weeping from several sites, with a fibrinoid exudate encasing the surface. The only operation feasible at this point is total colectomy. Whenever possible, the rectum should be spared.

2. **Discrete perforation** can occur in patients with mild to moderate amebiasis at the site of ulcer formation. This complication is ushered in by a sudden change in course, with the rapid onset of severe abdominal pain and signs of an acute abdomen. Such patients should be started on antiamebic therapy, such as emetine or intravenous metronidazole, if the diagnosis is known in advance, as well as broad-spectrum antibiotics against the intestinal flora. Exploratory laparotomy should be undertaken at the earliest possible moment. At operation, a discrete perforation usually can be identified, and the surrounding bowel is relatively healthy. The operation depends upon the extent and location of the perforation and the state of the intestinal wall; relatively conservative measures are recommended, since the mucosal ulcers will almost certainly heal with antiamebic therapy.

B. **Ameboma** can occur any time in the course of amebiasis, either during an acute episode or at a later period when the disease is apparently cured or at least quiescent. It is an active inflammatory reaction with granuloma formation, fibrosis, and scarring. It may present as a hard, smooth mass, with or without superficial ulceration. Multiple tumors of this type can be found throughout the bowel, but the commonest presentation is a single constricting mass, most often located in the cecum or sigmoid colon. Pain is a frequent, almost constant, feature, yet the patient often does not have symptoms of diarrhea or amebic dysentery. Fecal examination fails to reveal the amebic form in the majority of cases, particularly when the disease presents in the subacute or chronic phase. Complications of ameboma are stricture with obstruction, intussusception, and volvulus. The mass is often mistaken for a colon carcinoma.

1. The **diagnosis** can be established by colonoscopic biopsy, which displays typical ulcerations and amebic trophozoites. If the lesion is in the cecum, however, direct biopsy by colonoscopy is somewhat difficult. In this instance, a past history of amebiasis, along with a **positive amebic serology,** should suggest the proper diagnosis.

2. The preferred **treatment** of ameboma is antiamebic drugs, either metronidazole or emetine, which should cause a dramatic disappearance of the lesion within 1–3 weeks. Indeed, response to therapy is additional confirmation of the etiology.

   Two caveats should be entered: On the one hand, carcinoma of the colon can coexist with amebiasis, particularly in Western societies, although it is relatively uncommon in the tropics. On the other hand, scar and stricture forma-

Table 2-8. Treatment of amebiasis

Type	Agent	
Cyst Carrier	Diloxanide furoate (Furamide) Diiodohydroxyquin—second-line drug	
Intestinal Invasive		
Mild–moderate	Metronidazole Tetracycline or paromomycin	plus diloxanide furoate
Severe	Intravenous metronidazole or emetine, followed by diloxanide furoate	
Extraintestinal	Metronidazole Emetine and/or chloroquin followed by diloxanide furoate	

tion, particularly in the rectum, may not disappear with antiamebic therapy, so that operative intervention may be required to relieve obstruction. This procedure should be delayed if possible until adequate antiamebic therapy has been completed and the extent of resolution has been determined.

VIII. **Treatment.** There is no firm agreement about the management of asymptomatic individuals with cysts in their stools. Some authorities practice enlightened neglect and prefer not to treat. Others recommend specific chemotherapy be instituted in all cases (Table 2-8).

Diloxanide furoate (Furamide) is administered in a dose of 500 mg tid for 10 days.* Diiodohydroxyquin (Diodoquin), in a dose of 650 mg tid for 20 days, is a second-line treatment. There are occasional reactions related to the iodine contained in this compound. Of more serious import are the rare instances of optic atrophy and peripheral neuropathy which have been reported, especially with prolonged use.

A. **For mild-to-moderate intestinal amebiasis,** the preferred antimicrobial, in the view of most experts, is **metronidazole,** 750 mg tid for 10 days. (Many patients are unable to tolerate this dose because of vomiting or nausea; 500 mg tid can be given in these instances. Alternatively, antibiotics such as **tetracycline** (250 mg qid for 10 days) and **paromomycin** (250 mg qid for 10 days), can be administered. Diloxanide furoate should be used along with the antibiotics in order to eradicate the cysts.

B. **Severe amebic dysentery** is often associated with vomiting and/or ileus, thereby interdicting the use of oral preparations. In such instances, intravenous metronidazole (500 mg q8h for 10 days) or emetine (1 mg/kg/day [max 60 mg/day] IM for 5 days) should be employed, to be followed later by diloxanide furoate.

Surgical Complications of Typhoid Fever and Salmonellosis

I. **General principles.** Typhoid fever is a febrile illness of prolonged duration which is marked by hectic fever, delirium, enlargement of the spleen, abdominal pain, and a variety of systemic manifestations. Although caused primarily by **Salmonella typhi**, typhoidal disease occasionally is produced by other types of salmonellae. The portal of entry is the gastrointestinal tract, but typhoid fever is not truly an intestinal disease, having more systemic symptoms than those related to the bowel. In areas of improved sanitation and medical facilities, the mortality is 1–5%. The major causes of death are **intestinal perforation, hemorrhage,** and **severe toxemia.**

*In the United States this drug can be obtained from the Parasitic Diseases Division, Center for Disease Control, Atlanta, Georgia.

II. Pathogenesis. The pathologic events of typhoid fever are initiated in the intestinal tract following oral ingestion of typhoid bacilli. The organisms penetrates the small-bowel mucosa, sparing the stomach, making its way rapidly to the lymphatics and the mesenteric nodes, and, within minutes, enters the bloodstream. There is a paucity of local inflammatory findings, which explains the lack of intestinal symptoms at this stage.

Following the initial bacteremia, the organism is sequestered in macrophages and monocytic cells of the reticuloendothelial system. It undergoes multiplication and reemerges several days later in recurrent waves of bacteremia, an event that initiates the symptomatic phase of infection. Now in great numbers, the organism is spread throughout the host, infecting many organ sites. The intestinal tract may be seeded by direct bacteremic spread as, for example, to Peyer's patches in the terminal ileum. The gallbladder contains a large number of bacilli, and contaminated bile is another means of infecting the gut.

Hyperplasia of the reticuloendothelial system, including lymph nodes, liver, and spleen, is characteristic of typhoid fever. The liver contains discrete, micronodular areas of necrosis, surrounded by macrophages and lymphocytes. Inflammation of the gallbladder is common and may lead to acute cholecystitis. Patients with preexisting gallbladder disease have a penchant to become carriers, because the bacillus becomes intimately associated with the chronic infection and may be incorporated within the gallstones themselves. Lymphoid follicles in the gut, such as Peyer's patches, become hyperplastic, with infiltration of macrophages, lymphocytes, and red blood cells. Subsequently a follicle can ulcerate and penetrate through the submucosa to the intestinal lumen, discharging in its wake large numbers of typhoid bacilli. As the bowel wall is progressively involved, it becomes paper-thin and is susceptible to transmural perforation into the peritoneal cavity. Erosion into blood vessels produces severe intestinal hemorrhage.

III. Diagnosis. The definitive diagnosis is established by isolating the organism. During the 1st week, blood cultures are positive in 90% of patients. As bacteremia abates during the subsequent weeks, other sites become colonized. Stool cultures are positive in the 2nd and 3rd weeks, when the organisms are shed from the lymphoid follicles of the intestinal wall. During the 3rd week, urine culture yields typhoid bacilli in approximately 30% of patients. The specific skin rash of typhoid fever, "rose spots," harbors the organism, and they can be sampled by small skin snips of the lesions which are cultured in nutrient broth. These are positive in two-thirds of patients. A most useful source is the bone marrow, which is positive for **S. typhi** in 90% of patients, even when they have previously been treated with antibiotics.

The tier of agglutinins (Widal test) against somatic (O) and flagellar (H) antigens rises during the 3rd week of illness. An O titer of 1:80 or more in unimmunized individuals is suggestive of typhoid fever. Higher initial titers or a fourfold rise provide stronger evidence. The H antigen is nonspecific and is likely to be elevated from prior immunization or infection by other enteric bacteria. There are many false-positive and occasional false-negative Widal reactions, so a diagnosis based on titer rise alone is rather tenuous.

IV. Complications

A. Intestinal perforation. The ileum is the main site of bowel perforation. This complication occurs in approximately 3% of patients with typhoid fever and much less commonly in patients with other forms of salmonellosis.

Perforation usually occurs 3 weeks after onset of the disease or during convalescence. It is not related to severity of disease, nor is the incidence of perforation lowered by antibiotic treatment. The onset is usually sudden, with signs of an acute abdomen; an x-ray generally shows free air under the diaphragm.

The ulceration is generally small, measuring 0.5 cm in diameter, and is typically oval. In one-third of cases there are multiple perforations of the ileum. Most ulcerations are found between 10 and 40 cm proximal to the ileocecal sphincter, with an average distance of 25 cm.

A typhoidal perforation is unique in that it virtually never seals itself off by surrounding omentum or fibrous tissue. At operation, the abdomen is filled with pus and small-bowel contents. The perforation remains open and continues to flood the peritoneal cavity until surgically repaired or until the patient succumbs.

1. **Initial treatment** involves:
   a. Rehydration with fluids, electrolytes, colloid, and blood.
   b. Nasogastric intubation to decompress the small bowel.
   c. Antibiotic therapy. The recommended therapy for typhoid fever is chloramphenicol, 750–1,000 mg, q6h PO or IV, for 14 days.
   d. Additional antibiotic coverage is required in the setting of intestinal peforation to include the intestinal microflora contaminating the peritoneal cavity. The addition of an aminoglycoside (gentamicin, tobramycin, or amikacin) is usually sufficient to manage the remaining pathogens. (See Chap. 12 for doses of the aminoglycosides.)
2. **Early surgical intervention.**
   Because the perforation will not wall itself off, early surgical intervention is indicated. The procedures of choice are as follows:
   a. Simple closure of a single perforation is the treatment of choice. The indurated area is removed, including a margin around the perforation. Debridement and peritoneal lavage to remove pus and small-bowel contents is recommended.
   b. Resection and primary anastomosis is the required approach in the event of multiple perforations. Whenever possible, the distal ileum, which is not usually involved, should be preserved in order to maintain physiologic function.
   c. Exteriorization of the distal ileum occasionally is indicated when the patient is critically ill.

   Under optimal conditions, mortality of ileal perforation is 3–10%. In many areas of the world, however, where diagnosis and treatment are delayed, and where patients are often malnourished, the mortality from bowel perforation may be as high as 50%.

B. **Intestinal hemorrhage.** Since both hemorrhage and perforation share the same pathologic basis, their location and relationship to typhoidal ulcers in the ileum are similar. Bleeding may be sudden and severe or a slow ooze. Prior to antibiotic treatment, the incidence of intestinal hemorrhage was 10–20% in various series, but it is somewhat less frequent since specific therapy has become available. Many patients with hemorrhage can be managed by transfusions, and they cure themselves as the ileum undergoes repair during the 3rd and 4th week of the illness. In some cases, however, the blood loss becomes life-threatening, and surgical intervention becomes imperative. An angiogram may be useful to identify the source and amount of bleeding; in most patients the ileal location is fairly obvious and this procedure is unnecessary. The operative approach, when required, is resection and primary anastomosis, attempting to remove the areas of ulceration. Usually there are multiple ulcers, many of which are oozing blood.

C. **Acute cholecystitis.** Large numbers of typhoid bacilli accumulate within the gallbladder. When this organ becomes inflamed, the classic presentation of acute cholelcystitis is produced. The majority of patients with acute typhoidal cholecystitis can be managed medically with nasograstric suction and continuation of the antibiotic regimen. A small number, however, have an intense inflammatory response in the gallbladder that requires operative intervention.

V. **Treatment. Chloramphenicol** remains the standard therapy because of its proved efficacy and high activity against most clinical isolates of typhoid bacilli. The dose is 750–1,000 mg by mouth, administered in four equally divided doses daily, for 14 days. In the case of very sick patients it may be necessary to give the drug by the intravenous route; the same total daily dose should be used. Chloramphenicol is well absorbed in the intestinal tract but rather poorly absorbed from intramuscular sites. The response to such therapy is remarkably constant, as defervescence regularly ensues 3–5 days after initiation of treatment. Intestinal perforation and hemorrhage can develop during what is apparently successful treatment. Relapse, seen in 5–10% of treated patients, can occur following an otherwise uneventful course and should be treated again with the same drug.

Ampicillin is an alternative therapy but is somewhat less effective than chloramphenicol. The dose is 6 gm/day in four to six divided doses for 14 days. Amoxicillin, a closely related drug, provides better absorption and increased efficacy. The total dose is 4 gm/day in four divided doses. Sulfamethoxazole/trimethoprim has shown promising results in typhoid fever. The dose is four tablets/day (80 mg/400 mg per tablet).

VI. Management of typhoid carriers. A chronic carrier is defined as a person with positive stool cultures for at least 1 year following an episode of typhoid fever or, in some cases, positive stool cultures without a documented history of disease. The possibility of spontaneously aborting the carrier state is very unlikely after this time. Chronic carriers are most common in older age groups, in women (3:1 ratio of women to men), and in people with gallstones. The organism usually is harbored in the gallbladder, often forming part of gallstones, and persists in a symbiotic relationship with the host, causing neither local inflammation nor systemic symptoms. The bile contains enormous numbers of bacilli, up to 10^9/ml, and they are discharged in the feces in varying concentrations. The organisms are viable and fully infective, so that the carrier is capable of transmitting the infection. Curiously, the carrier does not infect him- or herself since the host is somehow protected from its own organisms. The organism can be eliminated, in some patients, with prolonged antibiotic therapy. A regimen that works in approximately two-thirds of patients is ampicillin, 6 gm/day in four divided doses for 6 weeks. Relapse of the carrier state generally are associated with stones and gallbladder disease. In individuals with gallstones or chronic cholecystitis, cholecystectomy cures the carrier state in 85% of patients. This procedure, however, is recommended only for individuals whose profession is not compatible with the typhoid carrier state, i.e., food handlers and health care providers.

VII. Other *Salmonella* infections. There are over 2,000 serotypes of *Salmonella*. Some cause disease in humans, but most are confined to animals and birds. The vast majority of human *Salmonella* infections are simple gastroenteritis, which require neither antibiotics nor surgical consideration. Occasionally a nontyphoidal *Salmonella* can cause the syndrome of typhoid fever. The same principles of management as for typhoid (see sec. **IV.A**) apply to these cases. Localized infections in bones, joints, and urinary tract can occur with *Salmonella,* and these are treated as if they were caused by other gram-negative bacilli, with the special considerations for antibiotic therapy of *Salmonella*. In general, the nontyphoidal salmonellae can be treated with ampicillin, amoxicillin, or sulfamethoxazole/trimethoprim.

3 Infections of the Biliary Tract, Liver, Pancreas, and Spleen

Biliary Tract Infections

Surgical diseases of the biliary tract and liver are frequently associated with infectious processes. Certain anatomic features are responsible for the septic conditions. (1) The rich lymphatic system that interconnects these structures facilitates the movement of microorganisms; (2) the liver is subjected to portal vein bacteremia with intermittent incursions of microorganisms from the bowel; and (3) the biliary tract can be colonized in a retrograde fashion directly from the lumen of the upper intestine.

I. Acute cholecystitis. This condition refers to severe biliary tract symptoms resulting from obstruction of the cystic duct. Ninety-five percent of cases are caused by a gallstone, and the "acalculous" remainder presumably are related to bile sludge. Obstruction of the cystic duct leads to increased intraluminal pressure, obstruction of bile flow, chemical inflammation, and, in some instances, bacterial infection.

The initial **clinical symptoms** are those of **biliary colic.** If the stone is dislodged from the cystic duct, either falling back into the gallbladder or passing into the intestine, the acute symptoms promptly subside.

A. Gallstones

1. Acute cholecystitis affects approximately 5% of all patients with gallstones. A past history of postprandial distress, nausea, belching, fatty food intolerance, and intermittent biliary colic is a useful clue to the presence of gallstones. Stones in the gallbladder or biliary tract are extremely common, being found in approximately 10% of white Americans over age 30. The incidence increases with age, so that approximately one-half of 80-year-olds have gallstones, many of them silent throughout life. Certain epidemiologic features have been associated with gallstone formation: (1) The incidence of stones in women is twice that in men. There is considerable question whether parity increases the incidence. (2) Racial differences are quite prominent. Blacks have a low incidence, whereas American Indians of certain tribes have a high incidence. Orientals have a propensity to form hepatic duct stones.
2. **Formation** of gallstones and acute cholecystitis are related to underlying diseases. The incidence is high in patients with diabetes mellitus, pancreatitis, cirrhosis, and chronic hemolytic diseases such as sickle cell anemia and hereditary spherocytosis. The correlation with obesity is not well established, although underweight individuals appear to have a low incidence of gallstones. Gallstone formation also is increased in ulcerative colitis, Crohn's disease, and in patients who have undergone intestinal bypass operation for obesity.

B. Bacteriology of the gallbladder and bile

1. The predisposing cause of biliary tract infection is bacterial contamination of bile, known as **bactibilia.** Each of the following risk factors associated with chronic calculus disease increases the risk of bactibilia and postoperative infection:

a. Previous history of jaundice, or jaundice at the time of operation
b. Common duct obstruction
c. Recent history of fever and chills
d. Prior biliary tract surgery
e. Advanced age (over 70 years)

2. Bile from healthy individuals without gallbladder disease is generally sterile, although there may be transient retrograde contamination by organisms from the duodenum. Bile obtained during operation for chronic calculus cholecystitis has an incidence of bacterial colonization of approximately 25% Acute cholecystitis is associated with positive bile cultures in 50–70% of cases; the incidence of infected bile is increased to 90% with common duct obstruction. Biopsy of the wall of the gallbladder shows an even higher rate of bacterial contamination in all these circumstances.
3. In patients with uncomplicated acute cholecystitis, *Escherichia coli, Klebsiella,* and enterococci, often in combination with one another, are the most common organisms in bile. Anaerobes, such as *Bacteroides, Clostridium,* and anaerobic streptococci, are less frequently found, although in some situations the rate of isolation is increased. Anaerobic bactibilia can be expected in the following settings: elderly patients (over 70), severe symptoms, prior biliary-intestinal anastomosis or other complex biliary surgeries, and common duct obstruction. In these special cases *Bacteroides fragilis* is found in 40%, *Clostridium perfringens* in 30%, anaerobic streptococci in 10%, and *Fusobacterium* in 5%. Anaerobes are combined with aerobes (coliforms and streptococci) in 95% of cases. Overall, polymicrobial infections are found in two-thirds of cases. The microorganisms isolated from culture-positive bile in uncomplicated cholecystitis are as follows:

Microorganism	Percent of cases
E. coli	70
Klebsiella	30
Other coliforms	10
Enterococci	20 (usually in mixed culture)
Other streptococci	5
Pseudomonas	5
Bacteroides	10
Clostridia	10
Anaerobic streptococci	5

C. Diagnosis of acute cholecystitis

1. The most prominent local symptom is **biliary colic.** The pain often begins after a large evening meal, with a gradual onset in the right upper quadrant of the abdomen, radiating around the right costal margin to the angle of the scapula. The pain is constant and can become quite severe. It may be intensified by respiration and movement. In some patients the pain is referred to the back and right shoulder. Although the right upper quadrant is the most common site, localization of biliary tract pain is notoriously elusive. The pain may be most intensive in the midepigastrium, the lower quadrants of the abdomen, the chest, and even occasionally in the left upper quadrant. Biliary colic can also masquerade as cardiac pain, and in patients with heart disease, angina pectoris may be confused with biliary tract symptoms.
2. **Nausea, vomiting,** and **anorexia** are regularly associated with the pain. Those patients who venture to sample a morsel of food experience intensified pain and often vomiting.
3. The **presence of gallstones** is suggested by a previous history of biliary colic, a positive x-ray in the past, or an underlying disease or racial background that favors the formation of gallstones.
4. **Physical findings** include tenderness just below the right costal margin with some voluntary guarding of muscles in this area. Occasionally, a smooth, tender gallbladder can be palpated, but more often there is fullness in the

right upper quadrant, which represents inflammation of surrounding tissues. The abdomen may be slightly distended, with hypoactive bowel sounds due to impending ileus.

5. **Leukocytosis** is present in a **minority** of patients in the early stage of disease and is generally below 15,000 WBC/mm^3.
6. **Liver function tests** show a slight rise in serum bilirubin, generally less than 2 mg/100 ml, accompanied by mild elevations in alkaline phosphatase and amylase and often normal or slightly elevated levels of transaminase. These chemical parameters may, however, remain normal in the early phases, when the diagnosis is enigmatic.
7. Plain **x-rays** of the abdomen show a mild, and nonspecific, ileus. Calculi can be visualized in the right upper quadrant in approximately 10% of patients. Positive findings of oral or intravenous cholangiography are nonvisualization of the gallbladder in the face of a normal common duct; a dilated common duct, suggesting obstruction; the presence of gallstones in the gallbladder; and nonvisualization of the biliary tree. However, it is unlikely that these techniques will be revealing when the serum bilirubin is greater than 3.5 mg/100 ml. Ultrasound has become extremely useful in demonstrating dilatation of the biliary tree and/or gallbladder enlargement. Radionuclide scans, such as HIDA, are also helpful in displaying the biliary tract.

D. Management

1. Early vs. late intervention

a. A polemic has raged for many years concerning early or late operative intervention in acute cholecystitis. The advocates of **early intervention,** generally within 1–2 days of onset of symptoms, argue that the procedure is safe for the following reasons: (1) It entails the same morbidity as late operations; (2) surgical resection is easier before the development of fibrosis and scar formation; (3) the hospital stay is substantially reduced, allowing the patient a more rapid recovery and return to work; (4) any delay in operation can mask a silent perforation or empyema of the gallbladder, which may be difficult to diagnose in older patients; and (5) a second attack or perforation can occur during the waiting period.

b. On the other hand, the adherents for **delay in operation,** generally 6–12 weeks following the onset of symptoms, offer the following arguments: (1) the patient would be in optimal condition at a later time, fully hydrated and in normal electrolyte balance; (2) additional time allows the diagnosis to be established beyond doubt; (3) the acute inflammatory process has completely subsided, thus making surgical resection easier; and (4) the incidence of postoperative complications during an elective procedure at a later time is considerably reduced.

c. Both schools of thought have their ardent spokesmen, but in recent years the pendulum seems to be shifting toward early surgical intervention. In actual clinical practice, however, basic surgical principles are observed by advocates of either school, and the patient's clinical course, rather than the surgeon's philosophy, dictates the necessary management.

2. Principles of management

a. The following approach, divided into three stages, can be applied to the management of acute cholecystitis. It is obvious that some patients move rapidly from one stage to another, so considerable clinical judgment is necessary.

Indications	**Therapy**
Stage 1: Initial Therapy and General Support Measures	
Biliary colic with persistent pain, requiring hospitalization.	Nothing by mouth. Insert Levine tube, if vomiting and distention are present. IV fluids and electrolytes. Analgesics. Antispasmodics.

Stage 2: Control of Infection

Fever Leukocytosis Ileus Tenderness or a mass in right upper quadrant.	Antibiotics: Cefazolin (or another cephalospo- rin), 1.5 gm IV q6h **or** Ampicillin 2–3 gm IV q6H **plus** Gentamicin/tobramycin.

Stage 3: Relief of Obstruction (decision should be made rapidly)

Progression of sepsis: persistent or rising fever, shaking chills, hypotension, rising WBC. Increasing signs in right upper quadrant: rigidity, rebound tenderness, or an enlarging mass. In some cases, a smooth mass becomes irregular in shape, with surrounding peritoneal signs in the region. Progressively abnormal liver function tests. Diabetes or advanced age increases the risk of perforation, empyema, and other complications.	Surgical removal of the gallbladder; common duct exploration, when indicated. Continue antibiotics.

b. The preferred operation is **cholecystectomy.** However, either because c serious deterioration in the clinical course, advanced age, or signs suggesting imminent perforation of the gallbladder, an emergency **cholecystostomy** can be life-saving. This operation is performed under minima general, or even local, anesthesia. The gallbladder is decompressed t relieve intravisceral pressure and a Pezar or Foley catheter is inserte into the gallbladder. Any calculi immediately in sight should be removec but extensive exploration is not recommended. Even impacted stone may have to be left behind at this stage in order to complete the procedur with great dispatch and minimal trauma.

3. Antibiotic therapy. Selection of appropriate antimicrobial drugs in biliar tract sepsis depends on the clinical situation and the achievable antimicrc bial levels in the bile. Penetration of these drugs into bile is greatly impaire in the setting of obstruction, thereby attenuating the therapeutic margir This emphasizes the need to relieve obstruction by surgical management i a patient unresponsive to antibiotics.

In acute cholecystitis without signs of septic shock or severe toxicity, therap can be directed at the aerobic pathogens. Since therapy is initiated befor cultures are available, and since the microorganisms are often multiple an may involve resistant strains, it is virtually impossible to select an antibioti regimen that will encompass all potential pathogens. The following is a reasonable approach to therapy.

a. Uncomplicated (no hypotension or systemic toxicity): Cephalospori (cefazolin, 1.5 gm q6h); **or** ampicillin 3 gm q6h plus gentamicin tobramycin 1.0 mg/kg q8h.

b. Severe disease, common duct obstruction: Ampicillin **or** ticarcillin **o** cefoxitin, 2 gm q6h, plus gentamicin/tobramycin.

c. Suspect anaerobes (see sec. **I.B.B**): Cefoxitin; **or** clindamycin, 600 m q6h, plus gentamicin/tobramycin.

d. Antibiotic therapy may **fail** for several reasons:

(1) Obstruction, which does not permit entrance of the drug into th infected area.

(2) Enterococci, which are resistant to cephalosporins, including cefoxitin, as well as to clindamycin and aminoglycosides.

(3) *Klebsiella,* which are resistant to ampicillin.

(4) *B. fragilis,* which are resistant to ampicillin and aminoglycosides as well as to conventional cephalosporins.

(5) Prior biliary surgical procedures, leading to colonization with resistant organisms, such as *Pseudomonas, Serratia,* and *Proteus.* These organisms are resistant to many conventional antibiotics.

e. **Following operation,** antibiotics can be distcontinued within 2–3 days if the procedure has gone without complications. For patients with extensive local infections, perforation, or gangrene, antibiotic treatment should be continued for at least 7–10 days, or as long as the clinical conditions dictate.

f. **Complications** of acute cholecystitis include gangrene of the gallbladder and perforation; empyema of the gallbladder; pancreatitis; generalized septicemia and shock: and spreading infection involving the liver or the subhepatic space (Morison's pouch).

II. **Empyema of the gallbladder.** Prolonged obstruction of the cystic duct by a stone can lead to a large collection of pus within the gallbladder, a condition referred to as **empyema.** Increased intracystic pressure, along with infection and disintegrating leukocytes, causes necrosis of the gallbladder wall. The major complications of empyema are perforation and generalized peritonitis.

A. **Signs and symptoms.** Initially the disease resembles acute cholecystitis. Within 48 hours, however, the abdominal distress has escalated. Right-sided abdominal tenderness is marked and is associated with tachycardia and a fever of 39°–40°C. The physical examination, if the patient can tolerate it, usually reveals a distinct mass in the right upper abdomen. Signs of generalized peritonitis would indicate perforation or leakage of the empyema, i.e., rebound tenderness, absent bowel sounds, and abdominal rigidity. While these signs are classically found, older patients have a more cryptic course, with a paucity of abdominal findings. Persistent systemic toxicity, hypotension, or renal failure, in the setting of cholecystitis, should raise the suspicion of empyema.

B. **Laboratory findings.** Laboratory findings are similar to those of acute cholecystitis, except that the white blood cell count may become markedly elevated, often above 20,000 WBC/mm^3.

C. **Diagnosis is** usually established by x-rays or scans. Flat plates can show an enlarging mass in the right upper quadrant. Gas is often visible in the wall of the gallbladder or in its contents. Ultrasound and CT scan are very helpful in establishing the diagnosis.

D. **Treatment.** Treatment is **early surgical drainage** and removal of the gallbladder. Preoperative stabilization should include appropriate fluid therapy, parenteral antibiotics, hypothermia, and expansion of the intravascular volume. This resuscitation should be done rapidly, however, so as to accomplish surgical removal of the gallbladder before rupture and generalized peritonitis occur. Cholecystectomy is preferred to tube drainage, because the gallbladder wall is frequently gangrenous and necrotic. However, a temporizing cholecystotomy may be necessary in critically ill patients who could not survive a prolonged procedure.

Obstruction of the cystic duct in the absence of infection leads to massive swelling of the gallbladder, known as **hydrops.** While this condition may require surgical management, it does not need emergency intervention. Hydrops of the gallbladder can be a secondary phenomenon associated with serious medical illnesses. Surgical drainage is not obligatory in such cases, but it is very difficult to differentiate between this benign condition and empyema.

III. **Emphysematous cholecystitis (pneumocholecystitis)**

A. This severe, although relatively rare, variant of acute cholecystitis is diagnosed by an **x-ray of the abdomen.** The findings include air in the biliary or gallbladder lumen, blebs in the wall, and collections of gas in the pericholecystic tissue. Alternatives to consider in differential diagnosis of this x-ray appearance are communication with the gastrointestinal tract; lipoma of the gallbladder (a benign condition); and incompetence of the sphincter of Oddi, which produces gas in the common duct as well as in the gallbladder and biliary tree.

B. Several **clinical features** serve to distinguish acute cholecystitis from the emphysematous variety.

Feature	Acute cholecystitis	Emphysematous cholecystitis
Male–female	1 : 2.5	2.5 : 1
Without stones	10%	30%
Gangrene	2%	75%
Perforation	4%	20%
Mortality	4%	15%
Clostridia in bile	10%	50%

C. The gas is presumably produced by microorganisms, and there is a higher incidence of positive cultures in the emphysematous condition. Coliforms, especially **E. coli** and **Klebsiella,** are most frequently found, followed by *Clostridium,* an organism noted in 50% of cases (*C. perfringens* is the most common species.) The emphysematous form occurs more often in males and is seen with unusual frequency in **diabetics.** It is highly likely to produce gangrene and perforation.

D. Because it is highly lethal, it is important to diagnose emphysematous cholecystitis. X-rays of the abdomen are required in all patients with acute cholecystitis. If gas is recognized in the gallbladder, the surrounding tissue, or the biliary radicles, early operative intervention is clearly indicated.

IV. Acute cholangitis

A. Cholangitis is defined as **infection within the bile ducts**—the common duct and/or the hepatic radicles. The milder form of acute cholangitis is associated with partial obstruction and an inflammatory reaction within the biliary tree. A further extension of the process, **suppurative cholangitis,** produces pus in the bile ducts and can be diagnosed only upon operation. Such purulent collections are associated with a more fulminant course and a higher mortality.

Partial obstruction, caused by stones or benign stricture, is likely to produce cholangitis, whereas complete obstruction due to tumor is rarely associated with biliary sepsis. This difference may be related to the colonization of the biliary tract by intestinal organisms that occurs with partial obstruction.

B. There are two opinions concerning the **route of entry** of microorganisms in cholangitis: (1) from the lower intestine, carried via the portal vein, with excretion through the bile and subsequent colonization of the bile duct; or (2) by retrograde extension to the biliary tract from the upper intestine, in the setting of partial obstruction.

C. Most patients with cholangitis have had prior operative procedures on their biliary tract. The **common clinical settings** are

1. A common duct stone, retained from a recent cholecystectomy. The hiatus between the original operation and the onset of new symptoms is generally less than one year.
2. A common duct stone, formed as a primary concretion within the hepatic or common duct; such patients have undergone cholecystectomy 5–10 years, or even longer, prior to recurrence.
3. Benign strictures following biliary tract or intestinal surgery.
4. Malignant tumors of the head of the pancreas, sphincter of Vater, or bile duct.
5. Biliary-intestinal reconstructive procedures.
6. Abnormal connections or fistulae between the biliary tract and the intestine.

D. Signs and symptoms: The classic presentation of acute cholangitis is known as **Charcot's triad:** fever, abdominal pain, and jaundice.

1. **Fever** affects 95% of patients with cholangitis, although it may be observed in only two-thirds at the time of hospital admission. Fever is sudden in onset and paroxysmal, often associated with shaking chills, and rarely lasting for more than 1–2 days.
2. **Abdominal pain** and/or right upper quadrant tenderness is seen in the majority of patients during the course of cholangitis. The degree of local tenderness with cholangitis usually is less than that observed with acute

cholecystitis. The pain may be constant or colicky, often radiating to the back or right shoulder. It can persist for several days, even after the fever has subsided.

3. **Jaundice** is noted clinically in two-thirds of patients and by measurement of serum bilirubin in over 90%. It is generally of a mild character, although it may be pruritic. The jaundice progresses to a peak over 3–5 days and then gradually returns to a baseline level.
4. The **precentage of other signs and symptoms is as follows:**
   - **a.** History of fever in 95% of cases
   - **b.** Fever on admission in 65% of cases
   - **c.** RUQ tenderness in 80% of cases
   - **d.** Abdominal pain in 80% of cases
   - **e.** Jaundice in 80% of cases
   - **f.** Nausea and vomiting in 50% of cases
   - **g.** Peritoneal irritation in 45% of cases
   - **h.** Shock in 5% of cases
5. **Attacks** of cholangitis, consisting of a constellation of signs and symptoms, occur intermittently and can persist for several years, if appropriate treatment is not instituted. Some patients, however, develop severe infection and septic shock, and may succumb in the acute episode.

E. Laboratory findings

1. One or more liver function tests almost invariably yield abnormal results during an attack of acute cholangitis. On the other hand, the white blood cell count is quite unpredictable, normal in some cases and inordinately high in others, even in the range of a leukemoid reaction (> 30,000 WBC/mm^3). It is important to obtain blood cultures before initiating antibiotics, since the yield of positive cultures is 40%.
2. Progressive elevation of the serum alkaline phosphatase to moderate levels, in the presence of a normal serum bilirubin, suggests blockage of one of the main hepatic ducts. This complication usually occurs postoperatively when a stone has been pushed into a hepatic duct during exploration of the common duct.
3. The **percentage of cases with abnormal values** is:
   - **a.** Bilirubin in 90% of cases
   - **b.** Alkaline phosphatase in 90% of cases
   - **c.** Transaminase in 90% of cases
   - **d.** Positive blood cultures in 40% of cases
   - **e.** WBC (> 10,000/mm^3) in 60% of cases
   - **f.** Amylase (serum) in 35% of cases
   - **g.** X-ray (flat plate) in 15% of cases

F. Bacteriology. Cultures of bile are always positive in acute cholangitis. The bacteriologic findings are similar to those observed in acute cholecystitis. Coliforms, particulary *E. coli* and *Klebsiella,* are the most frequent isolates. *Streptococci* are next, and anaerobes such as *Clostridium* and *Bacteroides* are somewhat less common. In older patients or in patients with obstruction of the common duct, anaerobes are more likely to be present, in association with aerobes.

G. Diagnosis. The diagnosis of cholangitis is based on the typical triad of symptoms in the setting of prior biliary surgery or partial obstruction. Laboratory data support the diagnosis. If the bilirubin is only modestly elevated, an intravenous cholangiogram can be performed. Tomography is often useful to demonstrate dilatation of the common duct. Other approaches can be used when cholangiography is nonproductive, such as transhepatic cholangiography and transduodenal retrograde cholangiography. Ultrasound and HIDA scans are highly accurate and are becoming the preferred diagnostic procedures. A liver biopsy is extremely helpful to make the diagnosis in cryptic cases that present as fever of unknown origin. Characteristic findings are seen in the portal areas, including inflammatory changes, infiltration with PMNs, fibrosis, and proliferation of bile ducts.

H. Treatment. The appropriate choice of treatment of cholangitis depends on the severity of symptoms and the underlying cause. All patients should undergo initial medical therapy that includes

1. Initiation of antibiotics, similar to those advised for acute cholangitis (ampicillin and an aminoglycoside, or a cephalosporin; cefoxitin is useful when anaerobes are suspected)
2. Intubation of the upper intestine
3. Intraveous fluid and electrolytes
4. Relief of pain

Medical management is a delaying tactic so that the patient's condition can be improved in preparation for primary surgical treatment. As soon as the patient is stable, common duct exploration and choledocholithotomy, or repair, reconstruction or bypass of strictures should be performed, as dictated by the underlying pathology.

If the patient has not responded to initial medical management, it may be necessary to intervene in an emergency fashion to prevent life-threatening complications. Frequently, in these critically ill patients, only decompression of the common duct with a T-tube can be tolerated. Surgery to correct the underlying cause of the biliary blockage is postponed until the clinical condition has improved. If the patient's condition is less critical, the common duct should be explored, and stones, if present, should be extirpated. The gallbladder, when present, is removed, and a T-tube is placed in the common duct, thus obviating the necessity for a second operation. The liver should be examined for evidence of abscesses, which should be drained.

A common error in the surgical treatment of patients with suppurative cholangitis is to drain only the gallbladder. This procedure does not produce proper drainage of the common duct, the actual site of the suppurative infection.

I. **Complications** of acute cholangitis include unrelenting sepsis and septic shock, liver abscess, and recurrent, relapsing cholangitis. Mortality is approximately 15%, and the usual cause of death is uncontrolled sepsis.

Pyogenic Liver Abscess

I. **General Principles.** The incidence of liver abscess has remained unchanged over the past 50 years, representing approximately 0.5% of autopsies in a general hospital. There has been a shift in the predisposing causes of this infection, but regardless of the forms, the mortality remains high, reported as 25–50% at leading surgical centers. The reasons for the high fatality rate are **cryptic presentations,** with diagnosis made only at autopsy, **severe underlying illness,** and **inability to perform adequate surgical drainage** due to technical problems or multiplicity of abscesses.
The location of liver abscesses is as follows:

Solitary, right lobe	50%
Solitary, left lobe	5%
Multiple, single lobe	35%
Multiple, both lobes	10%

II. **Clinical features**
Liver abscesses are seen at all ages, although most frequently in patients 60–80 years old. The presentation may be **acute** or **chronic.**

A. **Acute presentation,** defined as fewer than 5 days of symptoms, is characteristic of patients with multiple, often small, abscesses. The condition usually follows an **acute abdominal catastrophe** such as bowel perforation or appendicitis or is associated with **septicemia.** The patient is generally jaundiced and complains of right upper quadrant pain. A high mortality is associated with acute presentations.
B. A **chronic** course is seen in 70% of patients with liver abscess, and the symptoms have a mean duration of 5 to 7 weeks. The patient is often hospitalized with a diagnosis of "fever of unknown origin" or "cholangitis."

C. Symptoms

Fever	90% (often 40°C)
Chills	40%
Abdominal pain	70%
Anorexia	40%
Nausea and vomiting	30%
Weakness	30%
Weight loss	25%
Pulmonary symptoms	25%

D. Signs

Enlarged liver	60–80%
Tenderness	60–80%
Pulmonary findings	50%
Jaundice	25%

E. Most patients have fever and some abdominal or pulmonary findings that raise the suspicion of **hepatic infection.** Clinical jaundice suggests multiple abscesses, which may be associated with pylephlebitis; this setting carries a grave prognosis. The clinical course may be insidious and highly cryptic. In some series, over 50% of the cases are diagnosed at autopsy, although this percentage has decreased in recent years with the advent of scanning techniques.

F. Abnormal laboratory findings

Leukocytosis	90%
Anemia (HCT < 35%)	50%
Alkaline phosphatase	95%
Transaminase	60%
Bilirubin	50%
Low albumin	75%
Elevated serum Vitamin B_{12}	90%

III. X-ray findings

A. The **chest x-ray** reveals abnormalities in the right thorax in 50% of cases, usually consisting of basilar atelectasis, pneumonitis, or small accumulations of fluid. A **flat plate of the abdomen** occasionally reveals air in an abscess cavity. An **intravenous pyelogram** may show depression of the right kidney. An **upper GI series** may show the stomach to be displaced laterally, and a **barium enema** can indicate an enlarged liver.

B. The preferred **scanning** method is computed tomographic scan (CT scan), which has a positivity of 95%. If CT scan is not available, a **^{99}Technetium liver scan** can be used. An abscess smaller than 1 cm in diameter may not be visualized, and even large abscesses can be missed, although this chance is reduced if the scans are done in several projections. **Ultrasound** is useful for demonstrating fluid in the mass in order to differentiate abscess from tumor. **Arteriography** also has a high yield of positivity, but this study is complementary to the other scans for localization and is not absolutely necessary for diagnosis. The **gallium citrate scan** has been highly touted, but our experience suggests that the CT and Technetium scans are more reliable.

IV. Sources of Infection

Biliary tract (usually obstruction due to pancreatic cancer, stones, or cholangitis)	20–30%
Portal vein (drainage from abdominal viscera, i.e., ruptured viscus, ulcer, leaking anastomosis, appendicitis, diverticulitis)	20–30%
Direct extension (gallbladder, kidney)	15%
Systemic bacteremia	10%
Nonpenetrating trauma	5%
Pylephlebitis	5%
Cryptic	20–40%

V. Microbiology. The types of microorganisms are related to the source of infection:

Biliary tract	Coliforms and streptococci, few anaerobes
Portal vein (abdominal viscera)	Mixed—coliforms and anaerobes
Systemic bacteremia	Staphylococci and streptococci

Overall, about 30% of the liver abscesses are caused by aerobic or facultative bacteria; 50% are due to mixed aerobes and anaerobes; and 20% are caused by pure anaerobes.

Bacteria	**Occurrence in abscess** (%)*
Aerobic and facultative	
Coliforms (*E. coli, Klebsiella, Proteus,* etc.)	40
Streptococci	20
Staphylococci	10
Pseudomonas	5
Anaerobic	
B. fragilis	20
Other *Bacteroides*	10
Anaerobic streptococci	40
Fusobacteria	30
Clostridia	20
Actinomyces	5

Bacteremia occurs in approximately 50% of patients with liver abscess. If the blood cultures are collected properly, half will yield anaerobes, usually anaerobic streptococci, *Bacteroides,* or fusobacteria, and the other half will contain coliforms or, in cases associated with endocarditis, staphylococci or streptococci.

VI. Antibiotic treatment

Optimally, antibiotics are selected after the pathogen is cultured and its sensitivity is known. However, this is rarely possible in liver abscess, since antibiotics usually have to be started before the abscess is drained and often before the exact diagnosis is established, i.e., for therapy of fever of unknown origin and sepsis. Several empiric drug regimens have been recommended, and all seem to be reasonable in light of the expected pathogens.

Clindamycin and an aminoglycoside (gentamicin, tobramycin, or amikacin)
Metronidazole and an aminoglycoside
Chloramphenicol and ampicillin
Cefoxitin (alone or with an aminoglycoside)
Cefazolin or cephalothin (for staphylococci or streptococci, or for coliforms related to the biliary tract; not good for anaerobes)

VII. Surgical management. An almost inviolable rule is that gross collections of pus within the liver must be drained. Drainage is somewhat urgent when the diagnosis is suspected or has been established, since rupture of the abscess can lead to irreversible complications. The preferred operative approach is **anterior transperitoneal** by a right subcostal incision in order to create maximum exposure and drainage. Occasionally, patients can be drained by an **extraserous transthoracic** route, if the abscess is in the right posterior region. This method avoids soiling the peritoneum, but it sacrifices full exposure and the opportunity to search for other abscesses.

At the time of laparotomy, an abscess is usually directly visualized or palpated on the liver surface. Some collections, however, are deep in the parenchyma, and they must be identified by means of an aspirating needle. Liver scans in several projections are very helpful in localizing the lesion, but the long aspirating needle may be finally required to define the precision location. The major consideration, once the abscess has been localized, is to ensure adequate drainage in the dependent position. Several intraperitoneal drains should be placed, including a **sump drain** at the

*Several different bacteria can be recovered from a specimen.

entrance of the tract, **Penrose drains** in the liver, and **catheters** for irrigation of the cavity.

At certain medical centers, liver abscesses are being drained percutaneously, by a catheter inserted into the cavity under guidance of ultrasound or CT scanner. A pigtail catheter is used that will stay in place in the abscess cavity. Small amounts of radiopaque dye can be instilled in order to follow the closure of the cavity. This technique should not be applied to deep, multiloculated abscesses.

Drainage is the ultimate management ploy, but additional factors should be considered. If there is biliary obstruction, or lesions in contiguous structures, they must be corrected in order to obviate recurrence of the infection.

Prevention of hepatic abscess should be considered when dealing with blunt abdominal trauma or perforation of an abdominal viscus; these events can lead to liver injury, subcapsular hematoma, and liver abscess formation. Appropriate surgical management involves removal of disintegrated or devitalized tissues, repair of bile leaks, possible T-tube insertion for adequate drainage of blood and bile, appropriate sump and Penrose drainage of the right upper quadrant, and adequate exploration to identify all damaged tissue. Such steps at initial laparotomy can prevent the subsequent development of liver abscess.

Amebic Liver Abscess

I. **General principles.** Although amebic infection of the liver comes from an intestinal site, most patients with liver abscess do not have an active intestinal infection, nor even a past history of this condition. Thus, an amebic etiology should be considered in any case of discrete masses in the liver, until an alternative diagnosis can be proved.

II. **Clinical presentation.** An amebic liver abscess usually develops over several months, but occasionally it has an abrupt onset, with fever and right upper quadrant pain, lasting less than a week. At the other extreme, the patient complains of dull, aching pain over the right side for many months before the diagnosis is established.

A. Symptoms	**Percent of cases**
Pain	90
Pain on right side	75
Pain on left side	25
Cough	45
Diarrhea	40
Previous history of dysentery	35
B. Signs	
Intercostal tenderness	93
Fever	80
Signs at right lung base	75
Liver enlarged and tender	75
Just enlarged, not tender	1

The disease has a marked predominance in males, being seven times more frequent than in females, and usually occurs after the second decade of life.

C. **Laboratory findings** are not specific. Two-thirds of patients have a mild leukocytosis, without eosinophilia (unless there is a concurrent worm infection), and 50% have anemia related to chronic infection. Liver function tests are quite variable. Most patients have no elevation of bilirubin, but mild increases in alkaline phosphatase and transaminase are rather common.

III. **Amebic serology.** A multiplicity of serologic tests are now available for diagnosing invasive amebiasis. Since there are high levels of precipitating, agglutinating, or complement-fixing antibodies, it is possible to demonstrate their presence by immunodiffusion, immunoelectrophoresis, counterimmunoelectrophoresis (CIE), latex fixation, and complement fixation. The most reliable test is the **indirect hemagglutination test** (IHA),when performed in a laboratory with appropriate standards and controls.

The IHA test measures mostly serum IgG (with some IgM). A **diagnostic titer is 1:128 or greater** (see p. 36). Liver abscess is associated with high titers, generally greater than 1:1024, although there is some variability. It should be recognized that a false-negative serologic result has been noted in approximately 5–10% of patients with proved invasive disease, either in the colon or in the liver. A high titer remains for many months or years following cure, although it has a tendency to decline over a period of time.

IV. Scanning procedures. A **liver scan** with ^{99}Technetium is extremely useful in identifying an amebic liver abscess. Approximately 90% occur in the right lobe, with the remainder in the left lobe. **CT scan** is now the most accurate scanning technique. **Ultrasound** helps to demonstrate a fluid-filled cavity. **X-ray of the chest** shows an abnormality at the right base in 75% of patients; the most common findings are atelectasis and/or a small pleural effusion.

V. Differential diagnosis. The diagnosis of amebic liver abscess has become simplified in recent years with the advent of liver scan, CT scan, ultrasound, and amebic serology. When a mass is noted by scan, the differential diagnosis lies between an abscess of amebic or pyogenic origin, a cyst, or a tumor. The most useful single test is **amebic serology.** The serologic test is positive (≥1:128 by IHA) in approximately 95% of patients with proved amebic liver abscess. The diagnosis of carcinoma, either primary or metastic, is suggested by an **ultrasound study,** which shows a solid mass, in the case of tumor, and fluid in amebiasis. It has been claimed that scanning with gallium 67 displays a rim around an amebic abscess, whereas a carcinoma or pyogenic abscess shows a uniform distribution of the isotope. This finding, related to central necrosis in an amebic abscess, is also seen in the other two conditions, so that differentiation with this scan usually is not possible.

- **A. Separation of amebic from pyogenic liver abscess** is the most perplexing problem. The chemotherapy and operative approach are entirely different for these conditions. Patients with amebic liver abscess tend to have an enlarged, tender liver. As a general rule, an amebic abscess is associated with less fever and toxicity, a lower white blood cell count, and a more chronic course. In patients with proved amebic liver abscess, the parasite cannot be found in the stool of 50% of patients, even with careful searching. Thus, the diagnosis of amebic liver abscess cannot be excluded by a failure to find the parasite or by a negative history of diarrhea.
- **B. Aspiration of abscess pus** may be required for diagnosis in difficult cases. The amebic abscess is filled with reddish brown material that on microscopic examination has few cellular elements. Trophozoites of *Entamoeba histolytica* are difficult to identify in pus, unless the material is aspirated from the abscess wall. On the other hand, pus from a pyogenic abscess is yellow or green; polymorphonuclear leukocytes and bacteria can be observed on microscopic examination; in about one-third of cases there is a distinctly foul odor.
- **C.** The **therapeutic response** is anathema to most surgeons, but there is some merit to this test in patients with amebic liver abscess. The response to appropriate treatment usually occurs within 2–3 days and is often very dramatic, with a decrease in pain, toxicity, and the size of the liver.

VI. Needle aspiration. Needle aspiration of an amebic liver abscess is not required for either therapy or diagnosis in the majority of cases. However, the following situations indicate a need for aspiration:

- **A.** A large abscess that, because of its copious volume of fluid, may resorb with great difficulty even with adequate chemotherapy.
- **B.** A left lobe abscess that may rupture into the pericardium with catastrophic results. Left lobe abscesses should be given careful consideration for open surgical drainage.
- **C.** Cases in which the diagnosis is in doubt and the patient's clinical condition requires rapid decision.
- **D.** Lack of response to initial therapy. This may require aspiration to verify the diagnosis and to examine the possibility of bacterial superinfection.

The major risks of needle aspiration are **infection** introduced by the procedure and **hemorrhage.**

VII. Treatment

A. Metronidazole is the treatment of choice for amebic liver abscess; it is used in doses of 500–750 mg PO tid for 10 days. There are well-documented treatment failures, with patients advancing from colitis to liver abscess while receiving this drug. However, treatment failures are noted with all antiamebic regimens, without exception, and metronidazole seems equally effective and probably less toxic than other available drugs. As acceptable alternatives, chloroquine (0.5 gm PO/day for 3 weeks), either alone or in combination with emetine (1 mg/kg/day for 10 days, with a maximum of 650 mg for a total course), can be used. Whatever the regimen, an additional drug should be added to kill cysts within the intestinal lumen, and the preferred agents are diloxanide furoate or diiodohydroxyquin.

B. The **response to treatment** of amebic liver abscess is judged largely on clinical grounds. The critical parameters are diminished fever and toxicity, a decrease in the size and tenderness of the liver, a fall in white blood cell count, improvement in the chest x-ray, and a reversal of abnormal laboratory findings. The liver scan may show surprisingly little change, even in the presence of apparent clinical cure. Large defects remain for at least 2–4 months, and for as long as 2 years in some patients, without signs of relapse. Similarly, the serology remains positive at high titer for months or even years.

C. Indications for **retreatment** are deterioration in the patient's clinical status with apparent reaccumulation of fluid within the abscess, as indicated by scans, radiographic changes in the chest, and physical findings. Since treatment failures are seen in approximately 5% of patients treated with any of the available therapeutic regimens, it is important to reinvestigate such patients by direct aspiration of abscess contents in order to rule out the possibility of bacterial superinfection. On the other hand, the parasite itself may cause relapse; in this setting an alternative drug—metronidazole, chloroquine, or emetine—should be selected.

D. Most amebic liver abscesses can be **aspirated** by a needle or trocar and only rarely require surgical exploration.

E. Indications for surgery in amebiasis are

1. Left lobe abscess, because of danger of pericardial perforation
2. Perforation into peritoneum, subdiaphragmatic space, pleura, or pericardium.
3. Secondary bacterial infection
4. Insecure diagnosis in abscess not approachable by needle aspiration

VIII. Complications of liver abscess. Perforation of the abscess is the major complication and can occur in the

A. Abdominal cavity, causing peritonitis, usually with secondary bacterial infection in the subdiaphragmatic space

B. Lung, causing amebic empyema, lung abscess, or bronchohepatic fistula

C. Pericardium, in the case of a left lobe abscess, resulting in constrictive pericarditis

Viral Hepatitis*

Recent progress in our understanding of viral hepatitis has increased our knowledge of its epidemiology. With the advent of an effective vaccine for hepatitis B and the use of blood screening for this entity, we are now able to decrease markedly its morbidity and mortality. Newer diagnostic tests have shown that posttransfusion hepatitis is primarily of the type called **non-A, non-B,** not hepatitis B. Hospital personnel (and surgeons in particular) should be aware of their substantial risk of contracting hepatitis B.

I. Types of hepatitis

A. Hepatitis A

Hepatitis A, formerly called **infectious hepatitis,** is caused by a 27-nm RNA virus that has not been fully characterized. Illness is usually abrupt in onset,

*This section was written by David R. Snydman, M.D.

Table 3-1. Estimated morbidity for hepatitis B in the United States

Condition	No. patients
New cases	200,000/yr
Jaundice with liver damage	50,000 (26%)
Hospitalization required	10,000 (5%)
Chronic HBs carriers*	12,000–20,000 (6–10%)
Chronic active hepatitis	3,000– 5,000 (2–3%)
Lethal fulminant hepatitis	250 (0.1%)
Cirrhosis with death	4,000 (2%)
Hepatic carcinoma	900 (0.4%)

*Defined by positive serology for HBsAG on two occasions separated by at least 6 months.

with fever, malaise, nausea, vomiting, abdominal pain, and jaundice. The group most commonly affected is young children and adolescents, since contact is primarily person-to-person. The major mode of transmission is through the fecal-oral route, in which close contact occurs with an infected person. There are rare common source exposures via contaminated food or water. The incubation period is 15–45 days (mean, 30 days). The virus can be demonstrated in the feces of individuals incubating infection 1–2 weeks before onset of jaundice. There may be a brief viremic period prior to the onset of jaundice, but a blood carrier state has not been shown, and hepatitis A is not a significant cause of posttransfusion hepatitis. A serum antibody has been described that measures immunity to the hepatitis A virus. This antibody appears to be long-lived, and it confers immunity to subsequent challenge with hepatitis A virus. The diagnostic test for hepatitis A is the presence in the serum of IgM antibody to the hepatitis A virus (HAVAB-M, Abbott).

B. Hepatitis B

Hepatitis B, formerly called **serum hepatitis,** is caused by the 42-nm DNA virus, which has been termed the **Dane particle.** In contrast to hepatitis A, the illness frequently has an insidious onset and is associated with extrahepatic manifestations such as arthritis and skin rashes. The disease is transmitted primarily by percutaneous inoculation, such as through blood transfusion or needle stick. Recent evidence suggests that contaminated saliva, semen or blood introduced onto mucosal surfaces can transmit the disease. Prospective studies of hepatitis B in homosexual males have confirmed that sexual transmission of the virus is very prevalent in this population. The incubation period for hepatitis B is 40–180 days (mean, 90 days). The virus can be demonstrated in the blood from 1–2 months before the onset of jaundice, to 1–2 months after the onset of jaundice. Other body secretions have been shown to contain the virus, in particular saliva, urine, semen, and bile. There is a chronic blood carrier state, which can affect up to 10% of normal patients. Several groups of patients are at higher risk of becoming chronic carriers, namely, patients on chronic hemodialysis, those receiving multiple transfusions (sickle cell anemia, hemophilia), and those with Down's syndrome. The course of the chronic carrier state is quite variable, ranging from total lack of symptoms to chronic active hapatitis with or without postnecrotic cirrhosis. Morbidity and mortality are variable but in general are more severe in this illness than in hepatitis A (Table 3-1).

Several antigen-antibody systems have been described in hepatitis B. The hepatitis B surface antigen, HBsAg, is found on the surface of the virus, and it is the clinical marker for hepatitis B infection. In addition there are antibody markers to this surface antigen, **anti-HBs.** Immunity to hepatitis B is usually specific and lifelong. In order to make a diagnosis of acute hepatitis B one needs to obtain a positive HBsAg determination (Ausria, Abbott).

C. Non-A, non-B hepatitis. The discovery of serologic markers for hepatitis A and B has led to the realization that other hepatitogenic viruses exist. Non-A, non-B hepatitis refers to these agents. The symptoms are indistinguishable from those of hepatitis B. The incubation period varies between 30 and 180 days. The mode of transmission appears to be primarily parenteral, i.e., through contaminated blood or blood products or through needle stick (particularly drug abuse). The advent of adequate screening for blood contaminated with hepatitis B has reduced posttransfusion hepatitis B; however, non-A, non-B hepatitis constitutes about 80% of posttransfusion hepatitis. A chronic blood carrier state can exist. Alternative modes of transmission exist, since this disease causes about 25% of sporadic cases of hepatitis. The consequences of infections with these agents are quite variable; morbidity and mortality are probably similar to those in hepatitis B. Chronic active hepatitis can occur as a result of infection. Thus far, no serologic determinants have been discovered for these viruses.

II. Prevention of spread of infection

A. General measures. Several general measures are applicable to prevent the spread of hepatitis in surgical units. Surgeons should be aware of several groups of patients who are at high risk of harboring hepatitis B, namely, patients maintained on chronic hemodialysis, patients from institutions for the mentally retarded, those receiving multiple blood transfusions, homosexuals, and intravenous drug abusers. Many of these patients are asymptomatic carriers and therefore should be screened for HBsAg upon admission.

B. Procedures on general medical, obstetric, and surgical units. Patients with acute hepatitis B or with HBsAg-positive blood should be cared for in rooms separated from patients without hepatitis or in semiprivate or ward accomodations in which blood and instrument precautions are observed. Staff should wear gowns and gloves when handling blood or blood-contaminated objects from HBsAg-positive patients, when doing venipunctures, and anytime a potential for contact with blood exists. Scrupulous handwashing should be observed by both staff and the hepatitis patient. Masks or other facial coverings should be worn during procedures that might result in splashing of infectious material into the face. Dishes and eating utensils need not be disposable, because commercial dishwashers are adequate to prevent dissemination of the virus. All blood and other specimens from hepatitis B patients should be labeled "hepatitis precautions"; however, laboratory personnel should handle both labeled and nonlabeled specimens carefully, because the absence of a label certainly does not denote a safe specimen. In addition, all charts of patients with hepatitis B should be flagged "hepatitis." Items such as razors, toothbrushes, and food should not be shared by other patients.

C. Disinfection. Thorough cleansing of instruments, before any sterilization or disinfection procedure, is important. Autoclaving at 121°C for 15 minutes, boiling for 30 minutes, or exposing to dry heat at 170°C for 60 minutes are the treatments of choice for eliminating hepatitis virus from contaminated equipment. Instruments that cannot be handled in this manner should be treated with chemical germicidal solutions. Sodium hypochlorite (Chlorox) is the most commonly advocated solution. Hypochlorite solution containing 5,000–10,000 ppm of available chloride should remain in contact with the contaminated equipment for at least 30 minutes. Since hypochlorite corrodes metal, it may be necessary to utilize formaldehyde or glutaraldehyde.

D. Immune serum globulin (ISG). Immune serum globulin (gamma globulin) should be administered to any household contact of a patient with hepatitis A. The dose is 0.02 ml/kg. IGS should not be administered routinely to hospital contacts of patients with hepatitis A. Rather, emphasis should be placed on sound hygienic practices, as already outlined.

E. Hepatitis B immune globulin (HBIG).

1. Hepatitis B immune globulin (HBIG) has recently undergone clinical trials in the United States. It is efficacious in certain circumstances such as needle stick exposure or mucosal exposure to blood containing HBsAg. Current recommendations are a dose of 0.05–0.07 ml/kg body weight within a 7-day period after exposure, with a second identical dose administered 25–30 days

after the first. If HBIG is not available, ISG may be beneficial if given in the same dosage range.

2. **Infants born to mothers HBsAg positive** in the third trimester or HBsAg positive at delivery should receive HBIG, the dose being 0.13 ml/kg body weight initially, then 0.06 ml/kg monthly for the first 6 months.
3. **Spouses of patients** with hepatitis B appear to be at higher risk of acquiring hepatitis B than the rest of the family contacts. One controlled trial did demonstrate prevention through use of HBIG. Although it is not a Public Health Service recommendation, it would seem prudent to administer HBIG in a single dose (0.07 ml/kg) for exposure of a spouse or "significant other" to a person with acute hepatitis B. Other family members are not at significant risk to develop hepatitis B, and they need not receive prophylaxis.
4. HBIG is **not recommended for epidemic settings,** such as dialysis units where hepatitis B transmission is known to occur. Rather, hepatitis B prevention should be based on routine serologic screening of patients and staff for HBsAg and antibody to HBsAg (anti-HBs) as well as hygienic measures. Cohorting HBsAg-positive patients with anti-HBs positive staff, and using separate dialysis areas for HBsAg-negative patients have been shown to be effective in preventing transmission.

III. Hepatitis B vaccine

A. A vaccine for hepatitis B **(Hepatavax B, Merck)** has been licensed recently and is currently available. The vaccine is a purified preparation of HBsAg that has been heat- and formalin-inactivated. It is a killed virus preparation that induces a protective antibody response when given in three successive doses at 0, 1, and 6 months. The vaccine is recommended for health care workers, especially surgeons, and for homosexual males, hemophiliacs, dialysis patients, and infants born to HBsAg-positive mothers. Side effects associated with the vaccine have been limited to fever (in about 2%) and sore arm (in about 15%).

B. Recommendations for vaccine

1. **Prevaccination serologic screening.** HBV carriers and those with HBV antibody are protected and do not need to be vaccinated. Routine screening is commonly advocated to detect either anti-HBc or anti-HBs.
2. The **serologic response rate** of healthy persons who receive the vaccine is 92%; these individuals are protected unless they are incubating the disease at the time of vaccination. The duration of protection is not known. There is no need to document serologic response after vaccination.
3. **Preexposure vaccination** is recommended for persons at substantial risk for HBV infection.
   - **a.** Health care workers, including medical, dental, laboratory and support personnel, who have contact with blood or blood products. Immunization strategies within hospitals vary due to the cost of the vaccine ($100 for three doses) and the extent of anticipated exposure. The hospital staff at highest risk are medical technologists, operating room staff, phlebotomists, intravenous therapy nurses, surgeons, pathologists, and dialysis staff.
   - **b.** Clients and staff of institutions for the mentally retarded
   - **c.** Hemodialysis patients
   - **d.** Homosexually active males
   - **e.** Users of illicit injectable drugs
   - **f.** Recipients of factor VIII or IX concentrates
   - **g.** Household and sexual contacts of HBV carriers
   - **h.** High-risk populations, including Alaskan Eskimos and immigrants or refugees from areas with high endemic rates of HBV—especially eastern Asia and sub-Saharan Africa
4. **Postexposure vaccination**
   - **a.** Infants born to HBsAg-positive mothers
   - **b.** Sexual and household contacts of patients with acute HBV infection
   - **c.** Health care workers who receive needle stick exposure from HBsAg-positive patients

IV. Therapy. No specific treatment is available for any of the forms of viral hepatitis. Patients with severe derangement of liver function need to be hospitalized. Severe liver dysfunction is most often reflected in a prolongation of the prothrombin time. No specific diet need be employed. If anorexia is severe, however, intravenous fluids may be necessary. Parenteral vitamin K should be given to hypoprothrombinemic patients, but those with severe hepatocellular disease usually do not respond. Bed rest need not be strictly enforced, especially for young and previously healthy patients. There are no indications for corticosteroids in early uncomplicated hepatitis. Indeed, the use of steroids has not been shown to be beneficial in acute fulminant hepatitis.

Pancreas: Acute Pancreatitis

I. General principles. Acute pancreatitis is associated with a diverse group of conditions, including biliary tract disease, alcoholism, reflux of duodenal contents into the pancreatitic ducts, hyperparathyroidism, trauma (either nonpenetrating or occurring during operative procedures), and hyperlipidemia. Infection can play an important role in the clinical course and is responsible in large measure for the 5–7% mortality associated with this disease.

II. Types of infection

A. Approximately 10% of patients develop infections, often multiple ones, coincident with an episode of pancreatitis. The types of infection are

Type	Percent of patients
Bacteremia	9
Pancreatic abscess	4
Empyema	2
Peritonitis	2

B. Approximately 20% of patients with acute pancreatitis have a hospital-acquired infection, usually related to their debilitated state and the necessity for Foley catheterization, nasogastric suction, and intravenous lines. The hospital-acquired infections are

Infection	Percent of patients
Urinary tract infections	8
Pneumonia	5
IV catheters	2

C. Hemorrhagic pancreatitis is a severe form of acute pancreatitis and carries a high mortality. It is often associated with infection within the pancreatic ducts that can lead to bacteremia. It is seen in 3% of patients with acute pancreatitis; 95% of such cases occur as the first attack of pancreatitis. Clues to the diagnosis of a hemorrhagic process are a high pulse rate, out of proportion to the temperature; early development of hypotension, which responds poorly to volume replacement; and hypocalcemia.

III. Microbiology. The source of bacteria that infect the pancreatic ducts and surrounding structures appears to be the intestinal tract. Potential routes of bacterial spread are via infected bile, through the lymphatics surrounding the gallbladder and colon, by hematogenous dissemination, and by penetration from the adjacent bowel, particularly the colon. The most common bacteria are *E. coli, Klebsiella, Proteus, Enterobacter,* and enterococci. Occasionally, patients with pancreatitis have bacteremia with pneumococci, presumably from the respiratory tract, or staphylococci, which are spread from other sources such as skin infections, heart valves, or infected intravenous catheters.

IV. Treatment

A. Indications for antibiotic therapy. Prospective studies have established that there is **no benefit to the use of prophylactic antibiotics in acute pancreatitis.** Antibiotics neither reduce the severity of an episode nor prevent the severe infectious complications. There are, however, situations in which patients with pancreatitis should receive therapeutic antibiotics.

1. **Coexisting infections.** The most common are pneumococcal pneumonia, aspiration pneumonia, and urinary tract infection.
2. **Clinical sepsis** without an obvious source. Such findings as high fever, rapid pulse, toxicity, and hypotension suggest a septic process, which may be within the pancreas or in a cryptic site.
3. **Hemorrhagic pancreatitis.** Bacteria are known to colonize the pancreatic ducts in this situation, and this can lead to bacteremia or suppurative pancreatitis.
4. **Associated biliary tract disease.** Antibiotics are indicated for treating obstruction and sepsis.

B. Antibiotic therapy. Several regimens have been used, and all appear to be equally effective.

Ampicillin	2–3 gm IV q6h
plus	
An aminoglycoside:	See Chap. 12 for dosage
Gentamicin	
Tobramycin	
Amikacin	
or	
Cephalothin or another cephalosporin	2–3 gm IV q6h
plus	
An aminoglycoside	

Ampicillin should not be used as a single agent, since patients may be infected by *Klebsiella, Enterobacter,* or *Proteus,* organisms that often are resistant to this agent. *Pseudomonas* is occasionally found in these infections, so an aminoglycoside is a desirable component of combination therapy. Our preference is a cephalosporin and an aminoglycoside in order to cover staphylococci, resistant coliforms, and *Pseudomonas.* To be sure, enterococci are not included in the spectrum of activity, and these organisms are occasionally pathogenic in pancreatitis. No regimen covers all potential pathogens, however, and one has to choose between adding drugs, with their attendant toxicities, and a less-than-universal regimen.

Pancreas: Pancreatic Abscess

I. General principles. A severe complication of acute pancreatitis is pancreatic abscess. Approximately 4% of attacks of pancreatitis are complicated by abscess formation, and this event is responsible for 15% percent of all deaths associated with pancreatitis.

II. Clinical features. The usual course is **subacute,** occurring 2–8 weeks (with a mean of 4 weeks) after the onset of what appears to be typical pancreatitis. The patient has improved initially from acute pancreatitis with conservative management, and the symptoms of abdominal pain, nausea, and vomiting have abated. After this brief respite there is a return of fever, abdominal pain, and toxicity, and the appearance of a tender abdominal mass. The WBC increases, and the patient appears severely ill. In some individuals there is a prolonged elevation of serum amylase that never declines during the initial improvement stage. But most patients have a normal or only slightly elevated serum amylase during the presentation of pancreatic abscess. There may also be an **acute** presentation; in this setting, which is rather uncommon, the patient is admitted with a severe attack of pancreatitis that progresses relentlessly over a 6–10-day period until the diagnosis of pancreatic abscess is apparent.

III. Pathogenesis

A. The **development** of this abscess is related to release of pancreatic secretions during acute pancreatitis (Fig. 1). The lesser sac fills with a transudate contain-

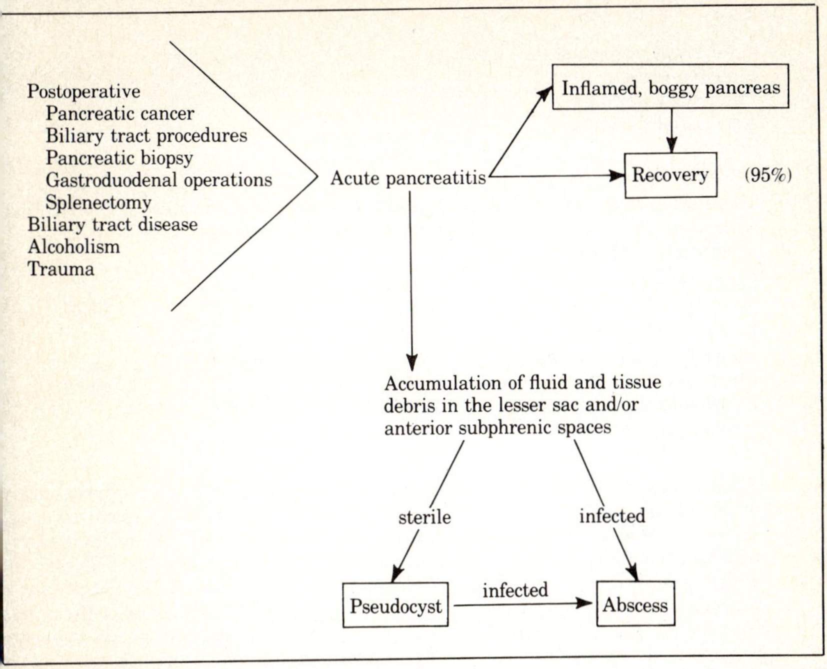

Fig. 1. Pathogenesis of pancreatic abscess. (After C. B. Jones et al., *Am. J. Surg.* 129:44, 1975.)

ing cytotoxic pancreatic secretions and necrotic tissue fragments from the pancreas, omentum, and surrounding structures. Since the lesser sac is in communication with the left subphrenic space, the process can spread to the left anterior, superior, or inferior subphrenic spaces, or it can remain entirely confined to the retroperitoneum. In the uninfected state this condition is known as a **pancreatic pseudocyst.**

B. The **route** of superinfection by microorganisms is cryptic. They may come from the pancreatic ducts, which are colonized by flora from the lumen of the bowel, or from lymphatics that are in communication with the GI tract. Alternatively, there may be direct extension of bacteria from the bowel wall or hematogenous spread into the rich cultural menstruum of pancreatitis secretions. In any case, the transudate is converted to an exudate by infection with enteric bacilli, and the contents turn to chocolate-brown pus interspersed with digested blood, fat, necrotic pancreas, and tissue debris.

C. The **anatomic boundaries** are difficult to ascertain due to destruction of surrounding landmarks. Depending on the direction of spread, the abscess may be contiguous with the left anterior subphrenic space, the lesser sac, or the retroperitoneal space. In approximately 25% of cases the entire pancreas is involved, with severe destruction; in the remaining cases the abscess is confined to either the head, body, or tail, in a fairly equal distribution.

IV. Symptoms

Abdominal pain	95%
Fever	85%
Nausea and vomiting	70%
Anorexia	50%
Weight loss	25%
Diarrhea	7%

V. Signs

Tenderness over mass	95%
Palpable mass	50%
Pulmonary findings	50%
Abdominal distention	45%
Shock	15%
Jaundice	10%

The **triad of fever, abdominal pain, and tenderness** over the abscess, in conjuction with acute pancreatitis, strongly suggests pancreatic abscess.

VI. Laboratory findings

Leukocytosis	90%
Anemia	80%
Low serum albumin	60%
Abnormal liver function tests	50%
Abnormal BUN or creatinine	45%
Elevated serum amylase	30%
Hyperglycemia	25%
Hypocalcemia	20%

While many of the laboratory tests are nonspecific, certain results raise the suspicion of pancreatic abscess. Persistently elevated serum amylase is a helpful sign but varies according to the underlying disease, the time course, and the amount of viable pancreas that has survived. In general, high serum amylase does not correlate well with the severity of pancreatitis. Prolonged elevation of serum amylase suggests pseudocyst or abscess formation. This finding is seen in 10–65% of cases in various reported series. A low serum calcium ($\leq$ 8 mg/100 ml) strongly points to severe pancreatic disease, either hemorrhagic pancreatitis or pancreatic abscess, and it connotes a serious condition associated with a high mortality.

VII. X-ray findings

A. Roentgenographic examinations are extremely helpful in indicating the presence of pancreatic abscess in 90% of cases. If the patient is able to undergo procedures, it is recommended that the following studies be obtained: flat plate and upright films of the abdomen, upper GI series, barium enema, and intravenous pyelogram. The major roentgenographic signs are:

1. **Displacement of extrinsic defects of the GI tract.** Anterior displacement of the stomach, widening of the duodenal loop, and gastric outlet obstruction due to extrinsic compression are the most frequent findings on upper GI series. These are noted in 70% of patients.
2. **Extraluminal gas,** the "soap-bubble sign," is found in 35% of patients. The gas bubbles are formed by metabolism of microorganisms and suggest a large abscess cavity.
3. A **persistently narrowed loop of small intestine** with a feathery pattern of the mucosa, associated with stasis of barium in the proximal and distal loops, is noted in 25% of cases.
4. **Pulmonary findings,** usually in the left chest but occasionally bilateral, are noted in 60% of patients. The most frequent abnormalities are basilar atetectasis, a paralyzed hemidiaphragm, and pleural effusion.

B. Ultrasound has been used with great success in the diagnosis of pancreatic abscess. This procedure can outline the boundaries of the abscess and aid in decisions concerning the operative approach. It can be used to guide a percutaneous needle drainage of abscess contents.

C. CT scan is a very helpful tool in diagnosing pancreatic abscess. However, it can give a false-positive result by indicating an abscess when there is only swelling and inflammation in the pancreas.

VIII. Predisposing causes

A. Pancreatic abscess develops in the following clinical settings:

Postoperative	35%
Biliary tract disease	20%

Alcoholism	20%
Abdominal trauma	5%
Unknown (cryptic or multiple causes)	20%

These percentages are approximations, depending greatly on the types of patients seen in a particular surgical clinic. For example, if alcoholism is a common problem among the population served by the institution, the percentage of alcoholics suffering pancreatic abscess is increased.

B. Pancreatic abscess is a complication of operative procedures that involve the upper gastrointestinal tract or biliary tract. The types of procedures at risk are resection of pancreatic carcinoma, biliary tract procedures (especially involving the common duct), biopsy of the pancreas, gastroduodenal operations, and splenectomy.

C. Uncommon predisposing conditions to consider in the differential diagnosis are periarteritis nodosa, serum lipid abnormalities, perforation of the duodenum by ulcer or foreign body, neonatal omphalitis, and necrotizing carcinoma of the pancreas.

IX. Differential diagnosis. Pancreatic abscess must be distinguished from a pseudocyst and a boggy edematous pancreas that may follow acute pancreatitis (see Fig. 1). In general, pancreatic abscess is associated with higher fever, leukocytosis, and signs of systemic toxicity. Although a pseudocyst may present with pain and a palpable mass, it causes less systemic toxicity and no signs of infection. The history is often more chronic with pseudocyst, and there may be elevated diastase in the urine. Ultrasound can be extremely helpful in differentiating a fluid-filled mass from an inflamed, boggy pancreas.

X. Microbiology. The types of bacteria isolated from pancreatic abscess are similar to those infecting other parts of the biliary tract and liver. Approximately 50% of cultures of abscess fluid yield a **polymicrobial flora,** while the other half are **monocontaminated.** In about 10% of cases the culture yields no growth, but it is unclear whether this indicates sterilization with antibiotic treatment, misdiagnosis of a pseudocyst, or failure to use anaerobic techniques. Parenthetically, anaerobic bacteria have been isolated only on rare occasions and probably play little role in pancreatic abscess.

Microorganisms	**Occurrence in abscess** (%)
E. coli	35%
Proteus	20%
Klebsiella	20%
Enterobacter	15%
Pseudomonas	15%
Enterococci	20%
Other streptococci	15%
Staph. aureus	15%

XI. Treatment

A. Antibiotics. The goal of antibiotic treatment of pancreatic abscess is to reduce complications, not to cure the abscess, which requires drainage. Antibiotics can control septicemia, extension into adjacent spaces, and recurrences. On the basis of the expected bacteriology and clinical experience, the following two-drug regimen appears to be most useful:

A cephalosporin	
Cephalothin	3 gm IV q6h
or	
Cefazolin	1.5–2.0 gm IV q6h
plus	
An aminoglycoside	See Chap. 12 for dosage
Gentamicin	
Tobramycin	
Amikacin	

Some surgeons prefer chloramphenicol in this setting. This drug has excellent penetration into abscesses, but its spectrum is limited with regard to *Klebsiella, Enterobacter, Proteus,* and *Pseudomonas,* all of which may appear in pancreatic abscess.

B. Surgical management

1. **Drainage** of the abscess is the most important therapeutic modality, since virtually all patients with undrained pus in the pancreas will expire, despite antibiotics or other medical management. The preferred approach is external drainage by a transverse incision over the abscess. The transperitoneal route usually is required, since the abscesses tend to be multiloculated. The lesser sac is often involved, and this area should be approached from either above or below the transverse mesocolon. In selected cases an extraserous, retroperitoneal approach may be attempted. While some surgeons have recommended marsupialization, there has been a general disenchantment with this technique, so that it is not applied in most cases of pancreatic abscess.
   The abscess cavity should be widely exposed, taking great care not to soil the peritoneal cavity. Necrotic tissue within the pancreas, omentum, or surrounding structures should be gently debrided. Overzealous debridement can injure or unroof major vessels in the area, promoting what may be a severe bleeding episode.
2. **Sumps and rubber drains** should be applied to all dependent areas and left in place for at least 1 week. More extensive use of hard drains can erode exposed vessels, so these drains should be advanced progressively, as drainage decreases.
3. Pancreatic **abscess** may be secondary to **biliary tract obstruction.** The primary lesion should be corrected during the operative procedure, whenever possible, by removal of stones, T tube drainage, or Roux-en-Y procedure.
4. **Percutaneous drainage,** under ultrasound or CT scan guidance, has become an accepted modality. The patient must be observed closely for bleeding associated with the drainage tube.
5. It has been recommended that operations for pancreatic abscess be accompanied by a **gastrostomy tube,** in order to empty the stomach and diminish the chance of pulmonary complications by nasogastric suction, and by insertion of a **jejunostomy tube** for feeding. This approach has not gained wide acceptance, particularly in centers where intravenous hyperalimentation routinely is used. By whatever method, it must be appreciated that maintenance of nutrition is a key factor in recovery of patients with pancreatic abscess. The ordeal is long and energy-consuming, exhausting the patient's nutritional reserves and stamina. Adequate supplements should be administered, either intravenously or via jejunostomy, to all patients with this condition, in order to promote wound healing and reduce the devastating effects of prolonged illness.

XII. Complications

A. The mortality with pancreatic abscess is awesome, approaching 100% in patients who are not diagnosed preoperatively and who remain undrained.

Patients	**Mortality** (%)
Diagnosed preoperatively and undergoing surgery	40
Undrained	100
Overall	70–80

The poor survival in this infection is related to the multiple complications that can occur. Virtually all patients sustain one or another of these complications, and their severity determines the chance of survival.

Complications of pancreatic abscess	**Percent of patients**
Pleural effusion or pneumonia	80
Extension and dissection	35
GI bleeding	30
Renal insufficiency	30
Recurrence	25

Pancreatic fistula	20
Diabetes	20
Arterial erosion	15
Intraperitoneal rupture	15
Septicemia	10
Gastric or duodenal ulcer	10
Wound dehiscence	5

B. Pulmonary complications, principally insufficiency and/or pneumonia, arise frequently and form a significant segment of mortality. The most common finding is pleural effusion, usually on the left but occasionally bilateral. Pneumonia may be present as well, related either to atelectasis or to aspiration. Pulmonary embolism is a rare event since these patients often have associated coagulation defects.

C. The pancreatic abscess may **dissect** into the thoracic cavity, subhepatic or suprahepatic spaces, left suprarenal space, abdominal wall, or scrotum.

D. Gastrointestinal bleeding, another potentially lethal complication, is caused by stress ulcers of the stomach or duodenum, or by perforating ulcers caused by dissection of the abscess into the stomach, small bowel, or even large bowel. Although relatively less common, **major arterial erosions** are a near-lethal event; a clue to this occurrence is the appearance of bright red blood in the drainage tubes.

Splenic Abscess

I. General Principles. A solitary splenic abscess is relatively uncommon; the incidence in routine autopsies is 0.26–0.67%. The disease can occur at any age but is most frequent in young males, possibly because trauma and heroin usage are important predisposing factors.

II. Clinical features

A. Pain, usually in the left upper quadrant, left flank, or radiating to the left shoulder, is found in most patients.

B. Chills and fever affect virtually all patients sometime during the clinical course.

C. A friction rub is occasionally audible at the left lung base or over the spleen. If the abscess is fluid-filled—a rare event, to be sure—a tympanic note can be heard upon percussion.

D. Laboratory findings are nonspecific. Approximately two-thirds of patients have leukocytosis, and the majority are somewhat anemic.

III. Predisposing Causes. Although some cases of splenic abscess arise "spontaneously" without a precipitating cause, over 90% fall into one of the following groups:

A. Trauma, either blunt or associated with surgical procedure. The mechanism appears to be a subcapsular hematoma that becomes organized and is somehow seeded via the hematogenous route to form an abscess.

B. Septicemia. The underlying circumstances can be bacterial endocarditis, heroin usage, a *Salmonella* infection with seeding in the spleen, or hematogenous spread of infection from other organ sites, such as the abdomen, pelvis, lungs, and skin.

C. Direct extension from an infection in a contiguous site within the abdomen.

D. Hemoglobinopathies. The most common are SC, AC, S-thalassemia, and, in children, SS. The mechanism appears to be splenic infarction with subsequent seeding by the bloodstream. In older patients with SS, asplenia occurs, so that abscess is uncommon in this age group.

IV. Pathology. The gross pathology in a solitary splenic abscess is a thick-walled, irregular, large abscess. There may be an associated subcapsular hematoma. In some cases a mycotic aneurysm is present in the adjacent vessels.

Splenic abscess can be induced in experimental animals by direct trauma to the spleen to produce a hematoma or by ligating the splenic artery; the animal is then subjected to an intravenous inoculum of bacteria, such as staphylococci, and a splenic abscess develops. Infarction of the spleen is the critical factor in the experimental setting.

V. Bacteriology

Bacteria	Percent of occurrence
Gram-negative bacilli (*E. coli, Klebsiella, Enterobacter, Pseudomonas*)	40
Staph. aureus	15
Anaerobes	10
Streptococci	10
Salmonella	10
"Sterile"	15

Blood cultures are positive in 30–50% of patients with splenic abscess. Some older reports note a high incidence of sterile splenic abscesses; in light of more recent information, many of these cases probably represent infection by fastidious anaerobic bacteria.

VI. X-rays and scans

A. The **chest x-ray** often demonstrates an elevated left hemidiaphragm, which may become more pronounced over several day's observation. On fluoroscopy, the diaphragm is fixed. A pleural effusion and atelectasis are noted frequently at the left base of the lung.

B. A **flat plate** of the abdomen occasionally shows small, extraintestinal gas bubbles, which indicate an abscess cavity. On rare occasions the cavity is massive, with an air-fluid level.

C. Barium x-rays of the bowel reveal a displaced stomach and splenic flexure.

D. The **Technetium Tc 99m scan** shows a large, irregular mass in the spleen in most, but not all, cases. Occasionally, nonspecific splenomegaly is reported.

E. Ultrasound can be quite helpful in demonstrating the location and size of the abscess cavity.

F. CT scan is probably the most useful technique for demonstrating a splenic abscess.

G. An **arteriogram** demonstrates a cavity when it has been missed with other scans. Under most circumstances, however, this study is not required, since the diagnosis can be made by noninvasive, scanning methods. The arteriogram also may reveal mycotic aneurysms in the splenic, hepatic, or superior mesenteric arteries.

H. Gallium scanning can be helpful in outlining the abscess. It may be difficult to interpret the gallium scan, since the spleen itself picks up the material and may show diffuse enlargement. In addition, there may be interference with the overlying splenic flexure of the colon.

VII. Therapy

A. The **preferred operative approach** to splenic abscess is splenectomy through an anterior incision. Splenotomy and percutaneous needle aspiration are not advised, since the abscess may be very large and the contents can be spilled inadvertently into the peritoneal cavity. In addition, there is often a vascular network surrounding the cavity due to tortuous, aneurysmal vessels.

B. Antibiotic treatment should be appropriate for the infecting organism. There may be an early clue from positive blood cultures or a Gram's stain of the material at operation. It is advisable, however, to initiate antibiotic treatment before undertaking the operation. An empiric regimen, which would be adequate for most of the expected pathogens, is as follows:

A cephalosporin, such as cefazolin, 1.5 gm q6h, plus
An aminoglycoside, such as gentamicin, tobramycin, or amikacin (see Chap. 12 for dosage)

VIII. Multiple splenic abscesses. A diagnosis often made by autopsy is multiple, small, focal abscesses riddling the spleen in a homogeneous fashion. Such cases are nearly always associated with abscess formation in other organs, and the spleen receives its share of the septic load through the hematogenous route. Such patients usually have endocarditis or septicemia from other causes. Heroin addicts are particularly predisposed to develop such complications. The disease has a very poor outlook because of the serious nature of the infection throughout the body. The diagnosis is usually made post mortem; even if it were established in advance, there would be no benefit to operating on the spleen due to the disseminated nature of the disease. The mortality in multiple splenic abscesses is over 90%.

IX. Complications

A. Perforation of the splenic abscess can occur into the abdominal cavity, the pleural space, or the lesser sac.

B. A splenic abscess can spread infection to other organs by the hematogenous route.

C. Unrelenting sepsis can lead to hypotension and shock, a common mode of exodus for undrained patients.

4 Gynecologic and Obstetric Infections

Pelvic Inflammatory Disease (PID)

I. General principles. Pelvic inflammatory disease consists of inflammation of the oviducts and ovaries with mucosal thickening, edema, suppuration, and even abscess formation. Infections of the upper female pelvic tract usually ascend from the cervix and vagina. The pathogens may be **exogenous,** introduced by sexual intercourse, or **endogenous,** part of the normal vaginal flora. Occasionally a pelvic infection arises from nongynecologic sources, such as appendicitis. The presentation can be acute or chronic. Symptoms range from mild, which can be treated on an outpatient basis, to severe, which require hospitalization.

PID is a major cause of morbidity among young, sexually active women. The recent statistics are awesome: 800,000 cases of PID occur each year in the United States. The incidence is 12–13 cases/1,000 women/year in the 15–24-year age group. Among women born after 1945, 15% will develop PID by age 30. Of all women in the United States, 15% have had one or more episodes of PID.

The sequelae are also imposing. The incidence of infertility is 15% among women with a single episode of PID and rises to 70% for women with three or more episodes. Ectopic pregnancy is 10-fold more frequent. Chronic abdominal pain afflicts 10% of women with PID.

The incidence of PID is similar among maried and single women, but divorced and separated women have a higher risk. No correlation can be made with the frequency of intercourse. Although it is true that prostitutes have a higher incidence of PID, it is a popular, and unfortunate, misconception that PID is necessarily associated with promiscuity.

II. Risk factors associated with increased incidence of PID. The factors relating to the increased incidence of PID in recent years include

- **A.** Increased sexual activity
- **B.** Use of intrauterine devices (IUD)
- **C.** Increase in pelvic surgery and cesarean sections
- **D.** Delayed diagnosis and inadequate therapy

III. Signs and symptoms.

- **A. Pelvic pain** is the most frequent complaint. The intensity may be mild to severe and in many patients is a relapsing event.
- **B. Nausea and vomiting** are often present.
- **C. Anorexia** is especially common during acute episodes. The **temperature** is elevated in 30–50% of patients.
- **D. Spiking fevers, shaking chills,** and **tachycardia** suggest a more severe form of disease.
- **E. Associated urinary tract symptoms,** such as urgency, frequency, and dysuria, are sometimes present. Bowel complaints, however, are uncommon.

IV. Physical examination

- **A. Abdominal examination** reveals bilateral or unilateral tenderness over the lower quadrant. It is uncommon to palpate a mass, except in the rare circumstance of a large pelvic abscess that projects anteriorly. The upper quadrants of the abdomen are usually benign.

B. Vaginal examination may reveal diffuse erythema of the mucosa and a purulent cervical discharge.

C. Bimanual examination demonstrates tenderness by manipulation of the cervix. There is frequently unilateral or bilateral adnexal tenderness. However, it is relatively uncommon to palpate a discrete mass in the adnexa or cul-de-sac. The presence of a mass in these sites suggests pelvic abscess.

It must be emphasized that physical findings are often at variance with those observed under direct vision at laparoscopy or operation. There is a tendency to overdiagnose "a pelvic mass" or to localize disease specifically to the tubes or ovaries on the basis of bimanual examination. Hence, diagnosis and subsequent therapeutic plan should be based on all features of presentation, including past history, symptoms, physical findings, and diagnostic studies.

V. Differential diagnosis. Major alternative diagnoses masquerading as PID include

A. Appendicitis

B. Ectopic pregnancy

C. Endometriosis

D. Twisted or ruptured ovarian cyst

VI. Microbiology. The incidence of various pathogenic organisms reported from different clinics varies with the age, socioeconomic background, and sexual habits of the patient, as well as with the means of obtaining material for diagnosis and the laboratory facilities for culturing the organism.

Pathogens	Percent of total cases
Mixed vaginal flora	40–60
Neisseria gonorrhoeae	30–50
Chlamydia trachomatis	20–40
Combined infections	40–60
Mycoplasma hominis	? (low)
Ureaplasma urealyticum	? (low)

A poor correlation exists between the type of pathogen and the symptoms, signs, or physical findings in patients with PID. When large groups of patients are compared, some generalizations can be made concerning the broad groupings of gonococcal and nongonococcal infection. It must be emphasized, however, that these findings do not necessarily apply to individual patients, and that the only definitive diagnosis is by Gram's stain or microbiologic culture.

Characteristics	Gonococcal	Nongonococcal
Course	Acute	Subacute, relapsing
Onset	During or shortly after menses	Throughout cycle
Fever >38°C	50%	30%
Vaginal discharge	More common	—
Cervical exudate	More common	—
Liver tenderness	More common	—
Response to therapy	More rapid	—

A. *Neisseria gonorrhoeae.* This pathogen is spread to the tubes and ovaries by ascending from a primary focus in the cervix or vagina. Gonorrhea may also involve the urethra, Skene's glands, and Bartholin's glands. Many females with gonorrhea have a prolonged latent period from the time of the original infection. Local defense mechanisms are diminished during menstruation; for this reason, many cases of salpingitis and disseminated gonococcal disease arise during or shortly after onset of menses.

The causative organism is a gram-negative diplococcus, kidney-shaped, with the flattened ends slightly indented and lying parallel. A Gram's stain preparation of cervical discharge or culdocentesis fluid generally reveals the diplococci, often lying within leukocytes.

The incidence of gonorrhea in pelvic inflammatory disease is variable, depending on the type of patients seen in a particular clinic or practice. In areas of high incidence, 50% of PID is caused by this organism; in other clinics, however, the incidence of isolation is about 10%. An average value for many institutions appears to be one-third of PID cases. Some clinics are reporting that *N. gonorrhoeae* is responsible for a declining incidence of such cases, as other organisms are increasing in prevalence. Mixed infections, comprising the gonococcus and other pathogens, are reported variously at 20–40% of all cases of PID.

B. Mixed vaginal flora. These pathogens arise from normal flora of the cervix and vagina. They are seen more commonly in relapsing cases of PID. It has been postulated that other organisms, such as gonococci or chlamydiae, cause acute damage to the tubes, and that the subsequent, relapsing process is endogenous (vaginal flora) as a result of impaired function within the oviducts. The most common pathogens are *Peptostreptococcus* (anaerobic streptococci) and *Bacteroides* species. In the milder cases, anaerobic streptococci appear to predominate. When there is discrete abscess formation, *Bacteroides* is particularly common.

C. *Chlamydia trachomatis.* This organism also ascends from the cervix. Positive cultures can be obtained during an acute attack from either the cervix or the tubes (by laparoscopy). No specific clinical features distinguish patients infected with this organism, although their symptoms are milder, as a rule, than those caused by gonococci or mixed flora.

There remains considerable controversy over the role of *Chlamydia* in acute salpingitis. Studies from Sweden, utilizing scrapings of the fallopian tube obtained at laparoscopy, have documented a high incidence of *Chlamydia* infections, on the order of 30%. On the other hand, gonorrhea is rather rare in Sweden. Workers in the United States have failed to culture *Chlamydia* from laparoscopy specimens, but these studies were done with swabs of purulent material from the tubes, not scrapings. Serologic studies from the United States, however, tend to corroborate the findings in Sweden, indicating a 20–30% incidence of *Chlamydia* in PID, especially the milder cases. Mixed infections have been documented as well.

D. *Mycoplasma and ureaplasma.* These organisms have been isolated from cervices of patients with PID and from healthy women. In a few instances, they have been cultured directly from the oviducts of women with acute salpingitis. Thus, they appear to be pathogenic in a small number of cases, although their true incidence is unknown due to their high carrier rate and the difficulty of diagnosing them with current techniques.

VII. Microbiologic diagnosis. All women with suspected PID should undergo a pelvic examination, both for physical findings and for material for Gram's stain and culture (vaginal and cervical discharge). Whether or not to perform the other tests listed here (**C–H**) depends on severity of symptoms (laparoscopy, blood cultures) and suspected pathogens (serology for *Chlamydia*).

A. A **Gram's stain** of material from the endocervical os is helpful in the diagnosis of gonorrhea. The presence of typical gram-negative diplococci in an intracellular location has a 98% correlation with positive culture; when the Gram's stain is negative, up to one-third of such patients may still yield a positive culture.

B. Culture of endocervical fluid is useful for gonorrhea but not for anaerobes or *Mycoplasma*. (Cervical discharge can also be used for *Chlamydia*, but such cultures are not available in most routine laboratories.) Since *N. gonorrhoeae* is highly fastidious, the organism should be grown on Thayer-Martin medium, which permits growth of pathogenic *Neisseria* while suppressing the normal flora. The culture should be placed in a CO_2 atmosphere for maximum yield. In clinical practices where a bacteriology laboratory is not readily available, the specimen should be inoculated into Trans-grow medium, which preserves the organism during transport. Since anaerobic streptococci and *Bacteroides* are part of the normal flora of the vagina, it is not useful to culture for these organisms from material obtained from the vagina or cervical os.

C. Culdocentesis. Aspirate is useful for culturing *N. gonorrhoeae* and other potential PID pathogens. The mucosa must be carefully cleansed with antiseptics such as iodine and alcohol before aspiration, in order to avoid contamination by normal flora. Even scrupulous cleansing may fail to dislodge the normal vaginal flora from the mucosa, however, so a positive culture of these types of organisms from an aspirate must be considered with some skepticism. *Chlamydiae* have a low yield of isolation from culdocentesis fluid.

D. **Serologic tests** are useful for identifying *Chlamydia* infections. A fourfold rise or decline in titer is diagnostic, although even a high initial titer is suggestive. Unfortunately a serologic diagnosis tends to be retrospective and is not particularly helpful in designing initial therapy.

E. In many clinics, **laparoscopy** is routinely performed on women with severe PID to exclude certain alternative diagnoses (ectopic pregnancy, pelvic abscess, appendicitis) and to obtain material for Gram's stain and culture. Aspirates from the tubes are useful for isolating all major pathogens. There is a good correlation between positive endocervical cultures and tubal cultures for gonococci. *Chlamydia* can be isolated best from scrapings of the tubes, rather than from fluid exudate. The isolation of *Ureaplasma* or *Mycoplasma* from this source is significant, although special facilities are required for such cultures.

F. **Blood cultures** are positive in a small percentage of patients with PID. Such cultures should be obtained from patients who are septic and require hospitalization.

G. **Urethral culture** of the male sex partner should be performed in suspected cases of gonorrhea. In 10–15% of cases, the symptomatic female has a negative culture but her male consort is positive. It is most important to treat the male contact in order to avoid relapse of the patient and potential spread to other contacts.

H. **X-ray films of the abdomen, pelvis, and chest** should be obtained of patients with severe PID. A white blood cell count and differential and a urine analysis are also helpful.

VIII. **Treatment.** In setting up a therapeutic regimen for PID, there are two major considerations: the diagnosis of gonorrhea, and the severity of the infection.

A. **Mild, uncomplicated gonorrhea** (cervicitis or asymptomatic carrier)

Penicillin G procaine	4.8 million units IM, divided between two sites, at one visit
plus probenecid	1 gm PO, just before injection
or	
Ampicillin	3.5 g PO, one dose
plus probenecid	1 gm PO
In penicillin-allergic patients:	
Tetracycline HCl	500 mg qid for 7 days

B. **Moderate-to-severe gonococcal pelvic inflammatory disease**

Penicillin G procaine	4.8 million units IM, in two sites, at one visit
plus probenecid	1 gm PO, just before injection
followed by ampicillin	500 mg PO qid for 10 days
In penicillin-allergic patients:	
Tetracycline HCl	500 mg PO qid for 10 days

Some strains of *N. gonorrheae* have high-level resistance to penicillin due to production of penicillinase. These organisms should be treated with spectinomycin, 2 gm IM as a single dose, in asymptomatic carriers, or with tetracycline (as just listed) in the symptomatic patients. Cefoxitin can also be used for resistant organisms.

C. **Mild undiagnosed PID.** It is important to treat gonococci, anaerobic bacteria, and chlamydiae. Tetracycline is satisfactory in this regard and is often the treatment of choice:

Tetracycline	500 mg qid for 10 days
or	
Doxycycline	100 mg PO bid for 10 days

Ampicillin has been used in many clinics with equal success, despite its relatively poor activity against *Chlamydia* and *Mycoplasma:*

Ampicillin	500 mg qid for 10 days

A 5–10% failure rate can be expected with either regimen; if the patient still exhibits mild symptoms, it may be advisable to convert to the alternative drug. However, hospitalization for intravenous therapy is a better choice at this stage. A single-dose injection of penicillin is not adequate therapy for pelvic inflammatory disease.

D. Moderate-to-severe undiagnosed PID. The same regimens for the milder cases, tetracycline or ampicillin, can be used theoretically in the more severe cases. A decision should be made early, however, regarding the necessity for hospitalization. Patients should be advised that treatment in the hospital will lead to a better outcome. It is important to treat such patients specifically for pathogenic anaerobes such as *Bacteroides* that may be complicating pyosalpinx or pelvic abscess. In these cases, clindamycin, cefoxitin, or metronidazole should be administered, but such therapy is impractical on an outpatient basis. It should be emphasized that clindamycin and metronidazole have poor activity against the gonococcus; hence, an appropriate drug such as penicillin should be included in the regimen when this organism is a potential pathogen.

Treatment for hospitalized patients with PID is as follows: (CDC recommendations. *MMWR* 31:43S, 1982).

Initial (hospitalization)	**Oral regimen, to follow**
Cefoxitin, 2 gm IV qid, **plus** doxycycline, 100 mg IV bid	Doxycycline, 100 mg bid
Clindamycin, 600 mg IV q8h, **plus** tobramycin or gentamicin, 1.5 mg/kg tid	Clindamycin, 450 mg qid
Doxycycline, 100 mg IV bid, **plus** metronidazole 500 mg IV qid	Metronidazole, 500 mg qid, + doxcycline, 100 mg qid

The parenteral regimen is given for at least 4 days and for at least 48 hours after the patient defervesces. The oral regimen is then continued to complete a 10–14 day course of treatment.

IX. Indications for hospitalization. Approximately 70% of patients with PID have been treated in the past as outpatients. Because of the high incidence of relapse, primarily due to noncompliance in younger women, hospitalization is now recommended in most cases. The absolute indications for hospitalization are for

A. Patients whose diagnosis is uncertain and for whom an acute surgical emergency, e.g., appendicitis or ectopic pregnancy, cannot be excluded

B. Patients whose physical examination raises a high level of suspicion of pelvic abscess or who are obviously septic

C. Patients who are unable to take oral medications due to nausea and vomiting or lack of compliance

D. Patients who fail to respond to oral or intramuscular antibiotics

E. Patients who are pregnant

Of those requiring hospitalization, over 70% are patients with nongonococcal PID. It should be emphasized that recurrent PID or "treatment failure" may be due to a sex partner who has remained untreated.

X. Risk factors for PID

1. **Contact with gonorrhea** may produce an asymptomatic carrier state in the female, which can subsequently blossom into acute PID.
2. **Menstruation,** in the case of gonorrhea, increases the risk.
3. **Previous attacks of PID** predispose to a chronic, relapsing state.
4. An **intrauterine device,** especially in a nulliparous woman, can cause endometritis and PID.

XI. Complications

A. Short-term complications involve a progression of the disease to abscess formation, pelvic peritonitis, septic pelvic thrombophlebitis, bacteremia, and septic shock.

B. **Long-term complications,** although not life-threatening, can produce considerable hardship and grief.

1. **Relapsing PID.** Within 1 year of the initial episode, 40% of patients have a recurrence. Gonococcal PID is often followed by nongonococcal disease. Each previous attack causes further damage to the bacterial clearance mechanisms of the fallopian tubes and sets the stage for relapse.
2. **Infertility.** A major cause of involuntary childlessness is PID. After three or more episodes of PID, 70% of patients are unable to conceive.
3. **Chronic pelvic pain and cervical discharge.** These symptoms can be so severe as to require subsequent hysterectomy for relief.
4. **Ectopic pregnancy.** The incidence is increased six- to tenfold.

Suppurative Disease of the Pelvis

I. **General principles.** Pelvic abscess and pelvic peritonitis are life-threatening infections. They may be acute or have a delayed and undulating course.

II. **Anatomic presentations**

A. Unilateral or bilateral parametrial abscess that points into either the vagina or the inguinal area.
B. Purulent collection in the cul-de-sac that points to the posterior fornix of the vagina; this may be associated with prolapse or fixation of the ovaries and tubes.
C. Tuboovarian or ovarian abscess that becomes fixed high in the pelvic lateral wall; this may point to the inguinal ligament.
D. Tuboovarian or ovarian abscess that presents as an abdominal mass and does not point to either the cul-de-sac or the inguinal ligament.
E. Catastrophic rupture of an abscess leading to pelvic peritonitis.

III. **Predisposing causes of pelvic abscess**

A. **Pelvic inflammatory disease** (PID)
B. **Vaginal hysterectomy.** A common form of suppurative pelvic infection is **vaginal cuff infection** following a vaginal hysterectomy. This may be a collection of pus or an infected hematoma.
C. **Abdominal hysterectomy**
D. **Cesarean section.** Cesarean section has a high incidence of infection, usually limited to the wound but occasionally associated with abscess formation in the pelvis. The lowest risk is with elective cesareans. The risk is especially high in emergency sections for premature rupture of membranes.
F. **Dilatation and curettage** (for diagnostic procedures, abortion, or to remove retained products of conception)
F. **Tubal ligation** (especially by the vaginal route)
G. **Nongynecologic abdominal operations**

IV. **Signs and symptoms.** Approximately one-third of patients present acutely with no past history of gynecologic illness. The remaining patients have **recurrent PID** or a recent surgical procedure.

A. **Pelvic pain** is the major symptom. Acute exacerbation of pain suggests rupture of the abscess. Approximately half the patients have chills and fever. Urinary complaints are common.
B. **Examination of the abdomen** may reveal a large mass rising from the pelvis or an abscess pointing to the flank or inguinal ligament.
C. **Vaginal examination** may show a discrete localization. Pointing of the mass into the posterior fornix of the vagina affords an opportunity to make a diagnosis by colpocentesis.

V. **Diagnosis.** The diagnosis of pelvic abscess often is apparent on abdominal and pelvic examination. In some cases, however, it is difficult to distinguish between salpingitis, a condition that can be managed with antibiotics, and abscess formation, a condition that may require operative intervention. The following laboratory and x-ray studies should be instigated:

A. Complete blood count with WBC and differential, urinalysis, serum electrolytes, and liver function tests.

B. X-rays of the abdomen and pelvis. These may reveal a mass lesion, ileus, or gas in the uterine wall or surrounding structures. (Small bubbles of gas are often visible in an abscess cavity.) X-ray films of the chest should be examined for the presence of pulmonary emboli.

C. Ultrasound study of the pelvis, which may reveal a fluid-filled abscess cavity. A computed tomography scan (**CT scan**) of the abdomen and pelvis is useful for demonstrating a mass lesion. Gallium scan can sometimes delineate an abscess; the full results of this scan cannot be read for 4 days, however, and false-positive readings result from isotope collected in the bowel or inflamed tissues. In our experience, gallium scanning is often unproductive in pelvic infections. (It should be emphasized that none of the scanning techniques should be taken as an absolute indication for surgery. An apparent "mass" can resolve with antibiotic management.)

D. Culdocentesis. This procedure can establish the presence of pus or blood in the cul-de-sac and furnish a specimen for bacteriology. If large quantities of pus are encountered, this approach can be employed for drainage.

E. Specimens for bacteriologic cultures should be obtained:

1. **Vaginal or cervical discharge**—useful for gonococci only (or *Chlamydia,* if facilities exist). Do not send for "routine" or anaerobe cultures.
2. **Blood cultures**—at least three sets before antibiotics are started
3. **Urine**
4. **Culdocentesis aspirate,** if obtained
5. **Laparoscopy aspirate or scrapings,** if obtained

VI. Microbiology

A. Sixty percent of such infections are associated with a **mixed aerobic-anaerobic flora,** usually derived from the normal vaginal flora; 35% of patients have pure anaerobic microorganisms; 5% of patients have aerobic organisms only.

1. **Aerobes in order of prevalence are as follows:**
   - **a.** *Escherichia coli*
   - **b.** *Klebsiella*
   - **c.** Streptococci
   - **d.** *Pseudomonas* (rare)
   - **e.** *Staphylococcus aureus* (rare)
   - **f.** *N. gonorrhoeae* (rare)
2. **Anaerobes in order of prevalence** are as follows:
   - **a.** *Bacteroides fragilis*
   - **b.** *Peptostreptococcus*
   - **c.** *Peptococcus*
   - **d.** *Bacteroides* species (*B. bivius* and *B. disiens*)
   - **e.** *Fusobacterium*
   - **f.** *Clostridium*

B. *N. gonorrhoeae* is an uncommon cause of pelvic abscess, although this organism causes severe salpingitis. Some patients with abscess have a mixed culture of gonococci with aerobes and anaerobes.

C. There is a high incidence of positive blood cultures among patients with suppurative pelvic disease. The most common bloodstream invaders are anaerobic streptococci, *Bacteroides, E. coli, Klebsiella,* and *Clostridium.* It is not uncommon to isolate more than one species of bacteria from a single blood culture, provided both aerobic and anaerobic media are used.

VII. Treatment

A. General principles

1. Immediate hospitalization and bed rest in semi-Fowler's position
2. High-dose parenteral antibiotics (see sec. **C**)
3. Intravenous fluids and electrolytes

4. Frequent monitoring of vital signs, with particular attention to blood pressure and urine output. Septic shock is a frequent complication of pelvic abscess.

B. Surgical management

1. **Indications for drainage of abscess:** About 70% of patients with "tuboovarian abscesses" respond to antibiotic treatment and do not require a drainage procedure. The diagnosis of abscess is not always well established in these cases, and many may actually represent a phlegmon. Such imprecision in anatomic diagnoses has led some authorities to use the appellation "tuboovarian complex." The specific indications for drainage are
   a. **Failure to respond adequately to medical management.** The time frame is variable, depending on the patient's clinical state. When the patient is septic and toxic the decision may have to be made within the first 1–2 days. Other patients show a partial response, but persistence of symptoms for 5–7 days may force surgical intervention.
   b. **Presence of a fluctuant mass.** If such a lesion is palpable, it generally has > 100 ml of pus. The diagnosis of a mass often is difficult. CT scan and ultrasound may demonstrate an "abscess." Clinical experience has shown, however, that such mass lesions can be cured by antibiotic therapy alone without direct drainage. (Presumably, these lesions can drain themselves through the uterus and into the vagina.)
   c. **Rupture of an abscess** or evidence of an intraperitoneal catastrophe. This event is heralded by a sudden change in the patient's course, with an increase in abdominal pain, often with rebound tenderness, associated with nausea and vomiting. There is exquisite pelvic tenderness. An elevated, often spiking, fever, with shaking chills and tachycardia, is present. On occasion, a pelvic mass appears to have changed in location, indicating partial rupture or dissection into fascial planes.
   d. **Septic pelvic thrombophlebitis,** when heparin therapy has failed (p. 79–81).
   e. **Elective procedures.** Some women have recurrent episodes of pelvic inflammatory disease, which may be accompanied by adnexal masses. Severe pelvic pain is often present. These symptoms are indications for elective hysterectomy.
2. **Surgical approach.** The definitive procedure for abscess is removal of pelvic organs. The most common circumstances are recurrent PID and post-cesarean section infection. A complete abdominal hysterectomy and bilateral salpingo-oophorectomy is the preferred operation. Appropriate drains for an abscess cavity should be applied. Many women would prefer to avoid this procedure, especially to preserve fertility. Whenever possible, a drainage procedure without resection (or even unilateral resection of a pyosalpinx) should be attempted.
3. **Colpotomy drainage** should be considered for patients who develop a fluctuant mass in the cul-de-sac. An abscess that dissects into the lower portion of the retrovaginal septum is particularly accessible through a vaginal cul-de-sac approach. A drain should be left in place. This procedure is useful in cases of pelvic abscess after hysterectomy, since there can be a complete resolution of the infection by colpotomy drainage alone when the uterus has previously been removed.

   It should be stressed that nearly half of patients who undergo culpotomy drainage have recurrence of symptoms that requires a more definitive surgical procedure. The reasons for failure with this limited form of drainage are
   a. A multiloculated abscess
   b. Additional abscesses in other pelvic organs
   c. Pyosalpinx

   Many women with recurrent PID are infertile. Of those who develop pelvic abscess that is successfully drained by culpotomy, a small percentage are subsequently able to conceive. This factor must be considered in the decision to perform a hysterectomy.

4. **Collections in the vaginal cuff** are managed with local drainage, usually without general anesthesia. The suture line is opened, and a small drain is inserted.
5. **Direct percutaneous drainage,** with a pig-tail catheter (to prevent slipping out of the cavity), can be attempted under ultrasound or CT scan guidance. This technique is being evaluated in several centers, and the initial results are favorable. The risks are bleeding, dissection of the abscess into other sites, and recurrence due to a multiloculated abscess.

C. **Antimicrobial therapy.** The appropriate choice of antimicrobial therapy can be a major factor in the successful management of suppurative pelvic infections. Nearly all such infections harbor anaerobic bacteria, usually in association with aerobes or coliforms. Antimicrobial therapy must be active against both aerobes and anaerobes. Several regimens have been recommended:

1. Clindamycin	600 mg Iv q6h
plus an aminoglycoside	
Gentamicin	1.5 mg/kg IV or IM q8h
Tobramycin	1.5 mg/kg IV or IM q8h
Amikacin	5 mg/kg IV or IM q8h
2. Metronidazole	500 mg PO or IV q8h
plus an aminoglycoside	
3. Chloramphenicol	750 mg–1 gm IV q6h
plus an aminoglycoside	
4. Cefoxitin	2 gm IV q6h

Cefoxitin can be used as a single drug, since it is active against anaerobes, including *B. fragilis,* most coliforms, and gonococci.

N. gonorrhoeae may be encountered in patients with PID, although it is not usually the cause of pelvic abscess. Since clindamycin and metronidazole have poor activity against gonococci, another antibiotic, usually **ampicillin** (1 gm q6h, IV), must be added to the regimen of patients suspected of being infected with this organism.

An old canard suggests that enterococci (*Streptococcus faecalis*) is important in the pathogenesis of suppurative pelvic infections. To be sure, these organisms can be isolated from pelvic infections, but the evidence for their inherent pathogenicity is virtually nil. None of the one- or two-drug regimens listed (**C.1.–4**) is effective against the enterococcus. Yet prospective therapeutic trials have shown these treatments to be effective, and it is not necessary to include specific therapy (such as ampicillin) for the enterococcus in this type of infection. We would strongly advise against the addition of penicillin or ampicillin for this express purpose.

Intrauterine Device (IUD) and PID

I. **General principles.** Use of an IUD increases the risk of endomyometritis and salpingitis. This device encourages colonization of the endometrial cavity by vaginal flora. The risk of acute salpingitis is increased three- to fivefold in IUD users. Nulliparous women appear to be at greater risk of complications with the IUD than multiparous women. Parenthetically, the birth control pill is associated with a lower risk of PID. On pathologic examination, IUD users have focal endomyometritis with a foreign body reaction and invasion by PMNs.

II. **Complications**

Complication	Increased risk of IUD users compared to nonusers
PID	3–5 times
Pelvic abscess	3
Infertility	7
Ectopic pregnancy	6

III. **Microbiology.** A mixed flora originating in the vagina colonizes the uterine cavity in

IUD users. The organisms involved in infection are similar to those in other forms of mixed pelvic infections (p. 75). *Actinomyces* (gram-positive, branching, anaerobic rods) has been found on the device itself and in the uterine cavity of IUD users; however, *Actinomyces* occurs in asymptomatic, as well as symptomatic women, and its role as a pathogen has not been established in this setting.

IV. Treatment

A. Mildly symptomatic women can be treated by removal of the device. Some women can be fitted with a device of different design at a later date. It is advisable, however, to recommend the use of another form of birth control when there has been an infectious complication.

B. Moderate symptoms, such as localized uterine pain, increased discharge, and low-grade fever, should be treated with an antibiotic, in addition to removal of the device. Either ampicillin (250 mg PO 4 times/day) or tetracycline (same dose) can be given for 10 days.

C. More serious complications, especially those that suggest spread of the infection into the fallopian tubes or the pelvis, require hospitalization and the administration of parenteral antibiotics. The regimens indicated for the serious forms of pelvic infection should be employed (see p. 77).

Ovarian Abscess

I. General principles. The ovaries may be involved by infection within their substance, even though the tubes are free of the septic process. This condition is usually associated with localized or diffuse peritonitis.

II. Predisposing causes

A. Pelvic surgery, especially vaginal hysterectomy

B. Postpartum infections, abortion, and cesarean section

C. Endometritis following a D&C

D. Diverticulitis or inflammatory bowel disease

III. Signs and symptoms include an episode of lower abdominal pain and fever for 3 days to 3 weeks, following an operative procedure such as vaginal hysterectomy. This is one of the few causes of postoperative infection with a normal early recovery phase. The pain is mild at first, but soon increases in intensity. An acute exacerbation, especially with high fever, suggests rupture of the abscess.

IV. Physical examination reveals lower abdominal pain with localized tenderness, muscle guarding, and, in many patients, rebound tenderness. Pelvic examination is difficult to perform, but in one-third of patients a discrete mass can be palpated.

V. Microbiologic agents are nearly always anaerobes, either alone or in combination with aerobic organisms. *Bacteroides,* anaerobic streptococci, *Clostridium, E. coli,* and *Klebsiella* are the major culprits, usually in association with one another.

VI. Treatment consists of initial antibiotic drugs and support measures (as indicated for pelvic abscess, pp. 75–77); however, this infection also requires surgery. The abscess is removed intact, but it is recommended that the pelvis be drained as well, otherwise a pelvic abscess will appear in the postoperative course. The major risk of ovarian abscess is delay in diagnosis and subsequent rupture of the abscess with catastrophic results.

Antimicrobial drugs are indicated in all cases of ovarian abscess. The regimens indicated for suppurative diseases of the pelvis should be used (p. 77).

Pyometra

I. General principles. Obstruction of the cervix leads to accumulation of pus and enlargement of the uterus, known as **pyometra.** Surprisingly, this condition can be insidious with relatively few systemic findings.

II. Clinical settings

1. **Carcinoma of the cervix or endometrium**—seen in approximately 70% of patients. Hence, malignancy should be suspected in all cases of pyometra.

2. **Radiation therapy** to the pelvis
3. **Previous cauterization**
4. **Spontaneous cervical stenosis** in postmenopausal women
5. **Polyps or myoma** that obstruct the cervix
6. **Tuberculosis,** a rare cause, leading to cervical stenosis

III. Microbiological agents of pyometra are derived from normal vaginal flora, and resemble those of pelvic abscess (p. 75).

IV. Treatment is initially antibiotics and conservative management. The specific antimicrobial agents are those recommended for suppurative diseases of the pelvis (p. 77). Since most of the women with pyometra are elderly and/or have serious medical problems, it is recommended that evacuation of the uterine cavity and tube drainage be instituted initially, to be followed at a later time by complete hysterectomy. However, if the patient can withstand the procedure, the definitive operation should be performed rather soon after stabilization with antibiotics, supportive care, and tube drainage.

Perihepatitis (Fitzhugh-Curtis Syndrome)

I. General principles. A perihepatitis, or inflammatory reaction involving the liver capsule, is seen occasionally in patients with salpingitis. In the past the causative agent was assumed to be the gonococcus. Recent studies, however, have implicated *Chlamydia* as the major culprit. The **pathology** consists of fibrous adhesions, known as "violin strings," forming between the anterior surface of the liver and the adjacent, parietal portion of the peritoneum, usually on the anterior surface.

II. Symptoms may be sudden and dramatic, with severe right upper quadrant pain that is exacerbated by deep breathing, coughing, or movement. The differential diagnosis includes cholecystitis, pyelonephritis, peptic ulcer disease, and acute hepatitis.

III. Physical examination reveals that the anterior abdominal wall is tender, and there is marked tenderness, often with rebound, in the right upper quadrant. The patient usually has active PID.

IV. Treatment. Most patients respond without specific therapy other than the antibiotics administered for the PID infection (see pp. 72–73). Since *Chlamydia* is a common cause, the preferred therapy is tetracycline, 500 mg qid for 10 days. In certain clinics, laparoscopy is used to make the diagnosis and even for treatment. The therapeutic procedure involves cauterization of the adhesions, which are then divided by blunt dissection or laparoscopic scissors. In most cases, however, conservative management is sufficient.

Septic Pelvic Thrombophlebitis (SPT)

I. General principles. Thrombosis of the pelvic veins represents a serious threat to the patient with pelvic infection. In addition to local suppuration, there is the danger of embolism to the lungs or kidneys.

II. Predisposing factors. Virtually all types of pelvic surgery and complicated obstetric events can lead to pelvic thrombophlebitis. The most common are

A. **Vaginal delivery,** particularly when associated with premature rupture of membranes and puerperal sepsis
B. **Septic abortion**
C. **Pelvic operations** such as hysterectomy
D. **Cesarean section**
E. **Pelvic inflammatory disease** and pelvic abscess

Multiple veins often are involved in the thrombotic process. The affected veins, in order of frequency, are the **ovarian, uterine, common iliac, hypogastric, vaginal,** and **inferior vena cava.** Pathologic findings include edema and induration of the vessel wall that progresses to suppuration and destruction of the vein by the infectious process.

SPT is a relatively rare disease. Its frequency in a major city hospital is reported as follows:

Surgical procedures	Number of cases of SPT per total events
Febrile abortions	1/200
Major gynecologic surgery	1/800
All deliveries (higher in cesarean section)	1/2,000

III. Signs and symptoms. SPT occurs in a setting of pelvic infection developing postpartum, postoperatively, or after abortion. The following features suggest the onset of this complication:

- **A.** Hectic fever with chills and extreme toxicity. The fever may have pronounced swings from normal to 41°C.
- **B.** Failure to respond to conventional antibiotic treatment and supportive care.
- **C.** Pleuritic chest pain, hemoptysis, and sudden onset of dyspnea. These findings indicate pulmonary embolism.
- **D.** Pelvic pain. This is an inconsistent feature and may be related to the primary suppurative disease in the pelvis rather than to the thrombotic process.

IV. Diagnosis. There is a paucity of findings that are directly attributable to the venous thrombosis.

- **A. Vaginal examination** may reveal some tenderness in the parametrium; only rarely can the thrombosed vessel be palpated. When there is massive thrombosis of both ovarian veins, there is an ileus and flank tenderness.
- **B. Blood cultures** are positive in only 5–10% of cases. This low figure may be due to the intermittent nature of the bacteremia or to the fastidious types of anaerobic bacteria that are involved.
- **C.** The **white blood cell count** is often normal or only slightly elevated.
- **D.** The **chest x-ray** shows patchy infiltrates in one-third of patients. Since these are septic emboli, associated with bacteria, the pulmonary infarct may become a metastatic infection, producing pneumonia, lung abscess, or empyema; these complications, however, are uncommon. The presence of multiple, small lung abscesses, without an air-fluid level, is a strong indication of septic pulmonary emboli.
- **E. Lung perfusion scans** are useful, since they show multiple, bilateral defects, even in apparently unaffected areas on chest x-ray. Pulmonary angiography has proved disappointing as a diagnostic tool, perhaps because the emboli tend to be dispersed as showers of very small particles.
- **F.** The **beneficial effect of heparin** strongly indicates SPT (see p. 81) and is an aid to retrospective diagnosis.

V. Microbiology. SPT is associated with those pelvic infections that are caused by a mixed aerobic-anaerobic or a pure anaerobic flora (p. 75). The actual organisms colonizing the vein are difficult to determine. In the few patients with positive blood cultures, the isolates are *Peptostreptococcus* (anaerobic streptococci), *Bacteroides,* and coliforms, in that order of prevalence. The antibiotics employed in therapy should cover at least these bacteria. (*Staph. aureus* is very rare as the pathogen.)

VI. Treatment

- **A. Antimicrobial therapy.** The appropriate choice of antimicrobial agents for suppurative diseases of the pelvis can avert the complication of SPT. When a patient is suspected of developing septic thrombosis, it is important to be sure that adequate drugs are employed.

  Since anaerobic bacteria such as *Peptostreptococcus* and *Bacteroides* are the major pathogens, the same regimens are recommended as for treating suppurative disease of the pelvis (p. 77).

  In some clinics, massive doses of penicillin (4 million units q4h) are added to the regimen in order to cover enterococci. It is our view that penicillin makes an insignificant contribution to these regimens (p. 77) and should not be used.

B. Anticoagulation therapy

1. Indications

a. Failure to respond to appropriate antibiotics after 4 days, on the part of a patient in a compatible clinical setting (postpartum, postoperative, or postabortal), is the major indication. Since continued fever and toxicity may be caused by undrained pus in the pelvis, appropriate surgical measures should be undertaken before the diagnosis of thrombophlebitis is made.

b. The **appearance of multiple pulmonary emboli** is another justification. This condition is suspected on clinical grounds with the onset of shortness of breath, chest pain, or hemoptysis. Confirmation is made by chest x-ray and lung scan.

2. Heparin. Heparin is the preferred drug for anticoagulation.

a. Administration

Intermittent injections, q1–4 h into an indwelling IV catheter, or
Continuous IV, at a constant infusion rate, with a pump

The intermittent IV method is a conventional approach often used in hospitals, but it may produce an infinite prolongation of the clotting time, just after the bolus injection. Although heparin is generally administered q4h, the half-life is in fact 1½ hours, so that by the end of the 4-hour interval most of the drug has been eliminated from the circulation. If available, continuous IV infusion is the preferred method, since it reduces the incidence of major bleeding episodes.

b. Initial dose. 5,000 units, administered as a direct bolus.

c. Subsequent doses. approximately 1,000 units/hr. The dose varies with the patient's weight and is influenced by a number of factors, including other drugs and individual responsiveness.

d. Monitoring. The activated partial thromboplastin time (PTT) should be prolonged by 1.5–2.0 times the baseline control values; or the clotting time should be prolonged to two to three times normal.

The dose of heparin has to be highest in the 1st 3 days of therapy. Bleeding and hemorrhagic complications are increased by the simultaneous administration of drugs such as aspirin, dipyridamole, phenylbutazone, and indomethacin. If the patient has thrombocytopenia due to severe sepsis, the heparin requirement is reduced.

If heparin therapy is successful, the patient becomes afebrile on an average of 2–3 days after initiation of therapy, although up to 7 days may be required in some cases. The total treatment period is 7 days after the patient has become afebrile, with an average total dose of 8–10 days. Heparin can be stopped abruptly, and it is not necessary to continue anticoagulation with warfarin (Coumadin).

C. Surgical management. The major objective of operative intervention is to remove or drain any persisting sites of infection in the pelvis. After adequate drainage, some patients, even with appropriate antibiotics, require additional surgery directed toward the thrombotic events. Indications for operation include

1. Persistence of fever and toxicity, despite appropriate antimicrobial therapy and anticoagulation, for at least 5–7 days of treatment with these two modalities combined.

2. Persistent pulmonary embolism. Since this is a life-threatening complication, it may force early surgical intervention.

The favored surgical procedure is transperitoneal ligation of the vena cava and possibly the ovarian veins. It is important to explore the pelvis in order to identify any sites of suppuration. A hysterectomy often is indicated in cases of uncontrolled pelvic infection.

Mortality in SPT is approximately 5%. Patients may die of septicemia and shock, progressive pulmonary infections with empyema and abscess formation, pulmonary insufficiency, or a catastrophic event in the pelvis such as ruptured abscess or severe hemorrhage. Massive pulmonary embolism is uncommon in this setting.

Vulvovaginitis

I. General principles. Four types of vulvovaginitis are noted clinically: monilial (*Candida albicans*), trichomonal, herpetic (Herpes simplex virus), and "nonspecific." The major symptom is vaginal discharge, which may be accompanied by pruritus, burning, dyspareunia, and dysuria. Certain conditions predispose to vaginitis:

A. Diabetes, which is associated with monilial infections and nonspecific vaginitis

B. Pregnancy, in which there is an increase in all forms of vaginitis, especially monilial

C. Foreign bodies, such as pessaries and IUDs

D. Certain drugs, such as antibiotics and hormones

Since treatment for each type of vaginitis is relatively specific, it is important to make an etiologic diagnosis.

II. Monilial (*Candida*) Vaginitis. Healthy women harbor small numbers of the fungus *Candida* as part of the normal vaginal flora; it is recovered in 25–50% of asymptomatic women. An overgrowth of *Candida* may occur from unknown causes, although it is rare in premenarcheal girls and postmenopausal women. The following conditions increase the chance that symptoms will develop:

1. Pregnancy
2. Diabetes
3. Hormone therapy, such as corticosteroids, birth control pills, and estrogens
4. Immunodeficiency disease
5. Antibiotic therapy

A. Signs and symptoms. The major symptom is severe itching. In addition, there may be dyspareunia, dysuria, and a profuse vaginal discharge. The discharge is often malodorous and has a typical creamy-white "cottage cheese" consistency. Examination of the vulva shows edema, erythema, and excoriations. The vaginal mucosa is erythematous, with overlying white patches that have a milky, curd-like appearance. There may be red patches on the skin surrounding the vulva.

B. Diagnosis. This condition is best diagnosed by direct observation of the vaginal discharge under the microscope. A wet mount, diluted with saline or 10% KOH, displays oval and budding yeasts and mycelial forms. If the wet mount is negative or questionable, a culture should be sent to the laboratory for growth on a specific medium, such as Mycosel.

C. Treatment.

1. The major remedy is direct application of an antifungal agent to the vulva and vagina. **Nystatin, clotrimazole,** or **miconazole** can be used, by vaginal application of cream or suppositories each evening for approximately 10 days. In the event of relapse, retreatment must be instituted for a longer period of time.
2. It may be necessary to consider **therapy of the male sex partner,** who may have monilial infection of the penis. Use of a condom or topical application of an antifungal agent to the glans penis are potential approaches.
3. An alternative regimen is local application of **1% gentian violet** solution. Patients are often reluctant to accept this therapy because it causes bright stains on clothing. However, it can afford dramatic relief.
4. Patients with severe irritation of the vulva may benefit from application of **tepid water** or direct use of **topical corticosteroid creams.** These creams should be used only during the hyperacute period, in conjunction with an antifungal agent.
5. Adjunctive therapy includes **topical anesthetics,** if pain is severe, and the recommendation that tight-fitting pantyhose or undergarments be avoided. Whenever possible, the predisposing cause should be eliminated: Antibiotics might be stopped, corticosteroids or other hormones reduced or deleted, and diabetes brought under control by medical management. Pregnancy may produce refractory vaginal moniliasis, which improves after delivery.
6. Rare cases of severe and unremitting vaginal moniliasis are associated with

generalized skin involvement. The patients often have immunodeficiency diseases or hypoparathyroidism. When the fungal disease becomes particularly difficult to manage in such individuals, relief can be gained from the use of **ketoconazole,** 400 mg/day, as a single dose, for 3 days. Extreme cases, in which ketoconazole has not succeeded, can be treated with small doses of intravenous **amphotericin B.** A dose of 10–20 mg/day IV, with a total dose of approximately 150 mg, often yields dramatic results. There is, however, a marked tendency to relapse, due to the underlying disorder.

III. *Trichomonas* vaginitis. This protozoan parasite can be demonstrated in vaginal secretions of 25% of American females in the reproductive years, although only a minority of individuals are symptomatic. Pregnancy predisposes to this infection. There is good evidence that the disease is sexually transmitted. It has a high incidence in prostitutes, a low occurrence in virgins, and an association with gonococcal infection. Furthermore, male consorts of infected females often harbor the protozoa in the urethra and prostate.

A. Signs and symptoms. The major complaint is profuse vaginal discharge. The exudate is grayish white or green, watery, and malodorous. In some individuals it is frothy and bubbling. Dysuria and dyspareunia are common symptoms. Examination of the vulva shows an erythematous, edematous mucosa. The vaginal epithelium is diffusely reddened, with inflammation and edema, the so-called strawberry appearance. A frothy, bubbly, watery exudate is clearly visible.

B. Diagnosis. Direct microscopic examination of the discharge reveals the motile parasite. A specimen is taken high in the vaginal vault, not from the endocervix. One drop of fluid, plus one drop of saline, is inspected under high magnification. The protozoa are motile, with a distinctive, undulating membrane; they are slightly larger than a white blood cell. In order to demonstrate motility, lubricants or douching agents should be avoided. It is not necessary to culture this organism. However, cultures for the gonococcus and monilia should be performed.

C. Treatment. The major therapeutic agent is **metronidazole,** which can be given by one of two regimens:

A single oral dose of 2 gm, or
250 mg tid for 4 days

It is important to treat the steady sex partner simultaneously with the same dose. *Trichomonas* infection in the male is usually asymptomatic, but failure to treat the male partner leads to a high incidence of relapse in the female. Metronidazole should be avoided in early pregnancy, since the drug passes the placental barrier. Acidifying douches can be used until the second trimester, when metronidazole can be administered. Some obstetricians prefer to avoid this drug altogether in pregnancy. Since this drug has an antabuse-like effect, alcohol should be avoided during its administration.

IV. Herpes vulvovaginitis. Herpes simplex virus (HSV) has two distinct types. Oral mucocutaneous infections are caused by **HSV type I.** Genital infections are caused by **HSV type II** in 70–90% of cases, and by type 1 in the remainder.

A. Epidemiology. The occurrence of genital herpes has increased in recent years, so that it now ranks second to gonorrhea as a cause of sexually transmitted infection in females. Venereal transmission is the rule. Sexual contact with an infected male has a 50–90% chance of producing disease in the female partner. There is rare nonsexual person-to-person transmission, especially among health professionals, and autoinoculation has been reported. HSV genital infection is uncommon in children and in nuns and is most frequent in adolescents and young adults. The highest incidence is found in prostitutes and in patients attending venereal disease clinics. In large surveys of healthy, asymptomatic females, 2–4% of vaginal cultures have been found positive for the virus.

B. Signs and symptoms. The disease occurs in **primary** and **recurrent** forms, which differ greatly from each other in clinical presentation (Table 4-1)
The incubation period for a primary infection is 2–20 days (mean, 6 days) after contact with an infected person. Approximately two-thirds of females who have

Table 4-1. Clinical presentation of herpes vulvovaginitis

Finding	Primary attack	Recurrent attack
Number of lesions	Multiple	Few
Location	Vulva, cervix, and perianal skin	Cervix; other sites less often
Inguinal adenopathy	Nearly 100%; painful	Less common, often symptomatic
Systemic symptoms (fever, headache, malaise)	Frequent	Uncommon
Severe pain	Frequent	Less common
Itching	Frequent, especially in later stages	Frequent
Duration	10–40 days	1–10 days

experienced primary herpes will develop relapses. The recurrent attacks are unpredictable, both in the interval and in the inciting event. They may be triggered by menses or trauma, e.g., sexual intercourse, but not generally by febrile episodes, as with oral herpes infections. Recurrent attacks tend to involve the cervix, and they present clinically with a mucoid, heavy discharge and itching. In some women recurrences are asymptomatic, since the lesions are on the cervix, but there exists the potential for viral transmission.

C. Diagnosis. Physical examination in the primary stage reveals multiple, tender vesicles and ulcers involving the vulva, perianal skin, and cervix. In recurrent attacks there is usually a paucity of lesions, with one to three vesicles on an erythematous base. A presumptive diagnosis can be made by scraping the vesicle onto a slide and staining the material with Giemsa, Wright's, or H&E stain (Tzanck test). Staining should reveal large, multinucleated epithelial cells with intranuclear inclusion bodies that are characteristic of this infection. Culture of this material in an appropriate tissue culture line grows the virus in virtually all active cases.

D. Treatment

1. A new agent has been introduced for treatment of **primary** herpes genital infections, **acyclovir.** This drug is used as a topical ointment (5%). Its mode of action is interference with viral DNA polymerase. Clinical trials have shown a beneficial effect in primary herpes simplex genital infections, with decreases in healing time, viral shedding, and duration of pain. It does not prevent recurrences, however. In **recurrent episodes,** although some patients have reduced pain and increased healing time, most patients are **unhelped by this drug.**

   The ointment is applied to all cutaneous lesions q3h, six times/day for 7 days. Therapy should be started as soon as possible for maximum benefit. A finger cot or rubber glove should be used to apply the drug to prevent autoinoculation to other sites or transmission to other persons. Oral and intravenous forms of acyclovir are currently being tested and should be licensed in 1984. Preliminary information suggests that the oral form may be useful in preventing recurrences of genital herpes infection. The intravenous form is employed in more serious primary cases of genital herpes infection and in disseminated herpes infection, especially in an immunocompromised host.

2. A number of other remedies have been recommended, but none is endorsed with enthusiasm. Among the questionable, and probably ineffective, topical therapies are idoxuridine, povidone-iodine, steroids, and Burow's solution. There have been recommendations for local application of tricyclic dyes, such as neutral red or proflavine, along with photoactivation by white fluorescent

or incandescent light. Recent studies have suggested that this technique does not work however; the theoretical issue has also been raised that the dye may transform the virus into an oncogenic agent.

3. An important consideration for the patient with primary herpes genitalis is to **maintain the vulva and perineum as dry as possible,** with frequent changes of cotton underwear and use of cotton wool. Gentle, **dry heat** can be provided by a light bulb placed at an appropriate distance so that overheating does not occur. **Topical anesthetics** can be used, but they should be avoided while the lesions are moist and weeping.

E. **Complications**

1. **Neurologic complications** can occur, such as severe pain and neuralgia; urinary retention due to bladder paralysis; meningitis; and transverse myelitis.
2. **Spread to a sexual partner** is possible during periods of viral shedding.
3. **Spread to the newborn** can occur at the time of parturition and lead to severe HSV infection of the neonate. Primary infection in the expectant mother is associated with stillborns, prematurity, and spontaneous abortions, albeit in low frequencies.
4. **Carcinoma of the cervix** has been linked epidemiologically to HSV genital infections. There is, however, considerable controversy over this and most authorities doubt the causative association between these conditions.

V. **Nonspecific vaginitis.** This is a milder form of vaginitis that is often diagnosed by exclusion, after the possibility of bacterial, viral, fungal, and parasitic infections has been eliminated. Nonspecific vaginitis is seen most often in women with many sex partners and is uncommon in young children and in nuns. However, it can occur in any woman, even those who are sexually inactive.

A. **Signs and symptoms.** The most common symptom is a grayish white or yellowish, watery **vaginal discharge.** It often has a foul, "fishy" odor, and this disagreeable feature may be the most distressing symptom for the patient. Examination of the vaginal mucosa reveals diffuse erythema with small erosions and punctate hemorrhages. Cervicitis is frequently present.

B. **Diagnosis**

1. The other forms of vulvovaginitis must be excluded.
2. A presumptive diagnosis of nonspecific vaginitis can be made by identifying **clue cells** in the vaginal discharge. These are epithelial cells to which large numbers of gram-negative bacilli have become attached. They can be seen in wet mount or, more vividly, by Gram's staining of the discharge.
3. pH of vaginal discharge exceeding 4.5 is characteristic.
4. Release of the fishy amine-like odor from the vaginal discharge can be accomplished by adding two drops of 10% KOH to a small quantity of discharge on a cover slip.
5. Abnormal amines in the discharge can be shown by gas-liquid chromatography (GLC).
6. A succinate–lactate ratio of ≥ 0.4 in the vaginal discharge can be measured by GLC.
7. Some laboratories have the facilities to culture *Gardnerella vaginale.* These fastidious organisms grow slowly on blood or chocolate agar when incubated in a CO_2 environment. A specific medium such as peptone-cornstarch-dextrose agar can be employed. The organism must be present in large concentrations in order to make the diagnosis. It must be emphasized that this organism can be isolated from vaginal cultures in asymptomatic women.

C. **Microbiology.** The causative organism is said to be *G. vaginale,* a small, pleomorphic, gram-negative bacillus. This bacterium is recovered from vaginal secretions in large numbers from women with this disease. It can be isolated from the urethra in 90% of male sex partners of infected women. Careful studies, however, have also revealed this organism in up to 50% of healthy women. Therefore, considerable doubt exists as to the intrinsic pathogenicity of *G. vaginale.*

Another striking feature of this disease is the abnormal composition of the vaginal flora; the normal constituents, such as lactobacilli (Döderlein's bacillus), are absent, being replaced by a variety of anaerobes, coliforms, and enteric bacteria

D. Treatment

1. Mild douching or application of anesthetic creams can give immediate relief of local pain and pruritus. Triple-sulfa cream has been recommended, one application intravaginally bid for 7 days.
2. A recent report has suggested that **metronidazole,** 500 mg PO tid for 7 days can cure this disease. In the event of relapse, it is advised to treat the steady sex partner with this drug as well. However, there have not been enough controlled clinical trials to establish absolute therapeutic recommendations in this disease.

Toxic Shock Syndrome

I. General principles. The toxic shock syndrome (TSS) was originally described in 1978 as a life-threatening disease caused by staphylococcal toxin and characterized by hypotension with multiple organ failure. It received little attention until 1980, when there were an alarming number of cases involving young adult women during menses. Within 2 years, over 1,500 cases were reported. The CDC,* which served as a repository for data collection, has provided most of the currently available information concerning epidemiology, diagnostic criteria, and management guidelines.

II. Requirements for diagnosis (case definition). Diagnostic criteria include **each** of the following:

1. **Fever** exceeding 38.9°C (102°F).
2. A diffuse, macular, erythrodermal **rash** that may resemble a sunburn.
3. **Desquamation** of the superficial epidermis, usually of the palms or soles, at 7–14 days after onset of symptoms.
4. **Hypotension,** with a systolic blood pressure of less than 90 mm Hg for adults, below the 5th percentile for children under 16, or an orthostatic drop of 15 mm Hg
5. Clinical or laboratory evidence for involvement of **at least three organ systems:**
   a. **Gastrointestinal** with vomiting or diarrhea at onset of illness.
   b. **Muscular,** with severe myalgias or creatinine phosphokinase, 2× normal.
   c. Hyperemia of **mucous membranes** of vagina, oropharynx, or conjunctiva.
   d. **Renal** failure, with BUN or creatinine 2× normal or pyuria (5 WBC/HPF) without urinary infection.
   e. **Hepatic,** with abnormal liver function tests including SGOT, SGPT, or bilirubin 2× normal.
   f. **Hematologic,** with thrombocytopenia (platelets < 100,000/mm^3).
   g. **CNS,** with altered consciousness and no focal neurologic findings.
6. Negative studies for alternative diagnosis, including negative blood, throat, and CSF cultures, although blood cultures may yield *Staph. aureus*.

It should be noted that these criteria do not include recovery of *Staph. aureus,* despite evidence implicating this microbe in the etiology. Similarly, menses and tampon usage are not mentioned, even though epidemiologic data show a clear association. The reason is that the CDC evaluated these factors as independent variables in patients who satisfied the clinical criteria defined above. The menstrual history, methods of menses control, and results of appropriate cultures are considered important components in total assessment, even though they are not mentioned in the case definition. It should also be noted that the diagnostic criteria are notably stringent; many suspect cases do not satisfy all criteria and are categorized as "probable TSS."

III. Disease patterns

A. Menstrual-associated cases. These account for 90–95% of reported cases.

1. Significant risks

a. Use of tampons. Noted in 99% of menstrual-associated cases. Most patients used tampons exclusively or extensively.

*Centers for Disease Control, Atlanta, Georgia.

b. **Fluid capacity or absorbency** of the tampon. A disproportionate number of patients used superabsorbent Rely tampons, which led to the withdrawal of this product in September, 1980.

2. **Presentation.** Most patients note onset of symptoms within 2–3 days of menses. Initial complaints are fever, diarrhea, and vomiting, followed by hypotension and mental status change.
3. **Mortality.** 3%.

B. Nonmenstrual-associated cases. These account for 5–10% of reported cases and result from staphylococcal infection.

1. **Most common sites of infection**
   a. Nonsurgical cutaneous wound
   b. Parturition or abortion
   c. Surgical wound
2. **Presentation.** Same findings as those noted in case definition (see Sec. **II**). The only differences compared to menstrual-associated cases are a staphylococcal infection and lack of association with menses. Nevertheless, the *Staph. aureus* infection is typically subtle. Patients with cutaneous wounds, for example, often show relatively few local findings indicating infection, although cultures from the wounds yield this organism. Patients with procedure-related TSS (surgical wound, abortion, delivery) usually have the precipitous onset of symptoms, including hypotension, within 2–4 days after the procedure.
3. **Mortality:** 9%.

IV. Diagnosis

A. The **diagnosis** is based on the previously noted criteria. Some patients fail to satisfy all criteria but are considered "probable TSS."

B. The **diagnostic evaluation** should include vaginal cultures in menstrual-associated cases and cultures of other appropriate sites in non-menstrual-associated cases. Additional laboratory tests in all suspected cases should include CBC, platelet count, DIC screen, liver function tests, electrolytes, calcium, CPK, renal function tests, chest x-ray, ECG, blood cultures, and sera for serologic tests for other potential causes (See **C**).

C. Differential diagnosis includes septicemia, rash-associated viral infections, adverse drug reactions, streptococcal scarlet fever, Rocky Mountain spotted fever, leptospirosis, Kawasaki's disease, and the scalded skin syndrome.

V. Microbiology. The agent of TSS is *Staph. aureus* located in the vaginal tract or in infected sites. This organism has been recovered from cervical or vaginal cultures in 95% of menstrual-associated cases; the vaginal carrier rate of the organism in healthy women is 2–9%. These strains presumably produce an extracellular toxin that is absorbed and causes massive vasodilation with third spacing of fluid, hypotension, and widespread organ damage. The large increase in TSS cases recorded in 1980 is variously ascribed to (1) a change in products for menses control, with increased usage of superabsorbent products; (2) widespread publicity, with increased recognition; and (3) a toxin-producing capacity that is a new property, or a property with increasing prevalence, of *Staph. aureus.*

VI. Treatment

A. Intravenous fluids to restore the intravascular volume and electrolyte balance. The relative merits of crystalloid and colloid fluids are debated.

B. Management of severe complications, which may include

1. Renal failure, sometimes requiring dialysis
2. Severe hypocalcemia
3. Severe thrombocytopenia with bleeding diathesis
4. Myocardial irritability
5. Acute respiratory distress syndrome

C. Removal of retained tampons or other foreign bodies. Some advocate vigorous local irrigation to facilitate removal of preformed toxin, although efficacy is not clearly established.

D. The utility of corticosteroids or naloxone is not established.

E. Antibiotic treatment directed against penicillinase-producing *Staph. aureus*—

usually nafcillin, oxacillin, or a cephalosporin such as cephalothin (2–3 gm q6h IV for 5 days). Efficacy in terms of clinical response is not clearly established, although patients receiving this treatment appear to have fewer recurrences.

VII. Prognosis. Mortality for menstrual and nonmenstrual cases is about 3% and 9%, respectively. Patients who survive usually recover completely. Major sequelae have occurred in a small number of patients, including loss of digits due to shock, permanent renal impairment, neuromuscular abnormalities, and neuropsychologic sequelae with decreased memory and concentrating ability. The risk of recurrences in menstrual-associated cases is 30–40%; the recurrent episodes are usually less severe, and the incidence is reduced among patients who receive antistaphylococcal antibiotics or discontinue tampon use.

Obstetric Infections

I. General principles. Infectious complications of childbirth can be extremely serious, threatening the life of the mother and the newborn and compromising the mother's future reproductive capabilities.

Puerperal morbidity is defined as an oral temperature of 38°C or greater on any 2 of the 1st 10 postpartum days, excluding the first 24 hours. While useful as a guideline, this definition often is an inadequate base for a diagnosis of endometritis or puerperal sepsis. Approximately one-third of patients develop low-grade fever shortly after delivery, and it usually resolves spontaneously. Among the noninfectious causes of fever are trauma, hematoma in the episiotomy incision, and infusion of fetal protein into the maternal circulation. In addition, endometritis can occur without fever, being manifested by increased lochia or pelvic pain.

II. Epidemiology. Postpartum infections arise in 1–8% of patients, with an average figure of 2–3%. In municipal hospitals, which care for patients with higher risk factors, the incidence of such infections is 5–15%.

Although obstetric deaths have shown a dramatic reduction in recent years, infection remains the second highest cause of mortality, accounting for 25–50% of maternal deaths. It is estimated that approximately two-thirds of the septic deaths are preventable.

III. Types of postpartum infection (in order of frequency)

- **A.** Endometritis
- **B.** Urinary tract infection
- **C.** Respiratory infection
- **D.** Mastitis or breast abscess

IV. Predisposing factors

- **A.** Cesarean section
- **B.** Prolonged labor (>18 hr)
- **C.** Premature rupture of membranes (>24 hr)
- **D.** Trauma at delivery
- **E.** Forceps delivery
- **F.** Anemia
- **G.** The use of vaginal, rather than rectal, examinations
- **H.** Intrauterine fetal monitoring
- **I.** Low socioeconomic status of patients

V. Puerperal sepsis. Although there has been a general reduction of puerperal sepsis, recent developments in obstetric techniques may be reversing this trend. For example, it is known that cesarean section (C-section) carries a higher risk for postpartum infection than vaginal delivery; more C-sections are being performed in recent years, mostly for fetal indications. There has been some controversy concerning intrapartum fetal and maternal monitoring; in high-risk situations, where these devices are most useful, there appears to be an increased incidence of amnionitis.

A. Cesarean sections. Cesarean section accounts for 50% of maternal deaths, many of which are related to sepsis. Emergency C-sections carry a far greater risk of infectious complications than elective procedures. The classic C-section has a higher incidence of infection than low-segment operations, probably because the uterine incision cannot be oversewn with peritoneum. Emergency C-sections are reported to carry a risk of 30–50% of wound infection; some patients develop more serious complications, such as pelvic abscess and septicemia. For this reason, many obstetricians recommend prophylactic antibiotics for emergency cesarean section. A cephalosporin, given before the operative procedure, is recommended:

Cefazolin, cephalothin, or cefoxitin, 2 gm IV, 2 hours prior to C-section, during the procedure, and 6 hours later.

It has been claimed that intraoperative antibiotics such as cephalosporins have reduced the risk of wound infection from 35% to approximately 10%. Recent studies have shown that the prophylactic cephalosporin can be given **after** the cord is clamped, with the same protection to the mother but sparing the infant a dose of drug.

B. Etiologic agents. The microorganisms responsible for postpartum endometritis and the more serious complication, pelvic abscess, are derived from the normal flora of the vagina. It is often difficult to establish an etiologic diagnosis, since cultures of vaginal discharge or those obtained through the cervix are invariably contaminated with normal flora. Such samples should not be relied on for bacteriologic diagnosis. Blood cultures are positive in approximately 10% of patients with severe endometritis or pelvic abscess. The organisms most commonly found in postpartum endometritis and pelvic abscess are as follows:

Aerobes	**Anaerobes**
E. coli	*B. fragilis*
Klebsiella	Other *Bacteroides* species (*B. bivius* and *B. disiens*)
Proteus	Anaerobic streptococci
	Clostridia

Mycoplasma and *Ureaplasma* have occasionally been isolated in deep wound infections and in blood cultures from patients with postpartum sepsis.

C. Antibiotic therapy. The usual patient with mild postpartum endometritis does not require antibiotic therapy, for such cases are self-limited and cure themselves.

1. **Moderately severe cases** of endometritis can be treated with ampicillin (250 mg PO q6h) or tetracycline (250 mg PO q6h). If the patient is unable to take oral therapy, ampicillin can be administered in larger doses (1 g q6h) by the intravenous route. It is unwise to administer tetracycline intravenously to women in the third trimester or immediately post partum.
2. **Serious infections** should be treated for a spectrum of aerobic and anaerobic bacteria. The choices of drugs are

Clindamycin	600 mg IV q6h
or chloramphenicol	750–1,000 mg IV q6h
or metronidazole	500 mg PO or IV q8h
plus	
An aminoglycoside	
Gentamicin	1.5 mg/kg IV or IM q8h
Tobramycin	1.5 mg/kg IV or IM q8h
Amikacin	5 mg/kg IV or IM q8h
or	
cefoxitin	2 gm IV q6h

D. Complications

1. **Septicemia and septic shock.** Postpartum women have a tendency to develop **disseminated intravascular coagulation (DIC)** during an episode of bacteremia. DIC may be associated with renal failure and irreversible hypotension.
2. **Septic pelvic thrombophlebitis** (see pp. 79–81).
3. **Pelvic abscess.** An abscess may rupture into the peritoneal cavity.

E. Prophylactic antibiotics. Prophylactic use of antibiotics is clearly indicated in certain situations, but remains controversial in others:

1. **Heart murmurs.** Patients with either rheumatic or congenital murmurs should receive appropriate antimicrobial coverage during vaginal delivery (see pp. 295–296).
2. **Emergency cesarean sections.** The bulk of opinion favors the use of intraoperative antibiotics, although some studies fail to show benefit (see sec. **V.A** for dosage).
3. **Prolonged rupture of membranes.** Since the greatest risk is after 24 hours, several authorities recommend an antibiotic such as a cephalosporin. Prospective studies have shown conflicting results, however, and some reports have indicated no benefit from prophylactic therapy.

VI. Group A streptococcal infections. The classic cause of childbed fever is the group A, β-hemolytic *Strep. pyogenes*. Since the organism is only rarely found on the cervix of pregnant women, most postpartum infections are thought to be spread by a physician or nurse in attendance, or occasionally from the nasopharynx or skin of the mother. Women in prolonged labor and those experiencing excessive blood loss are at greater risk of infection by this organism, although streptococcal infections can occur in apparently uncomplicated deliveries. Infection by *Strep. pyogenes* is the only epidemic form of puerperal sepsis still seen in modern hospitals.

A. Clinical features. The presentation is striking, with an abrupt onset of a high fever that may reach 41°C occurring very early in the course. Many patients have symptoms within 12 hours of delivery or surgical procedure; two-thirds of cases develop within the 1st day, and the additional ones by the 2nd day. Shaking chills and prostration are accompanying symptoms. There is pelvic pain, and the uterus is diffusely tender. A spreading erythema is occasionally visible on the skin of the lower abdomen or perineum; if present, the edges of erythema are elevated, with red streaking through lympathics in the skin. A thin, watery vaginal discharge may be present, although the lochia is generally rather scanty at this stage. Dehiscence of an episiotomy, cesarean, or operative incision is an early event.

Streptococcal peritonitis progresses rapidly as a diffuse erythema that forms few adhesions and has no localization of pus. Approximately 40% of patients have bacteremia, which may be associated with disseminated intravascular coagulation (DIC). The organism elaborates hemolysins, and the DIC, combined with bacterial hemolysis, produces a profound hemolytic anemia.

A single case of streptococcal puerperal sepsis should alert the ward team to the possibility of an epidemic situation. The affected patient must be completely isolated and mothers and newborns put under careful surveillance.

B. Treatment. The treatment of choice is high doses of penicillin G, 4 million units IV q4h. Besides antibiotics, support measures are critical to a good outcome. Patients often develop septic shock with a decreased intravascular volume. Fluid and electrolyte replacement is always indicated, along with administration of colloid. Many patients require transfusions due to hemolysis and DIC. There is usually no indication for surgery, except when necrotic tissue is present, and then only simple debridement is required. If appropriate treatment is instituted early, the outlook is favorable. Delay in recognition can lead to a rapidly fatal course, however.

VII. Group B streptococcal infection. This organism is a common cause of infection in the newborn and may cause a mild illness in the mother. Since group B streptococci are sensitive to penicillin, the neonate and/or the mother, depending on the presence of symptoms, should be treated with large doses of this drug. Table 4-2 compares group A and group B streptococci.

VIII. Staphylococcal infections. *Staph. aureus* is acquired from the patient's nasopharynx or from the physicians and nursing staff in attendance. Hospital staff have a high incidence, approximately 40%, of carriage of *Staph. aureus* in the anterior nares, throat, or anus.

Staphylococcal infections occurring in the skin produce a discrete abscess, a carbuncle, or a diffuse cellulitis (see p. 183). These organisms also can cause endometritis or

Table 4-2. Comparison of group A and group B streptococci in obstetrics

Setting	Group A streptococcus	Group B streptococcus
Vaginal carrier	Rare	Common (15–40%)
Occurrence of infection in newborns	Rare	Common
Mode of acquisition	Doctors, nurses, and attendants	Vaginal flora acquired during birth
Maternal disease	Severe	Mild
Prognosis in mother	Guarded	Good
Prognosis in neonate	Good	Poor (50% mortality)

wound infections. Staphylococcal pneumonia occasionally is seen as a result of aspiration of this organism during induction of anesthesia.

A. Mastitis. Nursing mothers are at risk for serious forms of staphylococcal mastitis and breast abscess. Bacterial infections of the breast must be differentiated from the physiologic engorgement that occurs on the second or third postpartum day. This natural event is associated with swollen, tender breasts and may be accompanied by low-grade fever. Such patients are not infected. The condition is benign, although it can be mistaken for sepsis.

1. **Clinical features.** Bacterial mastitis in the nursing mother is almost invariably due to *Staph. aureus*, coagulase-positive. The nursing mother is infected by her infant, who has been colonized in the hospital nursery. The disease often occurs 3–4 weeks after delivery. It is initiated by engorgement of the breast with an abrupt onset of fever, often reaching 40°C, accompanied by pain, firmness, and erythema in the affected breast. Septicemia is not generally a feature of the early stage, so systemic symptoms are not severe. Careful examination may reveal a fissure near the base of the nipple.

   The spectrum extends from cellulitis, to mastitis, to discrete breast abscess. These are benign diseases if properly treated. Delayed therapy or inappropriate use of antibiotics can lead to septicemia and even death.

2. **Treatment.** A semisynthetic **penicillin** or **cephalosporin** should be used, since the pathogen usually is resistant to penicillin G. Among the drugs that are recommended for oral therapy are nafcillin, dicloxacillin, oxacillin, and cephaloxin, in doses of 250–500 mg q6h. Mild cases can be treated with oral antibiotics, and breastfeeding is continued. Some patients, however, need to cease nursing, because it is painful; in addition, the infected milk continues to colonize the infant, who in turn reinfects the mother.

   Frank abscess formation requires **incision and drainage.** At times there are multiple interconnected abscesses. For this condition several incisions must be made under general anesthesia in order to break up the loculated walls.

IX. Clostridial infections. Over 25 species of clostridia are associated with pelvic infections. All the organisms have a characteristic appearance with Gram's stain, i.e., large, "box-car"-shaped gram-positive rods. The most common pathogen, *C. perfringens*, does not display spores when found in infected tissue. Several of the clostridia produce histotoxic substances, but the major threat in pelvic infections is the alpha toxin, a lecithinase, elaborated by *C. perfringens*. Most histotoxic clostridial infections are associated with unsanitary abortions, but there is an occasional example of clostridial myonecrosis accompanying a vaginal delivery.

A. Clinical conditions

1. **Simple contamination.** Histotoxic clostridia such as *C. perfringens* can be grown from the lochia of approximately 20% of women who present with **septic abortion** and occasionally in women with normal vaginal delivery. The vast majority of these bacteriologic isolations are not associated with clinical findings. It is important to recognize that clostridia are part of the

normal flora of the vagina and colon. Hence, the finding of clostridia in culture or on a Gram's-stained slide does not necessarily indicate severe sepsis; most commonly, these organisms reflect simple contamination.

2. **Bacteremia.** Clostridia can be isolated in blood cultures following septic abortion or even normal vaginal delivery. The event is often a transient bacteremia with no associated clinical manifestations. Obviously, all cases of clostridial bacteremia must be carefully scrutinized, but serious infection is not necessarily implicated.
3. **Suppurative infection without toxemia.** Various strains of clostridia can be isolated from suppurative diseases of the pelvis without the presence of gas gangrene or alpha toxemia. Approximately 10–20% of pelvic abscesses yield clostridia on careful culturing. Special anaerobic techniques are required, since several of the strains are highly fastidious. These organisms are invariably associated with a mixed infected flora of aerobes and anaerobes. Clostridia can also be noted in Gram's-stained slides of cervical discharges and culposcopy fluid from patients with severe pelvic infection.

   Since clostridia are so frequently associated with a complex mixed flora, it is unwise to proceed with surgical intervention merely because these organisms are found in the infected tissue. The most important guidelines are the clinical appearance of the patient and the presence of myometrial gas gangrene. If classic findings of toxemia and gas gangrene (see below) are not present, there is no need for specific therapy directed at the clostridia.
4. **Clostridial myonecrosis and alpha toxemia.** Gas gangrene is said to occur in approximately 1 in 800 septic abortions seen in the hospital. The exact incidence in normal deliveries or in cesarean sections is not known, but it is extremely low. The classic picture begins 2–3 days (occasionally < 24 hr) after the inciting event, either delivery or unsanitary abortion, and is heralded by the onset of jaundice and renal failure. The development of jaundice is extremely rapid, and within a few hours the patient's skin may be changed to a mahogany color. Hemoglobulinemia is present, and a dramatic fall in hematocrit becomes evident. The blood smear shows crinkled and shaggy erythrocytes due to the action of the lecithinase on the red cell membrane. Renal failure is rapid in onset. Oliguria is accompanied by port-wine urine due to hemoglobinuria. This progresses to complete renal shutdown due to acute cortical necrosis. Urine output diminishes to virtually zero. Pelvic findings may be minimal at this time. An x-ray of the pelvis aids in searching for gas in the uterine wall and surrounding pelvic structures. The term **gas gangrene of the uterus** is a misleading one, however, since the finding of gas in the tissues is often a late event, and the patient may have expired before gas has been discovered. Some patients have severe endometritis with pelvic pain. Hypotension is a regular feature of the syndrome and indeed may be the initial presentation. It is remarkable that patients with gas gangrene remain fully conscious and acutely aware of their surroundings. This keen mental awareness may persist up to the moment of death.

B. **Pathology.** Clostridia are obligately anaerobic organisms that require necrotic tissue for growth and toxin production. Two forms of pathologic process are recognized in gas gangrene.

1. **A superficial decidual infection limited to the uterine contents.** This infection may liberate large amounts of alpha toxin, so that the clinical features of gas gangrene are present. However, simple curettage often is sufficient to remove the necrotic areas and site of infection. In some cases the process can be recognized in the suppurative endometritis stage, before alpha toxemia or myometritis has ensued. Antibiotic therapy alone may be sufficient, although the decision to stay with it must be weighed carefully.
2. **Invasion of uterine muscles with myonecrosis and gelatinous destruction of tissue.** Remarkably few inflammatory cells are associated with this process. The infection can spread beyond the uterus itself into the surrounding muscles and soft tissues of the pelvis. This process requires a total hysterectomy, and it carries a grave prognosis.

C. Laboratory findings

1. Severe progressive **anemia** with accompanying hemoglobulinemia is present. The blood smear shows abnormal, crinkled red cell forms due to action of the toxin. Leukocytosis is common, and severe leukemoid reactions with WBC counts of 50,000/mm^3 may be seen.
2. **Renal failure** is prompt and progressive. It is accompanied by hemoglobinuria, oliguria, and progressive rise of the blood urea nitrogen (BUN) and creatinine. Because of cortical necrosis the kidneys cease to function altogether.
3. X-ray of the pelvis may reveal **gas** in the uterine tissues, although this may be a late finding. If gas is seen to be spreading up the abdominal wall and into other tissues, the outlook is grim.
4. Gram's stain of cervical discharge or culposcopy specimen demonstrates **gram-positive rods** with typical morphology of clostridia.

D. Treatment

1. Antibiotics should be administered immediately. Nearly all strains of clostridia are sensitive to penicillin G. The dose is 4 million units IV q4h. The dose should be reduced for patients with renal failure, i.e., 2 million units are administered IV q6h to patients with renal shut-down. Patients with penicillin allergy should be treated with chloramphenicol (750 mg–1.0 gm IV q6h). Some patients, especially those with septic abortion, have a mixed aerobic-anaerobic flora, in addition to clostridia. Besides penicillin, they should receive the antibiotics indicated for suppurative infections of the pelvis (see p. 77).
2. The severe anemia must be corrected. It is best to use fresh blood, administered by exchange transfusion of 4–5 units per cycle. Exchange transfusion accomplishes several goals: it removes unbound toxin and damaged red cells from the circulation, replaces clotting factors, and replenishes the circulating volume without overload.
3. A central venous catheter should be placed in order to monitor fluid administration.
4. Renal failure should be managed by hemodialysis.
5. The use of gas gangrene antitoxin is controversial. Furthermore, the antitoxin material is no longer being produced, so it may be unavailable. For those who care to use it and can procure it, it is important to give the patient a skin test before use (first by scratch test, then, if results are negative, by intradermal test), since the antitoxin is a horse serum. The dose is up to 50,000 units, depending on the severity of the disease. If a patient is in shock, the antitoxin should be administered by the intravenous route. This dose of antitoxin produces a high incidence of serum sickness, and it is generally felt that the benefit to the patient is marginal at best.
6. Hyperbaric oxygenation at 3 atmospheres is often recommended for gas gangrene of the limbs and abdominal wall, but it is felt to be of limited value for myonecrosis of the uterus.
7. Aggressive surgical intervention is often live-saving. When a patient has gas in the tissues, demonstrated by physical findings or x-ray, the decision for complete surgical extirpation of the uterus is obvious. Clinical findings such as progressive renal failure, jaundice, anemia, and severe hypotension also dictate immediate surgical intervention. In many cases, however, the patient has a milder form of the disease and may respond to initial antibiotic treatment and fluid replacement. Under these circumstances, a curettage and watchful waiting may avert a major operation. Clearly, careful monitoring of the clinical status is required if a less radical surgical approach is elected in the initial stages.

Septic Abortions

I. General principles. The majority of women requiring admission to the hospital following an unsanitary or "backroom" abortion have an uncomplicated course. About 15% develop sepsis, although only one-quarter of this infected group develop a serious complication. It should be emphasized, however, that this small minority may suffer a life-threatening complication. In former times septic abortion represented the major cause of maternal mortality.

II. **Clinical features.** The following features portend a **serious** outcome:
  A. High fever, and especially **shaking chills.**
  B. Marked abdominal findings with **rebound tenderness.** Although many patients have pelvic pain, the outcome is grave if the tenderness is beyond the confines of the uterus.
  C. **Significant hypotension.**
  D. **Low white blood cell count.** Normal or high WBCs are common and are not diagnostic or prognostic.
  E. **Disseminated intravascular coagulation (DIC),** i.e., low platelets, low fibrinogen, and the presence of fibrin split products.
  F. **Gas in the uterus or intraperitoneal space** on abdominal flat plate x-ray. This suggests perforation of the uterus and perhaps incipient gas gangrene. The presence of a foreign body is also a dangerous finding.
  G. A **history** of using soap, bleach, or other chemical agents as the abortive agent. Such cases have a grave prognosis.

III. **Microbiology.** The majority of infections associated with septic abortion are caused by the normal flora of the vagina or the large intestine. Anaerobic bacteria, such as anaerobic streptococci, *B. fragilis* and clostridia, are found in the majority of cases. Approximately two-thirds of these patients also have coliforms, such as *E. coli* and *Klebsiella*. Most infections are a mixed flora comprising both aerobes and anaerobes. There is a high incidence of bacteremia, and the same organisms are found in the bloodstream: anaerobic streptococci, *Bacteroides*, and coliforms. Approximately 1 in 800 cases is associated with *Clostridium perfringens* and alpha toxemia. There are rare cases caused by group A *Strep. pyogenes* and *Staph. aureus.*

IV. **Treatment.** The patient should be observed carefully, with frequent measurement of vital signs. Early warnings of complications include hypotension and reduced renal output.
  A. **Antibiotics** should be started immediately in patients who are febrile or who have other bad prognostic signs (see p. 77 for doses). The following regimens are suggested:
    1. Cefoxitin
    2. Clinidamycin and an aminoglycoside
    3. Metronidazole and an aminoglycoside
    4. Chloramphenicol and an aminoglycoside
  B. **Supportive care** including intravenous fluids and nasogastric suction, if ileus is present.
  C. **X-rays** of the chest to look for pulmonary embolism; x-rays of the abdomen and pelvis to look for gas and foreign bodies.
  D. **Complete blood count,** including **platelet count** if DIC is suspected.
  E. **Blood urea nitrogen** (BUN), **creatinine,** and **electrolytes** to monitor fluid and renal status. Urine output should be carefully watched.
  F. **Liver function tests.** These are often abnormal in the presence of septicemia and do not necessarily indicate intrinsic liver disease.
  G. **Blood cultures.**
  H. **Dilatation and curettage** (D&C) performed shortly after admission in order to remove infected necrotic tissue from the uterus. A Gram's-stained slide and culture should be performed on this material. The morphology of the microorganisms can often indicate the etiologic agents. An acute episode of fever and rigors may accompany the D&C, probably related to transient septicemia.

V. **Indications for surgery.** Many patients respond to early D&C, antibiotics, and general supportive care. Some patients persist with signs of sepsis, however, and for these high-risk patients aggressive surgery is indicated. Failure to perform a hysterectomy at the appropriate time is the usual reason for death in such patients. Indications for surgery include
  A. Gas in the uterine wall.

B. Progressive peritoneal signs suggesting uterine and/or bowel perforation.
C. Disseminated intravascular coagulation that does not respond to antibiotics and supportive care. Heparin may be indicated in these cases, but the best approach is to attack the septic focus directly by operative intervention.
D. Renal failure and/or hypotension.
E. Septic thrombophlebitis (pelvic veins) that does not respond to antibiotics and heparin.
F. Clostridial toxemia with myonecrosis.
G. X-ray appearance of foreign body or gas in the peritoneal cavity.

VI. Complications

A. Peritonitis from perforation of the uterus. There may be coexisting intestinal perforation.
B. Chemical abortions with soap or bleach are associated with a high mortality. Adrenal hemorrhage and necrosis, acute renal tubular necrosis, and pulmonary edema are the major findings.
C. Disseminated intravascular coagulation.
D. Renal failure and hypotension.
E. Pelvic abscess.
F. Septic thrombophlebitis of the pelvic and ovarian veins.

Infectious Complications of Abortions

I. General principles. The pregnant uterus is at great risk for infection. The performance of abortions under controlled aseptic conditions has greatly reduced the incidence of infection associated with early termination of pregnancy. However, such infections still occur, occasionally with dire consequences.

The risk of septic complications increases with the **age of gestation.** The technique for pregnancy termination is also related to infectious complications: Suction curettage has the lowest risk, whereas hysterectomy carries the highest. An additional factor that predisposes to infection is attempted tubal ligation at the same time as abortion.

II. Curettage

A. This technique has the lowest incidence of infection; the suction method appears safer, in terms of infectious complications, than sharp curettage.
B. The microbiology is related to the vaginal or fecal flora, consisting of both aerobes and anaerobes in a mixed culture. Rarely, the organism is introduced by a member of the operating team, i.e., group A *Strep. pyogenes* or *Staph. aureus.*
C. Endometritis and parametritis have been seen occasionally; these are usually related to retained products of conception and are associated with a late onset of symptoms.
D. The vacuum technique occasionally causes hemorrhage that can lead to an infected hematoma.
E. Perforation of the uterus and/or intestine is the major problem following sharp curettage. This may be immediately apparent due to excessive bleeding, abdominal distention, or herniation of a loop of bowel into the vagina. Such cases require emergency laparotomy and systemic antibiotics (see treatment of suppurative pelvic infections, p. 77).
F. Silent perforations may present in a delayed fashion with pelvic abscess or an infected hematoma.

III. Hypertonic saline injection

A. Low-grade postoperative fever has been reported in 10–20% of women undergoing this procedure. If blood cultures are obtained, a similar percentage are positive. The bacteremia is usually transient and does not lead to serious complications.
B. Intraamniotic injection can introduce numerous microorganisms, either from the environment, such as streptococci and staphylococci, or from the normal flora of

the vagina, such as *Bacteroides*, anaerobic streptococci, *C. perfringens*, and coliforms.

C. The major septic complications include endometritis, adnexal infections, peritonitis, and septicemia.

D. Patients with preexisting pelvic inflammatory disease seem to have a higher risk of infectious complications.

E. Pathologic changes include tissue trauma, especially to the blood vessels, and retained products of conception. Inadvertent injection into the myometrium may produce necrosis and sepsis.

F. Disseminated intravascular coagulation (DIC) has been described following this procedure.

G. Leukocytosis is not a useful sign, since many women have an increased white blood cell count as a result of the procedure itself. The dangerous signs are **hypotension, chills, and fever, DIC, renal failure,** and a **low WBC.**

H. All patients with septic complications should have a D&C within 8–12 hours; antibiotic therapy (see p. 77) and supportive care should be instituted. Failure to respond to initial therapy is an indication for surgical exploration.

IV. Hysterotomy

A. This procedure carries the highest risk of infection; in some series 20% of women have septic complications.

B. Infection is often related to persistent leakage of the fundal incision.

D. If tubal ligation is performed with hysterotomy, there is a marked increase in the incidence of infection.

E. The infecting organisms are a combination of aerobic and anaerobic bacteria, probably derived from the vaginal flora.

F. The main treatment is antibiotics (see p. 77) and supportive care; if these measures fail within 48–72 hours, a definitive operative procedure is indicated.

5 Urinary Tract Infections

Pyelonephritis, Cystitis, and Asymptomatic Bacteriuria

I. General principles. Urinary tract infections may involve any portion of the urinary tract from the renal cortex to the urethral meatus. Bacteriuria, defined as $> 10^5$ bacteria/ml urine (obtained by a "clean catch"), is the final common denominator of these processes. (Methods to evaluate urine cultures and to identify the site of involvement are reviewed in Chap. 15.)

II. Types of infection

A. Cystitis (Table 5-1) is a bacterial infection of the bladder. It may produce symptoms (**symptomatic bacteriuria**), or may be clinically silent (**asymptomatic bacteriuria**). The usual symptoms are dysuria, urgency, nocturia, and frequency; less often there is hematuria or pain (suprapubic, perineal, or low back). As these complaints are not diagnostic of urinary tract infection, however, they are of little value in localizing the site of involvement. As many as 50% of adult females with symptoms suggesting cystitis have negative urine cultures (**urethral syndrome** or **symptomatic abacteriuria**). Even when significant bacteriuria is present, it is uncertain that the infection is restricted to the lower tract. Involvement of the upper tract (kidneys) is suggested by fever, chills, flank pain or tenderness, and WBC casts in the urine. The absence of such symptoms does not rule out upper tract infection, since many patients with chronic bacteriuria harbor these bacteria in the renal pelvis. In young girls (6 years to puberty), symptoms restricted to the lower tract and absence of fever generally exclude upper tract infection.

B. Acute pyelonephritis (Table 5-1) is an acute bacterial infection with septic foci randomly distributed in the renal parenchyma and pelvicaliceal system. Clinical features are fever, chills, constitutional symptoms such as nausea and vomiting, flank pain, and tenderness in the costovertebral angle. There are often lower tract symptoms, such as dysuria, urgency, and frequency. Urinalysis shows WBCs, WBC casts, and proteinuria; bacteria are noted by Gram's stain of the unspun specimen. Anemia, roentgenographic evidence of reduced renal size, and impaired renal function suggest a background of chronic renal disease. The intravenous pyelogram (IVP) is generally normal in acute pyelonephritis; in **severe** cases studied in the acute phase the IVP may show renal enlargement, a narrowed collecting system (due to edema), and delayed excretion. Intravenous pyelography is regarded as safe during acute infection, although it is not usually indicated at this time. Retrograde studies and other forms of instrumentation can induce bacteremia in the presence of active infection and should be done only under appropriate antimicrobial cover.

C. Chronic pyelonephritis is a long-standing bacterial infection that may be **active** (continued bacterial growth in the renal parenchyma, with bacteriuria) or **inactive** (pathologic residue of previous infections). Histologically there is a segmental, interstitial, mononuclear infiltration with patchy wedge-shaped scarring. These histologic changes are nondiagnostic, since similar findings are noted with interstitial nephritis, obstructive uropathy, hypersensitivity nephritis, nephrosclerosis, hereditary nephritis, potassium deficiency, and several other condi-

Table 5-1. Types of urinary tract infection

Feature	Cystitis	Acute pyelonephritis	Urethral syndrome
Dysuria, frequency, suprapubic pain	+	±	+
Fever, chills, nausea, back pain, other systemic signs	±	+	±
Duration of symptoms (days)	1–2	1	2–7
Leukocytosis	–	+	–
Urinalysis			
WBC	+	+	±
WBC casts	–	+	–
Bacteria on stain	+	+	–
RBC	±	±	–
Cultures			
Urine	+	+	–
Blood	–	±	–

tions. When the diagnosis is limited to cases with corroborating clinical data, or when Enterobacteriaceae common antigen is required as a marker of infection, the incidence of chronic pyelonephritis in unselected autopsies is 1–3%.

Although histologic criteria are largely nonspecific, roentgenographic changes are likely to be more helpful. Caliceal dilatation (caliectasis) is particularly suggestive of chronic pyelonephritis. This type of defect also occurs with hydronephrosis. With the latter lesion, however, all calyces are involved. In pyelonephritis the process is characteristically asymmetric.

Chronic pyelonephritis occurs in patients with underlying structural defects, stones, or foreign bodies. Progressive renal failure is rare in patients with uncomplicated urinary tract infection, even when bacteriuria is chronic or recurrent. This observation has an important bearing on the indications for diagnostic studies and treatment of patients with bacteriuria.

D. Urethral syndrome (Table 5-1) refers to a symptom complex in females suggesting cystitis but with negative urine cultures. Possible explanations include vulvovaginitis (which should be apparent on inspection); urethritis (due to gonococci); intermittent or low-grade bacteriuria; and infection involving a nonbacterial pathogen, such as *Chlamydia*. Some females with the urethral syndrome harbor coliforms in the vaginal vestibule and subsequently will develop significant bacteriuria. Others have infection with *Staphylococcus saprophyticus,* an organism often ignored as a urinary tract pathogen.

Pelvic examination of some patients reveals an inflamed, tender urethra; these women generally respond to antimicrobial treatment. Other cases do not follow this pattern—introital cultures are negative, pelvic examination discloses no abnormalities, bacteriuria never develops, and there is no improvement with antibiotics. The etiology of this condition is cryptic. A variety of surgical procedures on the urethra have been performed in an attempt to quell the annoying symptoms. It is advised, however, that surgical intervention be restricted to patients who have an identifiable structural defect.

E. Necrotizing papillitis is a destructive process, localized to the terminal portion of the pyramid, which results in sloughing of renal papillae. The course is usually acute, fulminant, and highly lethal; occasional cases are more chronic, with a favorable prognosis. Necrotizing papillitis usually attacks patients with diabetes mellitus, obstructive uropathy, cirrhosis, sickle cell disease, or analgesic abuse. The disease is usually bilateral, although unilateral lesions can occur spontane-

Table 5-2. Incidence of urinary tract infection

Condition	Females (%)	Males (%)
Infants	1	1
School age children	1	0.04
Young adults	4	0.04
Pregnant females	3–7	—
Adults ≥ 50 years	10–15	4
Hospitalized patients	20–30	10–15
Single catheterization		
No serious illness	2	2
Debilitating disease	10–20	10–20
Pregnancy or postpartum	5–10	—
Indwelling catheter		
Open drainage—2 days	98	98
Closed drainage	5–10/day	5–10/day
Adult diabetics	15–20	10–15
Benign prostatic hypertrophy	—	10
Neurogenic bladder	80	80

ously or in patients with unilateral obstruction. Roentgenograms initially show erosion of the papillae; with progression, sequestered segments are sloughed to produce characteristic large, irregular calyceal defects. The diagnosis is based on typical roentgenographic changes and passage of sloughed tissue in the urine, especially when these occur in a susceptible patient.

In some instances the detached papillae can obstruct a ureter, causing renal colic, acute hydronephrosis, or suppurative pyelonephritis. Bilateral blockage results in acute oliguria. These complications represent urologic emergencies that require immediate urethral catheterization.

F. Emphysematous pyelonephritis is a severe, albeit uncommon, necrotizing form of parenchymal renal infection that has a predilection for diabetics. The patients are extremely ill, and gas is seen to extend from the perinephric space through the retroperitoneum to the flank, where it is clinically apparent as palpable crepitus. The hallmark is roentgenographically visible gas in the kidney or adjacent structures. The responsible pathogens are facultative aerobic, gram-negative rods, such as *Escherichia coli, Klebsiella, Proteus,* and *Pseudomonas.* Overall, the mortality is 40%. Those patients treated only with antibiotics have a higher mortality (70%); surgical therapy, with nephrectomy and/or drainage of the involved tissues, appears to offer a better chance for survival, with a mortality of only 33%.

III. Epidemiologic aspects

A. Neonates. Clinical evidence for urinary tract infection is generally lacking in newborns, and voided urine cultures are notoriously unreliable (Table 5-2). Only 1–10% of infants with significant bacteriuria in voided specimens yield a positive culture of urine obtained by suprapubic bladder aspiration. Using the latter specimen source, which is the most reliable, the prevalence of bacteriuria in neonates is 1% or less. They generally respond well to chemotherapy, but the relapse rate in the ensuing years is 25%.

B. Females. Approximately 1% of young females between the ages of 3 and 20 years have significant bacteriuria at any moment in time. Certain women, a susceptible subgroup of 5%, are subject to repeated infections alternating with periods of remission.

The incidence of urinary tract infections in **older females** (> 21 years) is determined by sexual habits and age. Among sexually inactive females, such as nuns, the prevalence of bacteriuria is only 0.5%. By contrast, about 4% of sexually active females have bacteriuria. This association has been ascribed to the transmission of introital bacteria into the bladder following urethral trauma occurring during intercourse. The quaint appellation "honeymoon cystitis" refers to symptomatic lower urinary tract infections following sexual intercourse. Approximately 50% of females with recurrent bacteriuria in childhood will again develop a urinary tract infection within 3 months of initiating sexual activity.

Several studies indicate that 3–7% of females develop bacteriuria during **pregnancy.** This incidence approximates that of nonpregnant females, but during pregnancy there is a propensity to develop symptomatic pyelonephritis. Such a relationship is possibly due to physiologic dilatation of the collecting system above the pelvic brim, which begins during the 3rd month of pregnancy and progresses until the last 2 months.

The incidence of urinary tract infection in adult females increases with age after 40 years. About 10% of females over age 50 have significant bacteriuria.

C. **Males.** Epidemiologic surveys of **boys and young adult males** (< age 30) show that only about 0.4% have bacteriuria. This reduced susceptibility of males as compared to females has been attributed to the longer urethra, the antibacterial properties of prostatic secretions, and the infrequent carriage of potential urinary tract pathogens in the distal urethra. Most urinary tract infections in males of this age group are associated with structural abnormalities of the genitourinary tract.

Approximately 4% of **middle-aged and elderly males** have bacteriuria. It is usually associated with chronic bacterial prostatitis, catheterization, instrumentation, or obstructive disorders such as benign prostatic hypertrophy.

D. **Associated conditions.** Conditions associated with an increased incidence of bacteriuria are diabetes mellitus, hypercalcemia, hypokalemia, nephrolithiasis, nephrocalcinosis, structural defects of the urinary tract, catheterization, instrumentation, and genitourinary surgery.

IV. **Recurrent urinary tract infections**

A. **Relapsing infection** is characterized by recurrence of bacteriuria with the same microorganism. Relapses usually occur within days or a few weeks after treatment has been discontinued. Patients with this pattern are likely to have a source of bacterial persistence, such as pyelonephritis, chronic prostatitis, or infected stones. Urologic conditions responsible for bacterial persistence are struvite stones, unilateral atrophic pyelonephritic kidney, vesicovaginal or vesicointestinal fistula, and infected ureteral stumps or urachal cysts. These conditions generally require surgical intervention to eradicate the infection.

B. **Reinfection** refers to recurrence of disease with a different microorganism, as indicated by the biotype, serotype, or antimicrobial susceptibility profile. Reinfection accounts for more than 85% of recurrent urinary tract infections in females. Most episodes involve different serotypes of *E. coli*. Reinfections, in contrast to relapses, tend to occur several weeks to years after chemotherapy has been discontinued.

V. **Underlying structural defects.** Urinary tract infections are considered **complicated** or **uncomplicated** on the basis of an underlying structural defect. A patient with a complicated infection is susceptible to relapses and, more importantly, to progressive renal involvement. The majority of patients with renal failure due to chronic pyelonephritis have anatomic defects, either obstructing lesions or vesicoureteral reflux.

Obstructing lesions occur at any point in the urinary tract. Those distal to the bladder compromise an important defense mechanism, regular and complete voiding of infected urine. Neurogenic bladders produce a similar problem. Obstructions in the renal parenchyma (nephrocalcinosis, medullary scars from previous infections, polycystic kidney disease) and ureteral obstruction apparently increase susceptibility to pyelonephritis by raising renal hydrostatic pressure. The initial site of infection is the renal parenchyma, rather than the static urine as in urethral obstruction or neurogenic bladder.

Obstruction per se does not cause urinary tract infection, but it does interfere with bacterial clearance. Instrumentation and catheterization represent major causes of microbial inoculation in the susceptible host.

VI. Bacteriology

A. Source. Bacteria reach the bladder or renal parenchyma by retrograde contamination, hematogenous dissemination, inoculation from contiguous infection, or lymphatic spread. Animal studies and clinical observations suggest that the **retrograde route** accounts for most urinary tract infections. The female urethra is short and located close to the perineum and rectum. Cultures of the vaginal introitus in women with recurrent urinary tract infections show a disproportionately high rate of antecedent colonization with coliforms. In contrast, the distal urethra in males harbors a flora composed principally of diphtheroids, *Staph. epidermidis,* and streptococci. Coliforms infrequently colonize the normal male urethra.

B. Pathogens. Over 90% of initial urinary tract infections are caused by strains of *E. coli,* which are susceptible to most antimicrobial agents. Antibiotic-resistant strains of *E. coli, Klebsiella, Enterobacter, Proteus, Pseudomonas, Serratia,* and enterococci are pathogens, as a rule, in urinary tract infections associated with multiple courses of chemotherapy, underlying structural defects, instrumentation, or catheterization. *Staph. saprophyticus* can cause cystitis and the urethral syndrome. Diphtheroids, lactobacilli, and anaerobic bacteria in cultures of voided urine usually represent contamination.

VII. Treatment. The decision to treat is based on symptomatology and realistic goals. The goals of therapy are eradication of bacteria from the urinary tract, control of symptoms, and protection against progressive renal insufficiency. Bacteriuria can serve as a harbinger of an underlying and potentially reversible lesion; in this event, urologic investigation may be more important to the ultimate prognosis than antibiotic therapy.

A. Symptomatic bacteriuria. All patients with symptomatic bacteriuria should be treated with antimicrobial agents. Choice of therapy depends on severity of symptoms.

1. **Mild infections** are usually treated on an outpatient basis. Antimicrobial therapy is less aggressive in mild infections, especially when bacteremia and underlying renal disease are not present. It is often difficult to distinguish between cystitis and pyelonephritis. For antibiotic selection, this question is moot, since the same agents are appropriate for both conditions. The major issue is duration of therapy.

   Women with cystitis generally respond to a **single dose** of an appropriate drug. The decision to try single-dose therapy is based on symptoms of urinary urgency, increased frequency of urination and dysuria, and bacteriuria as determined by culture or Gram's stain of unspun urine. The single-dose regimen is **not** recommended for males (of any age), pregnant women, patients with possible pyelonephritis (see **2**), and patients who are unlikely to supply follow-up urine for culture. Drugs for single-dose treatment in adults are as follows:

Amoxicillin	3 gm
Sulfisoxazole	2 gm
Trimethoprim/sulfamethoxazole	160/800 mg

   Treatment of young girls with a single dose is controversial. Sulfisoxazole (200 mg/kg) and amoxicillin (1–2 gm) have proved successful, but recurrences have also been seen with short-course regimens.

   Some authorities recommend a longer course of treatment (3–7 days), even in mild cases. Table 5-3 lists the appropriate oral drugs. The choice of parenteral vs. oral administration is determined by severity of systemic symptoms, the patient's ability to tolerate oral medication, and the antibiotic susceptibility pattern (some resistant bacteria are sensitive only to a parenteral drug).

2. **Pyelonephritis** should be treated with a longer course of therapy (10–14 days). The criteria for the longer course are high fever, chills, pain in the back or flank, or a past history of pyelonephritis. All males with acute urinary tract infection should be treated with this regimen, regardless of

Table 5-3. Oral antimicrobial treatment of urinary tract infections

Agent	Dose	Comment
Sulfisoxazole or sulfadiazine	2–4 gm PO, then 0.5–1.0 gm qid	Avoid in renal insufficiency; avoid in last 2 wk of pregnancy
Ampicillin	0.25–0.5 gm qid	
Amoxicillin	0.25 gm qid	
Nitrofurantoin	50–100 mg qid	Avoid in renal insufficiency
Tetracycline	0.25–0.5 gm qid	Avoid in pregnancy or in children < 8 yr
Cephalexin	0.25–0.5 gm qid	Restrict use to resistant pathogens, especially *Klebsiella*
Carbenicillin indanyl sodium	0.5–1.0 gm q6h	Restrict use to resistant pathogens, especially *Pseudomonas* and *Proteus*

symptoms, but special attention should be paid to the possibility of a structural defect. In mild cases, even when pyelonephritis is diagnosed, an oral regimen is used (Table 5-3). It is imperative to obtain urine for culture and sensitivities **before** starting treatment, since resistant organisms are more likely to occur in pyelonephritis.

a. Indications for hospitalization and parenteral antibiotic therapy are

(1) Inability to take oral medications

(2) Suspected bacteremia, as indicated by high fever, chills, severe toxicity, and hypotension

(3) Likelihood of a resistant pathogen, on the basis of recent hospitalization, previous cultures, or multiple courses of antibiotics

b. Parenteral regimens include

(1) Ampicillin, 1–2 gm IV q4h, plus an aminoglycoside (gentamicin, tobramycin, or amikacin)

(2) Cephalosporin, with or without an aminoglycoside

The parenteral regimen can be modified when culture reports become available. An early clue is provided by Gram's staining of unspun urine. Chains of gram-positive cocci suggest enterococci, for which ampicillin would be recommended.

As soon as the patient is afebrile, an oral drug can be used to complete the 10–14 day course. Some authorities recommend a more prolonged course (3–6 weeks), but proof of benefit for the longer course is lacking.

B. Asymptomatic bacteriuria. Significant bacteriuria, without symptoms, should be confirmed by a second urine culture before the diagnosis is established. The decision to treat is based on realistic goals and the predicted course without antimicrobials. Most authorities recommend routine treatment of asymptomatic bacteriuria only for young patients, pregnant women, and patients with stones infected with urea-splitting bacteria. Selection of an antimicrobial agent should await results of culture and sensitivity testing.

1. All **children and adolescents** with asymptomatic bacteriuria should be treated. These patients are vulnerable to subsequent symptomatic infections, and those with vesicoureteral reflux are likely to develop renal involvement. With each course of antibiotic therapy, long-term remissions are achieved in about 20% of young females, even among those with reflux. These patients are eliminated from the susceptible pool, and the total pool becomes progressively smaller with successive courses of therapy. The usual pathogens are strains of *E. coli,* which are susceptible to a variety of oral antimicrobial agents, including sulfonamides, tetracyclines, and ampicillin (Table 5-3). Tetracycline should be avoided in children under 8 years of age because of potential tooth discoloration. Duration of treatment is generally 10–14 days.

Continued treatment for 8 weeks offers no advantage over a short course. However, extended low-dose treatment for 6–12 months with sulfonamides, trimethoprim/sulfamethoxazole, or nitrofurantoin appears to reduce recurrences and may be administered to children with repeated attacks.

2. **Pregnancy.** Asymptomatic bacteriuria during the first trimester is a common precursor to development of pyelonephritis in the 3rd trimester or following delivery. Although the data are somewhat conflicting, there also appears to be an association between bacteriuria and both toxemia and prematurity. It is recommended that all pregnant females be routinely screened for bacteriuria and that those with positive cultures be treated, regardless of symptomatology, for 10–14 days. Acceptable antimicrobial agents are those with established safety during pregnancy, such as penicillin G, ampicillin, and nitrofurantoin. Sulfanomides are generally safe except during the final 2 weeks of pregnancy, when they may cause hyperbilirubinemia and kernicterus in the newborn. Tetracycline should be avoided; when given in the 1st trimester, it may cause the baby to develop discolored teeth, and when given in the 3rd trimester, it can create renal and hepatic abnormalities in the mother. Duration of treatment is 10–14 days. Treatment eradicates bacteriuria for the duration of pregnancy in 70–80% of cases, and repeat urine cultures are recommended. Some authorities suggest continuing an oral antibiotic until delivery, although the efficacy of prolonged treatment during pregnancy is not established.
3. **Middle-aged and elderly females** with asymptomatic bacteriuria generally have a favorable prognosis. Usually there is no demonstrable structural defect, and progressive renal failure is rare. Indications for antimicrobial therapy are arbitrary; most authorities restrict antimicrobial usage to symptomatic episodes.
4. **Adult males** with asymptomatic bacteriuria usually have underlying structural defects or obstruction, and the use of antimicrobials must be tempered by realistic goals. In general, treatment is given after the structural defect is repaired or for a symptomatic episode.
5. **Complicated urinary tract infections.** Bacteriuria is difficult to eradicate in patients with underlying anatomic defects or foreign bodies, such as an indwelling catheter, cystostomy, or nephrostomy. The usual result of short-term antimicrobials is recolonization by the original pathogen or reinfection by another, more resistant, organism. The most important factor in management is correction, if possible, of the predisposing defect. Short-term (7–10 days) use of an antimicrobial agent is suggested for symptomatic episodes and for patients with asymptomatic bacteriuria after the underlying cause has been eliminated. Extended courses of drugs are advised only for patients with obstruction associated with progressive renal impairment or frequent symptomatic episodes.

C. **Recurrent infections.** It is generally impossible to sterilize the urine of patients with chronic urinary tract infections after the usual 10–14-day course of antimicrobials. Although prolonged treatment has been advocated, controlled studies seldom show significant benefits. Prolonged use of antimicrobials is advised only in the following settings:

1. Frequent symptomatic reinfections (> 2–3/yr) in young girls and women can be treated with an extended course of prophylactic antimicrobials for months to years. Antimicrobial **prophylaxis,** used after sterilizing the urine with initial treatment, is intended to suppress potential pathogens in the introitus from entering the urethra and bladder. Desirable features of a prophylactic agent are
   a. Activity against likely urinary pathogens
   b. Ease of administration
   c. Minimal impact on the fecal flora (since the fecal flora serves as a major source of resistant organisms in reinfections)

   The preferred agent is trimethoprim/sulfamethoxazole, ½ tab (total, 40/200 mg) at bedtime. Another choice is nitrofurantoin, 50 mg once daily, but this drug has been associated with serious pulmonary side effects during prolonged use. Urine cultures should be monitored periodically. Prophylaxis should be discontinued if bacteriuria recurs or a symptomatic infection develops. The prophylactic drug is given for 6 months, although the course can be extended if the episodes recur.

2. Some females relate recurrent urinary tract infections to sexual intercourse. A prophylactic regimen of trimethoprim/sulfamethoxazole, ½ tab (40/200 mg) after intercourse, is prescribed. It is also recommended that the woman void after intercourse to clear the urethra of bacteria.
3. Relapsing infection, especially early recurrence with the same bacterium, suggests a structural defect, calculus, or pyelonephritis. An appropriate oral antimicrobial should be administered for 6 weeks to attempt eradication of the organism. Appropriate diagnostic studies should be undertaken (see p. 106). Relapsing infection in an adult male can be caused by chronic bacterial prostatitis. This diagnosis and the therapeutic approach are discussed separately (pp. 107–109).
4. Recurrent infection with progressive renal impairment should be treated for 4–6 weeks.
5. Children with vesicoureteral reflux should receive an extended course (6 wk–6 mo.) of an appropriate antimicrobial drug in an attempt to maintain bacteria-free urine.
6. Infected struvite stones should be treated for a prolonged period. Small stones may dissolve if the urine is sterile and acid. Since *Proteus mirabilis* is the usual urea-splitting organism in these cases, an appropriate oral agent for prolonged treatment is ampicillin.

VIII. **Response to treatment.** Appropriate antimicrobial agents usually render the urine sterile within 12 hours. Positive urine cultures after 48–72 hours of treatment indicate drug failure, and the antimicrobial agent should be changed according to susceptibility tests of the pathogen. Febrile patients often become afebrile within 24–48 hours but may take 3–5 days. Persistent fever beyond 3–5 days raises the possibility of acute urinary obstruction. Intravenous pyelography or, if necessary, retrograde pyelography should be performed, since such lesions require decompression to prevent renal destruction. Other considerations are a nonurinary tract source of fever, renal abscess, perinephric abscess, and necrotizing papillitis (Table 5-4).

IX. **X-rays.** Routine intravenous pyelography (IVP) is not warranted in most cases of urinary tract infection. Indications for IVP (and possibly other studies, as necessary) are

A. Girls, 6 years or younger, with bacteriuria
B. Females with recurrent infections
C. Males, any age
D. Failure to respond to appropriate intravenous antibiotics after 3–5 days; persistent fever, chills, or positive culture
E. Suspicion of obstruction, stones, or necrotizing papillitis

In the 1st three categories the IVP can be delayed until the acute phase is past, generally 3–5 weeks. It is not advised to repeat an IVP when a previous study is judged to be unrevealing, unless there are compelling issues such as **D** and **E.** IVP should be avoided in pregnancy; ultrasound is preferred if diagnostic studies cannot be delayed until after delivery.

Structural Defects in Children

I. **Types of congenital anomalies of the urinary tract**

A. Ureteral defects: ureteropelvic junction obstruction; ureterovesical junction obstruction; ureteral strictures; megaureter; retroiliac or retrocaval course; external compression
B. Vesicoureteral reflux
C. Vesical outlet obstruction
D. Urethral defects: prostatic valves, meatal stenosis, strictures, duplications

Table 5-4. Lack of response in patients with urinary tract infection

Cause	What to do
Inappropriate antimicrobial drug	Check sensitivities; repeat urine culture
Obstruction	Intravenous pyelography; if necessary, cystoscopy or retrograde pyelography
Abscess: renal or perinephric	Intravenous pyelography with nephrotomograms; inspiration-expiration films for renal fixation, arteriography, ultrasound, computerized tomography
Necrotizing papillitis	Examine urine for sloughed tissue; intravenous pyelography

E. Neurogenic bladder

II. Diagnosis. Important clues can be noted during physical examination of the abdomen (hydronephrosis or extrarenal masses) and genitalia. A high incidence of obstructing anomalies is found in children with cryptorchidism and hypospadias.
All infants and male children with significant bacteriuria should be given an IVP and a voiding cystourethrogam. The cystourethrogram should be delayed until the urine has been bacteria-free for 6 weeks, to evaluate reflux. Urethral and bladder neck abnormalities on cystourethrography should be confirmed with cystoscopy. For young females the diagnostic workup is reserved for those patients with a delayed response to treatment, pyelonephritis, or a recurrent infection.

III. Bladder neck obstruction. This condition was once a popular explanation for recurrent urinary tract infections in children. Careful scrutiny of the reports indicates that obstruction was seldom documented and that urinary tract infections recurred despite attempts at surgical correction. Presently it is recommended that operative intervention be restricted to patients with obstruction confirmed by cineradiographic studies, bladder-urethral pressure gradient, the presence of residual urine or bladder trabeculation, and a characteristic cystoscopic appearance at the vesicle neck.

IV. Vesicoureteral reflux. This condition has been shrouded in misconception and has given rise to countless unnecessary urologic procedures. Several important facts are pertinent:

A. Most children with x-ray evidence of chronic pyelonephritis have vesicoureteral reflux. There is a direct correlation between the degree of reflux and the incidence of calyceal clubbing. Urinary tract infections in patients with reflux are most likely to be associated with flank pain and fever. Vesicoureteral reflux may well be the result rather than the cause of urinary tract infections.

B. The incidence of vesicoureteral reflux is inversely related to age. Reflux is so common under age 3 that some regard it as a normal variant. Vesicoureteral reflux is unusual after age 3 but is present in 50% of young females with benign urinary tract infections. Approximately 80% of these patients have **spontaneous** disappearance of the anatomic abnormality by adulthood. The rate of spontaneous correction is related to the degree of reflux and the adequacy of antimicrobial therapy. Voiding cystourethrograms that show incomplete filling and only moderate dilatation of the ureters will usually reverse with adequate medical treatment.

C. Bladder neck obstruction is rarely a cause of vesicoureteral reflux.

D. Surgical tunneling of the ureter prevents reflux in more than 80% of patients. In the presence of only mild-to-moderate preoperative reflux, however, this maneuver does not significantly alter the natural course of the disease. More than 50% of patients have recurrence of bacteriuria, but pyelonephritis is rare. The incidence is similar in patients with reflux treated medically.
As a result of these observations it is recommended that **operative intervention for vesicoureteral reflux be based on the degree of the anatomic abnormality.** Patients who have reflux into the ureter (grade 1) or reflux into the ureter and

renal pelvis without ureteral dilatation (grade 2) should receive a trial of extended antimicrobial treatment. These situations account for 90% of cases. Approximately 10% of patients have reflux combined with dilatation of the ureter and pelvis (grade 3); such patients respond poorly to antimicrobial therapy and generally require surgery. There should be careful postoperative bacteriologic follow-up with a rigorous attempt to maintain sterile urine.

V. Distal urethral stenosis. This term refers either to a ring of "resistance" when a bougie or a boule is drawn through the urethra or to stenosis according to bougie calibration. These same "defects" have been observed in children without urinary tract infection. Without precise documentation of obstruction, it is not surprising that the response to urologic surgery has been variable. Urethral dilatation is generally unsuccessful, and there are conflicting reports regarding the efficacy of urethrotomy.

VI. Meatal stenosis. The normal caliber of the urethral meatus is difficult to define in young males. It is a "pin point" by visual inspection in 10–30% of males under 10 years of age.

VII. Indications for surgical procedure. A precautionary note should be inserted concerning indications for operation. Children, particularly females, have frequently been subjected to operations on the basis of nebulous criteria. Lesions of greatest controversy are vesicoureteral reflux, bladder outlet obstruction, and distal urethral "stenosis." Although improvement after a surgical procedure has been noted occasionally, results are variable, and there are few studies using a control group of subjects that receive optimal medical treatment. It is now estimated that **only a small percentage of young females** with recurrent urinary tract infections derive benefit from a surgical procedure.

Structural Defects in Adults

I. Types of acquired structural defects

- **A.** Urolithiasis
- **B.** Ureteral stricture: ureteritis, calculi, tuberculosis, posttraumatic stricture, external compression (extraureteral mass or retroperitoneal fibrosis)
- **C.** Urethral stricture: trauma (instrumentation or catheterization), urethritis (especially gonococcal)
- **D.** Benign prostatic hypertrophy
- **E.** Cystocele
- **F.** Tumors: renal, bladder, prostate, uterine, urethral
- **G.** Neurogenic bladder: diabetes mellitus, spinal cord injury, primary neurologic disease

II. Evaluation

IVP for bacteriuria should be restricted to the following groups:

- **A.** Adult males with persistent bacteriuria not related to instrumentation
- **B.** Adult females with recurrent bacteriuria, pyelonephritis, or bacteriuria combined with renal impairment
- **C.** Females with difficult-to-eradicate or recurrent bacteriuria during pregnancy. These women should be further evaluated by pyelography after delivery. IVP is optimally delayed until 3 months postpartum, since physiologic urethral dilatation has normally subsided at this time.

IVP for urinary tract infection should be accompanied by postvoiding films to determine bladder retention. In azotemic patients it may be necessary to use a high dose of contrast material in combination with tomography; this technique permits visualization in as many as 90% of patients with azotemia. Additional procedures (cystoscopy, cystourethrograms, residual urine measurements, cystometric studies) are performed as dictated by abnormalities on IVP and by renal function.

III. Indications for surgery. Surgical intervention is appropriate for precisely defined lesions that bear a probable relationship to renal disease. The ability of the patient to tolerate the procedure is an additional issue. A few conditions merit further consideration.

A. **Benign prostatic hypertrophy.** A residual urine volume greater than 50 ml is associated with significant bacteriuria in only 10% of males, provided there is no history of instrumentation or catheterization. It is advised that a postvoiding intravenous pyelogram be used to evaluate residual urine in these cases. Instrumentation should be avoided, since it is a major means of introducing bacteria into the bladder. The demonstration of residual urine or bacteriuria is not sufficient indication for operative intervention. This decision should be based on the frequency of acute attacks, the degree of renal impairment, and the presence of hydronephrosis and hydroureter.

B. **Infection stones.** Infection stones are caused by long-standing urinary tract infections involving urea-splitting bacteria such as *Proteus*. Such stones consist of precipitated magnesium ammonium phosphate and calcium phosphate. The responsible bacteria are buried in the depths of the stone, remaining inaccessible to antimicrobial drugs and serving as a persistent source of bacteriuria. Small infection stones may dissolve if the urine is kept sterile and acid for extended periods. With large stones, eradication of the infection requires surgical removal. This is technically difficult because of the common persistence of residual fragments. In some studies the excision of these calculi by routine methods was followed by recurrence of infection with the same organism in 50–70% of cases. The following guidelines are suggested:

   1. Antibiotics should be administered preoperatively for at least 1 week and continued postoperatively. In most instances ampicillin or penicillin G is suitable for infections involving *Pr. mirabilis*.
   2. At operation there should be a maximum attempt to remove all stone fragments.
   3. The renal pelvis and collection system should be irrigated through a nephrostomy tube with an infusion rate of about 100 ml/hr. Tomograms are taken to detect residual fragments. If any are detected, a nephrostogram is done to ensure that the irrigation is in contact with the residual fragments. Irrigation is continued until the fragments are no longer detected.
   4. Urine cultures are obtained daily, and the infusions are discontinued immediately if there is bacteriuria, fever, or flank pain.
   5. When a patient is a poor operative risk, the same approach may be employed with urethral catheters.

C. **Neurologic diseases.** With certain neurologic diseases, particularly traumatic spinal cord lesions, the bladder is either spastic or flaccid. Indwelling catheters are often used for extended periods of time. The result is a high rate of urinary tract complications, including pyelonephritis, hydrophrosis, renal calculi, penoscrotal abscesses, and fistulae. Indwelling catheterization of such patients for 3 years causes significant bacteriuria in 80%, periurethral abscesses in 25–30%, and renal calculi in 10%. (See pp. 313–314 for alternative approaches.)

   1. External sphincterotomy is considered for patients with detrusor–external sphincter dyssynergia following intermittent catheterization. Prequisites are cystometogram evidence that bladder contraction has returned, and cystourethrographic studies showing a narrowed external sphincter without bladder neck obstruction.
   2. Transurethral bladder neck resection is considered for patients with bladder neck obstruction.

Prostatic Infections

I. **Chronic prostatitis.** The prostate gland is remarkably resistant to infection, despite its direct continuity with the urinary tract. This is possibly explained by a component of normal prostatic fluid that inhibits growth of both gram-positive and gram-negative bacteria. Some persons lack this antimicrobial factor, and in these individuals the prostate becomes a reservoir of chronic infection that proves extremely refractory to antimicrobial therapy.

Table 5-5. Distinguishing features of prostatitis (acute and chronic) and prostatosis

	Acute prostatitis	Chronic prostatitis	Prostatosis
Age group	20–50 years	40–65 years	40–65 years
Symptoms	Constitutional symptoms and dysuria	Symptoms of cystitis	Perineal pain and dysuria
Prostate examination	Extreme tenderness	Normal	Normal
Pathology	Polymorphonuclear leukocyte infiltration	Mononuclear infiltration	Mononuclear infiltration
Culture	Bacteriuria usually present	Bacteriuria often present; partition urine cultures following therapy indicate prostatic infection	Partition urine cultures negative
Treatment	Parenteral antimicrobials	Oral antimicrobials	No adequate therapy
Relapse after therapy	Infrequent	Common	Common

Chronic bacterial prostatitis has been implicated as a major cause of recurrent urinary tract infections. This diagnosis should be suspected in all males with recurrent cystitis that cannot be attributed to anatomic defects, instrumentation, or catheterization (Table 5-5).

A. Symptoms. The dominant symptoms are often attributable to an associated cystitis: frequency; dysuria; and dull, persistent pain in the low back, perineum, genitalia, or suprapubic regions. The clinical spectrum extends from asymptomatic bacteriuria to chronic symptoms interrupted by bouts of acute prostatitis characterized by chills, fever, and systemic toxicity.

Repeated infection is highly characteristic of chronic bacterial prostatitis. Usually it represents true relapse, in that the same bacterial strain (with the same antimicrobial susceptibilities) is recovered on repeated samplings over extended periods despite intervening courses of chemotherapy.

B. Diagnosis. The chronically infected prostate usually appears normal by rectal or cystoscopic examination. The diagnosis is established by localizing bacterial infection to the prostate with quantitative cultures of partitioned urine and prostatic secretions (see p. 337). These specimens must be carefully collected during periods in which significant bacteriuria has been cleared. The number of bacteria in prostatic fluid is small, and contamination by the urethral flora must be avoided. Repeat cultures are often required. It should be emphasized that

1. Prostatic secretions in patients with bacterial prostatitis show oval fat bodies and more than 10 leukocytes per high-power field. There is no consistent relationship, however, between infection and cell count. Large numbers of leukocytes in prostatic secretions may be found in normal men without urologic disease.
2. Owing to the focal nature of prostatitis and the possibility of perineal contamination, needle biopsy of the prostate is generally unsatisfactory for bacterial culture. (Perineal contamination may be detected by control cultures obtained from the perineal area.)
3. Prostatic tissue chips are an unreliable culture source due to preoperative antimicrobial drugs, contaminating urinary bacteria, and the natural antibacterial action of the homogenized gland.
4. Histologic changes are nonspecific in biopsy specimens or resected tissue. A

chronic inflammatory response with mononuclear infiltration may be noted in the absence of infection.

C. Bacteriology. The usual pathogens are gram-negative bacilli. *E. coli* is the most common, followed by *Pr. mirabilis, Klebsiella,* and *Pseudomonas.* Enterococci are occasional pathogens. Other gram-positive organisms, such as *Staph. epidermidis,* diphtheroids, and α-hemolytic streptococci, usually represent contaminants.

D. Treatment

1. Antimicrobial agents are **notoriously ineffective** in eradicating bacteria from the chronically infected prostate, probably because the plasma-prostate barrier excludes nearly all such drugs. Erythromycin penetrates well but is ineffective against many gram-negative bacteria. Trimethoprim, however, is active against most pathogens (except *Pseudomonas*), and prostatic fluid levels of this agent actually exceed those of serum.
Recommended treatment is

   Trimethoprim/sulfamethoxazole 2 tabs (160/800 mg) bid for 6–12 weeks

   An alternative therapy is

   Doxycycline 100 mg bid for 6–12 weeks

   If these regimens fail to eradicate the infection, chronic suppressive therapy can be used for several months or years:

   Trimethoprim/sulfamethoxazole 1 tab (80/400)/day

2. Patients with symptoms of **cystitis** should be treated for lower urinary tract infection with an oral agent (see Table 5-3) with activity against the pathogen for 7–10 days, to eliminate bacteriuria. Although antimicrobial drugs can control symptoms, the prostatic focus of infection persists as a source of repeated bouts of cystitis.
3. **Surgical treatment.** Total prostatectomy is curative. However, the morbidity associated with this procedure, particularly impotence, is a major contraindication. Transurethral prostatectomy (TURP) is sometimes successful, but again, this represents a rather radical approach to a benign disease. TURP should be reserved for patients who cannot be controlled with long-term antimicrobial suppressive therapy. A maximum amount of prostatic tissue should be resected, since most bacteria reside in the peripheral zone of the prostate. Two or three operations may be required to achieve cure.

II. Prostatosis

A. Diagnosis. Prostatosis is clinically and pathologically similar to chronic prostatitis. Common complaints are perineal or low back pain and urinary discomfort. Expressed prostatic secretions show WBCs and oval fat bodies. The differentiating features are (1) patients with prostatosis are not subject to recurrent bouts of cystitis, and (2) partition urine cultures fail to reveal bacterial infection (Table 5-5). There is no evidence that fastidious organisms such as gonococci, mycoplasmas, and anaerobes are related to prostatosis.

B. Treatment. Antimicrobials and surgery play no role in prostatosis. Occasional patients respond to hot sitz baths, anticholinergic drugs, or periodic prostatic massage. All therapeutic modalities fail in most cases, however, and the patient either settles for reassurance or goes from physician to physician in an unsuccessful search for a cure.

III. Acute prostatitis.

In contrast to chronic prostatitis, acute infections tend to occur in young adults, the diagnosis is more easily established, and the pathogen is eradicated with antimicrobial treatment (Table 5-5). Acute and chronic infections of the prostate occasionally occur in the same patient.

A. Symptoms. The diagnosis of acute prostatitis is relatively straightforward, although there may be confusion when local complaints are minimal and the rectal examination is neglected.

1. Most patients complain of **rectal, perineal,** or **genital pain,** which may be accentuated with defecation or urination. Sympathetic enervation of the

prostate extends from the T-10 to the S-3 level, so referred pain can occur almost anywhere below the diaphragm. Occasional cases simulate acute cholecystitis or acute appendicitis.

2. There is usually an associated **urethritis** and **cystitis,** causing dysuria, frequency, urgency, terminal hematuria, or urethral discharge. Acute urinary retention can occur.
3. Some patients present with severe **systemic toxicity** including chills and spiking fevers.

B. Physical examination. Rectal examination reveals a prostate that is exquisitely tender, swollen, firm, or boggy. The gland may be so distorted and indurated as to suggest carcinoma. Vigorous massage is contraindicated, since it may cause bacteremia.

C. Laboratory findings. Urine culture usually yields the pathogen because of the associated cystitis. Any spontaneous urethral discharge should also be sent for Gram's stain and culture. However, **prostatic massage to obtain these secretions is contraindicated,** due to the possibility of inducing bacteremia or extending the infection to the epididymis. Massage is considered safe only after 2–3 days of antimicrobial therapy.

D. Bacteriology. The pathogens are those commonly involving the urinary tract, such as *E. coli, Proteus, Klebsiella,* and *Pseudomonas.* This grouping suggests retrograde passage of bacteria to the prostate via the urethra. The frequent association with instrumentation or indwelling catheters also implicates this route. Occasional cases, especially those involving *Staph. aureus,* result from hematogenous dissemination from a nonurinary site.

E. Treatment

1. Local heat with sitz baths.
2. Relief of urinary retention with suprapubic drainage. Some urologists prefer to insert a thin urethral catheter for 2–3 days and to perform suprapubic drainage only if there is persistent sepsis during catheterization. Instrumentation and repeated urethral catheterizations are contraindicated.
3. Antimicrobial drugs. Antimicrobials are usually curative, presumably because the plasma-prostate barrier breaks down in the presence of acute inflammation. Agents are selected on the basis of cultures of blood, urine, or urethral discharge (see Table 5-3). Gram's stain of urine or discharge is an early means of differentiating gram-negative bacilli from gram-positive cocci (*Staph. aureus* or enterococci). Drug selection is also tempered by the clinical setting and severity of symptoms:
   a. Uncomplicated gram-negative infections acquired outside the hospital environment are likely to respond to ampicillin or cefazolin.
   b. For seriously ill patients or those with hospital-acquired infections, gentamicin plus a cephalosporin is appropriate.

   In all cases the initial choice of drugs should be modified by results of cultures and sensitivities. Drugs are continued for 7–10 days.

F. Response to treatment. Most patients respond to appropriate antibiotics within 48 hours. Persistence of fever suggests inappropriate drug selection or possible abscess formation. Operative intervention is seldom required unless an abscess is present. Follow-up cultures of partitioned urines and expressed prostatic secretions are required to ensure eradication of the organism. Occasional cases progress to chronic prostatitis, which should be managed as previously described (see sec. **I.D**).

IV. Prostatic abscess. Prostatic abscess is an uncommon condition but is important to recognize, because it requires surgical intervention. Delay in drainage may lead to a fatal outcome. Formerly, most cases were caused by direct extension of gonococcal urethritis or *Staph. aureus* septicemia. During the past decade the majority of cases have been associated with a mixture of coliforms and anaerobic bacteria.

A. Diagnosis. Patients may present with symptoms suggesting acute prostatitis, including fever, leukocytosis, dysuria, and perineal or rectal pain. Alternatively, the process may be indolent, with minimal systemic toxicity. In the latter case, lower urinary tract symptoms are the dominant complaint, and the initial impression may be benign prostatic hypertrophy. Factors that specifically suggest prostatic abscess are

1. A **fluctuant gland** on rectal examination is considered diagnostic, but it may be difficult to detect due to exquisite tenderness. Occasionally the abscess is small and deep in the gland, and there is no abnormality on physical examination.
2. **Failure to respond** to appropriate antimicrobial therapy or early **recurrence** of symptoms when chemotherapy is discontinued is a strong indication of abscess.
3. **Perineal pain and acute urinary retention** occur more frequently with abscess than with acute prostatitis.
4. **Spontaneous drainage** of an abscess, either into the urethra or, less commonly, into the rectum. Rupture into the ischiorectal fossa is rare due to the barrier of Denonvilliers' fascia (septum rectovesicale). Drainage into the urethra results in a urethral discharge that is frankly purulent and may be voluminous. Spontaneous drainage is usually accompanied by a dramatic relief of symptoms.

In many cases the abscess is not appreciated until it is demonstrated by endoscopy or prostatectomy.

B. Treatment

1. **Antimicrobial agents.** Empiric antimicrobial therapy should be directed against suspected pathogens—coliforms, *Staph. aureus,* and anaerobic bacteria. Clindamycin with an aminoglycoside or cefoxitin with or without an aminoglycoside (depending on the suspicion of *Pseudomonas*) is likely to be effective.
2. **Surgical procedure.** Spontaneous rupture requires a surgical procedure to ensure complete drainage. Transurethral resection is the procedure of choice in most cases. Open perineal drainage is occasionally preferred, if the abscess is periprostatic and there is no urethral discharge. Perineal needle aspiration may be used initially as a diagnostic and therapeutic maneuver in cases of severe illness. A more complete drainage procedure is usually required at a later date.

Urethritis

Urethral discharge is a common complaint related to multiple etiologies (Table 5-6). Urethritis is classified as gonococcal or nongonococcal, and the cases seen in venereal disease clinics are approximately equally divided between the two types. Of the nongonococcal cases, a small percentage are due to *Trichomonas,* but the remainder are labeled "nonspecific," since pathogens cannot be identified by the usual diagnostic procedures.

I. Gonococcal urethritis

A. Symptoms. The usual incubation period in the male is 3–5 days after contact. Initially there is anterior urethritis with dysuria and a milky, purulent discharge. Systemic symptoms are unusual. Late in the course there may be extension to the posterior urethra, prostate, seminal vesicles, and epididymis. Involvement of these contiguous sites often results in local pain and fever. Asymptomatic gonorrhea (carrier state or incubating disease) has been detected by culture of the urethral meatus in males. Urethral infection in females is rarely associated with gonococci. (Gonococcal infection of the female genital tract is discussed in Chap. 4.) Gonorrhea can also occur in extragenital sites by direct inoculation of the columnar mucosal epithelium: in the pharynx, rectum, and eye. Disseminated gonococcal infection produces arthralgias, tenosynovitis or septic arthritis, and erythematous or hemorrhagic skin lesions (arthritis-dermatitis syndrome).

B. Diagnosis

1. **Gram's-stained smear** of urethral exudate showing typical gram-negative diplococci is virtually diagnostic. This finding requires culture confirmation

Table 5-6. Differential diagnosis of urethral discharge

Urethritis
Gonococcal
Nongonococcal
Trichomonas
Nonspecific
Chlamydia
Ureaplasma
Urinary tract pathogens
Prostatitis
Structural defects
Urethral diverticulum
Urethral stricture
Foreign body
Carcinoma
Irritation (topical chemicals, contraceptive creams, etc.)
Trauma
Systemic conditions
Reiter's syndrome
Stevens-Johnson syndrome
Behçet's disease

in females, since other *Neisseria* species reside in normal cervical flora. However, when the organisms are intracellular, they are almost surely gonococci.

2. **Cultures** of the genital tract should be performed on patients with suspected gonorrhea. In **males** who have insufficient discharge for culture (even with penile stripping), a specimen is obtained by inserting a calcium alginate swab 2–3 cm into the urethra and scraping the anterior portion. Approximately 2% of smear-negative males have positive cultures. In homosexual males the anal canal should also be sampled. Cultures in **females** should be routinely obtained from the endocervical canal and anus. Throat cultures for gonococci are obtained when there is evidence of pharyngitis or disseminated gonococcemia. Specimens for culture are immediately inoculated onto Thayer-Martin medium or held on Transgrow medium for transport to the laboratory.

C. Treatment

The treatment recommendations are summarized in Table 5-7. Amoxicillin is given as an initial dose, followed by tetracycline for 7 days. The tetracycline is included to eradicate *Chlamydia trachomatis,* which often coexists with gonococci. The principal concern with tetracycline is that it requires compliance to the regimen after leaving the clinic.

Patients with infections involving penicillinase-producing *Neisseria gonorrhoeae* or those who are likely to have acquired this infection in areas where the strains are prevalent should receive spectinomycin (2.0 gm IM). The sexual partners of these patients should be treated similarly. Alternative recommendations, or therapy for the patient with positive cultures after spectinomycin treatment, are

cefoxitin, 2 gm IM, plus probenecid, 1 gm PO
or cefuroxime (1.5 gm IM) plus probenecid, 1 gm PO
or cefotaxime 1 gm IM alone.

Follow-up cultures should be performed at 7–14 days. Sexual consorts should also be treated. A serologic test for syphilis is recommended.

Recurrence or persistence of symptoms may indicate therapeutic failure, reinfection ("ping-pong" gonorrhea), or concurrent nonspecific urethritis. A common cause of reinfection is failure to treat sexual partners. True therapeutic failures should be treated with spectinomycin, 2 gm IM or the alternatives (Table 5-7).

Postgonococcal urethritis (persistent discharge that is negative for gonococci on smear and culture) is treated with tetracycline (see sec. **II.D**).

II. Nonspecific urethritis

A. Symptoms are dysuria and/or urethral discharge. Compared with gonorrhea the discharge is less profuse and less purulent; symptoms are likely to be more prolonged; recurrence rates are high; and penicillin therapy often is ineffective. In some instances the two conditions coexist, and nongonococcal urethritis is the principal cause of "postgonococcal urethritis." Complications of nonspecific urethritis include prostatitis, epididymitis, and, possibly, urethral stricture.

B. Microbiology. Epidemiologic studies suggest the route of infection is venereal transmission. *C. trachomatis* accounts for 50–70% of cases. It is an obligate intracellular organism that is cultivated in tissue culture, so that routine smears and bacterial cultures are unrewarding. *Ureaplasma urealyticum* (formerly called **T-strain *Mycoplasma***) also causes this disease. Both organisms are sensitive to tetracycline, which is the antimicrobial drug of choice. Female partners of men with gonococcal urethritis due to *Chlamydia* often harbor this organism without symptoms. (Females can also develop salpingitis due to *Chlamydia;* see p. 71.) This supports venereal transmission as the mechanism of infection and indicates that sexual partners should also be treated.

C. Diagnosis. Specialized culture techniques are required to cultivate *Chlamydia* and *Mycoplasma*. In most instances the diagnosis of nonspecific urethritis is made by excluding gonococcal infection. This is most easily done by Gram's stain of the discharge (Table 5-8).

D. Treatment. Tetracycline, 500 mg PO qid for 7 days. As an alternative for patients who cannot tolerate tetracycline, erythromycin, 500 mg qid for 7 days, can be given. **Relapses** are treated with tetracycline for 14–21 days. **Refractory cases** require cystoscopy to detect urethral strictures. The sexual partner should be treated concurrently with oral tetracycline (same dose as just specified). The male patient should use a condom for sexual intercourse during treatment.

III. Trichomonal urethritis

1. **Symptoms.** Although *Trichomonas vaginalis* usually produces no symptoms in the male, it can cause urethritis, prostatitis, or balanoposthitis. Symptoms, when present, are dysuria and urethral discharge. (For infection in females, see p. 83.)
2. **Diagnosis.** A fresh wet smear of urethral discharge is placed under a coverslip and examined with high dry microscopy under reduced light. If no urethral discharge is available, scrapings from the anterior urethra are mixed with a drop of saline for immediate examination. Typical organisms are motile, globular protozoan parasites, 10–30 μ in diameter, with five lashing flagella, an undulating membrane, and an ovoid nucleus.
3. **Treatment.** Metronidazole, 2.0 gm as a single oral dose, or 250 mg tid for 7 days. The disease is venereally transmitted, and sexual consorts should be treated concurrently.

IV. Nongonococcal bacterial urethritis

A. Symptoms are dysuria and urethral discharge, which can be acute or chronic. The character of the fluid is purulent, milky, serous, or sanguineous. Antecedent urethral trauma is common, especially from instrumentation, catheterization, foreign body, or masturbation. Possible underlying structural abnormalities include urethral diverticula, strictures, or carcinoma. These associated conditions can cause a urethral discharge in the absence of infection; the fluid is thin or sanguinous, and cultures are negative.

B. Diagnosis is based on partitioned urine cultures, which yield disproportionately high counts of bacteria and WBCs in the first voided specimen (VBI) as compared to the midstream collection (VB2) and the post-prostatic massage specimen (VB3) (see p. 337 for details). The smears and cultures of the discharge also reveal the etiologic agent. The usual pathogens are *E. coli,* other enteric gram-negative bacilli, and *Staph. aureus*.

C. Treatment. Antimicrobial drugs are based on the results of cultures and should follow the guidelines for lower urinary tract infections: an oral agent for 7–10

Table 5-7. Treatment of gonorrhea

Type or stage	Drugs of choice	Dosage	Alternatives
Urethritis or Cervicitis	Amoxicillin **plus** probenecid **followed by** tetracycline HCl[b]	3 gm PO once 1 gm PO once 500 mg PO qid × 7 days	Penicillin G procaine, 4.8 million units IM[a] once **plus** probenecid 1 gm PO once Spectinomycin, 2 gm IM once Cefoxitin, 2 gm or cefuroxime 1.5 gm IM once **plus** probenecid 1 gm PO once Cefotaxime, 1 gm IM once
Anal			
Women	As for urethritis or cervicitis	—	—
Men	Penicillin G procaine **plus** probenecid	As for urethritis	Spectinomycin, 2 gm IM once
Pharyngeal	Tetracycline HCl[b]	As for urethritis	Trimethoprim-sulfamethoxazole, 9 tablets[c] daily × 5 days
	or Penicillin G procaine **plus** probenecid	As for urethritis	
Ophthalmia (adults)	Penicillin G crystalline **plus** saline irrigation	10 million units IV daily × 5 days	Cefoxitin, 1 gm or cefotaxime 500 mg IV qid × 5 days **plus** saline irrigation
Bacteremia and arthritis	Penicillin G crystalline **followed by** amoxicillin	10 million units IV daily × 3 days 500 mg PO qid × 4 days	Tetracycline, 500 mg PO qid[b] × 7 days Spectinomycin, 2 gm IM bid × 3 days Erythromycin, 500 mg PO qid × 7 days Cefotaxime, 500 mg or cefoxitin 1 gm IV qid × 7 days
Meningitis	Penicillin G crystalline	At least 10 million units IV daily for at least 10 days	Cefotaxime, 2 gm IV q4h for at least 10 days Chloramphenicol, 4–6 gm/day for at least 10 days

Endocarditis	Penicillin G crystalline	At least 10 million units IV daily for at least 3–4 wk	
Neonatal			
Ophthalmia	Penicillin G crystalline **plus** saline irrigation	50,000 units/kg/day IV in 2 doses × 7 days	
Arthritis and septicemia	Penicillin G crystalline	75,000 to 100,000 units/kg/day IV in 4 doses × 7 days	
Meningitis	Penicillin G crystalline	100,000 units/kg/day IV in 3 or 4 doses for at least 10 days	
Children (under 45 kg)			
Urogenital, anal, and pharyngeal	Amoxicillin	50 mg/kg PO once	Spectinomycin, 40 mg/kg IM once
	plus probenecid	25 mg/kg (max. 1 gm) once	Tetracycline (over 8 years old), 10 mg/kg PO qid × 5 days
	or Penicillin G procaine	100,000 units/kg IM once	
	plus probenecid	25 mg/kg (max. 1 gm) once	
Arthritis	Penicillin G crystalline	150,000 units/kg/day IV × 7 days	Cefoxitin 100 mg/kg/day or cefotaxime 50 mg/kg/day IV in divided doses × 7 days
			Tetracycline (over 8 years old) 10 mg/kg PO qid × 7 days
			Erythromycin 50 mg/kg/day PO in 4 divided doses × 7 days
Meningitis	Penicillin G crystalline	250,000 units/kg/day IV in 6 divided doses for at least 10 days	Cefotaxime 200 mg/kg/day IV for at least 10 days
			Chloramphenicol 100 mg/kg/day IV for at least 10 days

[a]Divided into two injections at one visit.
[b]Or doxycycline 100 mg PO bid.
[c]Each tablet contains 80 mg trimethoprim and 400 mg sulfamethoxazole.
Source: *The Medical Letter* 26 (658):5, 1984.

Table 5-8. Therapy according to Gram's stain of urethral discharge

Gram's stain result	Usual treatment	Diagnosis and rationale
Typical gram-negative diplococci within polymorphonuclear leukocytes	Tetracycline Penicillin G Amoxicillin	Virtually diagnostic of gonococcal urethritis
No gram-negative diplococci, atypical gram-negative diplococci or other organisms present extracellularly	Tetracycline	Usually due to *Chlamydia* or *Ureaplasma*. Occasional cases caused by gonococci respond to tetracycline
		Alternative diagnoses to consider 1. *Trichomonas*—do hanging drop 2. Urinary tract infection—3 glass urine culture 3. Traumatic urethritis—usually due to excessive milking efforts 4. Reiter's disease—symptom complex of urethritis, balanitis, conjunctivitis, arthritis, and mucocutaneous lesions

days (see p. 101). Instrumentation is contraindicated during bacterial urethritis, since it may induce bacteremia. Cystoscopy and urethrograms to detect underlying lesions should be performed after the infection has been eradicated.

Infections of the Male Genitalia

I. Penis

A. The differential diagnostic features and therapy of common infections involving the penis are summarized in Table 5-9.

B. These infections must be distinguished from noninfectious processes such as the following:

1. Primary dermatologic diseases that may involve the genital area, including psoriasis, lichen planus, eczema, neurodermatitis, and drug eruptions. In most instances the nature of the lesion and involvement of other areas of the body serve to distinguish these conditions.
2. Carcinoma and precancerous lesions (leukoplakia, Paget's disease, and Bowen's disease). Biopsy is required to establish these diagnoses.
3. Balanitis associated with systemic diseases of unknown cause, including Reiter's disease and Behçet's syndrome.

II. Scrotum

A. Abscess. Primary abscess of the **scrotal wall** is associated with infected hair follicles, sweat glands, or abrasions, and is analogous to soft tissue infections in other areas of the body. **Secondary** abscess occurs as an extension of infection from the periurethral tissue (especially after instrumentation of an infected urethra or prostatic surgery), or from the anorectal area, epididymis, or testes. Secondary infection is more common in diabetics. Occasional cases follow vasectomy. *Staph. aureus* is the most frequent cause of primary abscess, whereas coliforms are more common with the secondary infections. Treatment includes incision and drainage of superficial abscesses and debridement of any necrotic tissue. Secondary abscess may necessitate an orchiectomy. Systemic antibiotics are given according to Gram's staining and culture of the drainage.

B. Fistulae. Infected fistulae of the scrotum usually occur in association with a periurethral abscess or urethral stricture. They may also follow the passage of sounds for urethral dilatation. The infecting organisms are usually urinary tract pathogens, especially coliforms. Antimicrobial agents are selected on the basis of Gram's stain and culture of exudate carefully collected from the depths of the tract. The surgical procedure consists of excision of the entire fistular tract—including periurethral, inflammatory tissue—and closure of the urethral defect. Less common causes of scrotal fistulae to be considered in the differential diagnosis are tuberculous epididymitis, tertiary syphilis of the testes, schistosomiasis, and actinomycosis.

C. Erysipelas. This condition is an acute lymphangitis of the scrotal skin due to group A *Streptococcus pyogenes* (see p. 186). It may follow surgical incisions, minor abrasions, or open wounds. The lesion begins with a small area of erythema, which enlarges to produce an erythematous, indurated, raised area of inflammation with a sharply demarcated, advancing margin that eventually involves the entire scrotum. Vesicles and bullae may form. Extension through lymphatic channels produces cellulitis, adenopathy, and bacteremia. In most cases the pathogen is difficult to recover, even with needle aspiration of the advancing edge of inflammation; the diagnosis, however, is readily apparent on clinical grounds. The antibiotic of choice is parenteral penicillin G for 10 days. An alternative agent for patients with penicillin hypersensitivity is erythromycin, clindamycin, or a cephalosporin.

D. Gangrene. A severe necrotizing infection can involve the scrotum and adjacent structures. It is associated with significant mortality. Scrotal gangrene follows urinary extravasation or surgical procedures or may occur spontaneously. Characteristic findings are severe local pain, an acutely inflamed scrotum, and profound constitutional symptoms, including fever and prostration. In some cases there is gas formation with crepitation. When the disease has gross gangrene of the scrotum, it is known as Fournier's gangrene (pp. 195–196). The common pathogens are anaerobic bacteria, either alone or combination with coliforms. Occasional cases are due to *Strep. pyogenes*. This condition must be differentiated from erysipelas, acute epididymitis, orchitis, and torsion of the testicle. Treatment includes

1. Parenteral antibiotics:

Clindamycin	600 mg IV q6h
or chloramphenicol	3–4 gm/day
or cefoxitin	2 gm IV q6hr
plus	
An aminoglycoside	

2. Surgical drainage with multiple incisions and wide debridement of devitalized tissue.
3. If there is an underlying urinary extravasation, diversion of the urinary stream as soon as possible.

E. Venereal disease. Several conditions may involve the scrotal wall, including chancroid, granuloma inguinale, and syphilis (see Table 5-9).

F. Elephantiasis. Chronic obstruction of scrotal lymph flow causes transudation of fluid with edema and progressive hyperplasia of connective tissue.

1. **Filarial lymphangitis** is a tropical disease resulting from mosquito transmission of *Wuchereria bancrofti* or *Brugia malayi*. Orchitis or lymph varix of the spermatic cord occurs early. The lymph varix ruptures into the scrotal sac (lymphocele) or urinary tract (chyluria). Elephantiasis is a late and unusual complication. The diagnosis is based on typical findings of hydrocele or elephantiasis in a patient who has spent several years in an endemic area. Microfilariae are rarely found, except early in the course (hydrocele fluid, chylous urine or nocturnally collected blood smears). Treatment consists of diethylcarbamazine, 2 mg/kg tid daily for 2–3 weeks, to suppress micro-

Table 5-9. Differential diagnosis of penile infections

Condition	Agent	Usual location	Character of lesion	Regional adenopathy	Diagnostic studies	Treatment
Syphilitic chancre (primary syphilis)	*Treponema pallidum*	Glans or prepuce	Papule → shallow, painless, indurated ulcer Usually solitary	Discrete and firm No matting or suppuration unless secondarily infected	Express serous fluid from chancre or lymph node Aspirate for dark-field exam VDRL and FTS + in 25% early, 100% after 4 weeks	1. 4.8 million units penicillin a. Procaine penicillin, 600,000 units/day × 8 days b. Procaine penicillin in aluminum monosterate, 2.4 mil units, then 1.2 mil units × 2 at 3rd & 6th days c. Benzathine penicillin, 2.4 mil units, repeat at 7 days 2. Tetracycline, 500 mg po qid × 5 days
Chancroid	*Hemophilus ducreyi*	Parafrenular area, coronal sulcus, or shaft	Vesicopapule → soft, ragged, painful ulcer that bleeds easily Multiple lesions common May cause balanitis or phimosis	50% of cases have adenopathy, usually unilateral Periadenitis with matting and suppuration, rupture through one osteum	Express fluid from cleaned surface of recent lesion or node aspirate for Gram's stain Culture: inoculate specimen into 3 ml clotted blood (Do not biopsy node)	1. Trimethoprim/sulfamethoxazole, 2 tabs (80/400 mg) bid × 14 days 2. Tetracycline, 500 mg PO qid × 7–14 days 3. Erythromycin, 500 mg qid × 14 days Needle aspiration of suppurative bubos
Granuloma inguinale	*Donovania granulomatis*	Penis, groin, or perineal area	Nodule or papule → superficial irregular ulcer with vivid pink velvety, granular base → lesions extend with cicatricial healing	Uncommon unless secondarily infected	Excise fragment from edge (or aspirate of pseudobubo); spread on slide for Giemsa stain	1. Tetracycline, 500 mg qid × 14 days 2. Erythromycin, 500 mg qid × 14 days Local hygiene

		urethra	is seldom noted	may form multiple sinus tracts or extend to pelvic nodes and cause proctitis with rectal stricture (within 10 cm of anus)	Culture: difficult and seldom used Biopsy: nondiagnostic	mg qid × 21 days 3. Drain fluctuant nodes with large-bore needle
Herpes progenitalis	*Herpesvirus hominis*	Glans, prepuce, or shaft	Multiple vesicles that tend to burn or itch Often recurrent at same site	Common only with first infection Tender, discrete	Scrapings for cytology; note multinucleate giant cells and intranuclear inclusions	Initial attacks: Acyclovir topically 4–6x/day, 7 days; severe initial attacks: Acyclovir 5 mg/kg IV q8h*
Scabies	Mite: *Sarcoptes scabiei*	Penis and other cutaneous creases	Intensely pruritic papule or vesicle	None, unless secondarily infected	Scrapings to demonstrate mite or magnifying lens exam of a burrow site	Single topical application of 10% sulfur ointment or 25% benzyl benzoate
Condylomata acuminata (venereal wart)	Virus	Glans, coronal sulcus (may occur anywhere, including urethra)	Small nodules or pedunculated protuberances	None, unless secondarily infected	Appearance of lesion	1. Topical podophyllin 2. Cauterization 3. Circumcision may be required 4. Excision occasionally necessary to exclude carcinoma
Condylomata lata (secondary syphilis)	*T. pallidum*	Anogenital area	Hypertrophic granulomatous lesions	Often as part of generalized adenopathy Nontender, firm, discrete	VDRL and FTA always positive	Same as for primary syphilis
Balanitis	Variable: coliforms, streptococci, or *Staph. aureus*	Glans and prepuce	Erythema, weeping erosions	Variable; when present—tender, may suppurate	Typical appearance, associated with poor hygiene in uncircumcised male Gram's stain and culture of carefully collected exudate	Local hygiene Systemic antimicrobials if febrile or local adenopathy Dorsal slit to relieve balanoposthitis Circumcision when infection controlled
Gangrene	Usually anaerobic bacteria ± coliforms	Glans, prepuce, shaft, and anogenital area	Rapidly progressing necrotizing lesion extending along fascial planes with extensive sloughing Systemic symptoms may be severe	Variable	Typical appearance Gram's stain and culture of carefully collected exudate	Systemic antimicrobials such as gentamicin, in combination with cefoxitin, chloramphenicol, or clindamycin Early and extensive debridement of devitalized tissue

*This treatment does not prevent recurrences.

filaria and possibly affect the adult worms. There is no treatment for the anatomic abnormalities, however.

2. **Pseudoelephantiasis** is the same type of process but arises from causes other than filariasis. These include chronic infections, metastatic carcinoma, lymph node excisions, hernia repair, and venereal diseases with lymphatic involvement. Therapy is directed at the underlying cause. Surgical excision is seldom required for elephantiasis.

III. Orchitis

A. Mumps. Approximately 20% of postpubertal males with mumps develop orchitis. Symptoms begin abruptly with fever and severe testicular swelling, pain, and tenderness. These usually occur 4–9 days after the appearance of parotitis. In about one-third of cases salivary gland involvement is minimal or inapparent, making the diagnosis less obvious. Orchitis is bilateral in 20–40% of cases. Some degree of testicular atrophy occurs in about half of involved testicles, although bilateral atrophy with sterility is rare. Mumps orchitis accounts for 2–3% of sterility in males. An additional concern is an increased incidence of testicular neoplasms in patients with testicular atrophy following mumps, although this association is not firmly established. Symptoms of orchitis generally subside spontaneously within 4–8 days, but some degree of pain and swelling may persist for weeks.

1. **Diagnosis** is supported by an appropriate contact history, associated parotitis, and an elevated serum amylase. A serial rise in mumps complement-fixation titer is diagnostic. The mumps skin test is of limited value due to cross-reactions with other viruses (false-positive) and has variable antigenic potency (false-negative).

2. **Treatment** is bed rest, scrotal support, and ice packs. Scrotal support is achieved by wide adhesive bandages across the thighs ("Bellevue bridge") or pads of cotton wool to nest the scrotum gently from below. Following the acute period, an athletic supporter can be used until all inflammation has subsided. Controlled studies have failed to show any benefit from corticosteroids or diethylstilbestrol, and these drugs are not recommended. Similarly, gamma globulin and hyperimmune gamma globulin are of no value once orchitis has started. Anesthetic block of the spermatic cord may successfully relieve the pain of severe orchitis. Some urologists advocate incision of the tunica albuginea testis to release severe pressure, but results are difficult to evaluate because of anticipated spontaneous improvement by the time the procedure is performed.

B. Pyogenic orchitis. This is a relatively rare complication of hematogenous dissemination of bacteria, epididymitis, catheterization, prostatectomy, or instrumentation. There is high fever, sudden testicular pain, and tender local swelling. The bacteria usually responsible are coliforms or *Staph. aureus.* **Treatment** is scrotal support and systemic antibiotics (such as an aminoglycoside in combination with either a cephalosporin, nafcillin, or oxacillin). Aspiration of an associated hydrocele often provides considerable relief. Abscess formation is rare, but when present usually requires orchiectomy.

IV. Epididymitis. Epididymitis is the most common cause of acute scrotal swelling and pain. There is marked unilateral or bilateral tenderness along the course of the spermatic cord. In patients with exquisite tenderness, it may be necessary to infiltrate the spermatic cord with lidocaine to permit a more thorough examination. Rectal examination should be deferred, since this may produce contralateral involvement. Acute hydrocele is a common complication; hydroceles can be aspirated to facilitate examination of the scrotal contents. The differential diagnosis includes other causes of a painful, scrotal mass: orchitis, hemorrhage into a testicular tumor, trauma, and torsion of the testicle or spermatic cord. The infectious causes of epididymitis include the following.

A. Gonorrheal epididymitis. This has become a rare entity in the chemotherapeutic era. Most cases at present represent simple neglect, inadequate chemotherapy of gonococcal urethritis, unorthodox therapeutic maneuvers (such as urethral irrigations or instrumentation), or urethral strictures.

Treatment consists of scrotal support, analgesics, and aqueous penicillin G (4.8 million units IM) or amoxicillin (3 gm PO) plus probenecid (1 gm PO). Failure to respond indicates nongonorrheal infection, abscess formation (requiring drainage), or an underlying urethral stricture.

B. "Nonspecific" epididymitis is caused by coliforms, especially *E. coli* or, less commonly, *Pseudomonas, Staph. aureus,* or streptococci. Most cases occur in the course of a urinary tract infection or prostatitis in men over 45 years of age. Additional predisposing factors are instrumentation, catheterization, urethral stricture, and urologic surgery. Straining may also be an important factor, forcing infected urine into the vas. Symptoms are acute, chronic, or recurrent. The etiologic agent is usually detected with a midstream urine culture.

Treatment:

1. **Bed rest.**
2. **Scrotal support** (wide adhesive tape across thighs) until acute pain and swelling subside, then athletic supporter when patient is ambulatory, until inflammation has totally subsided.
3. **Analgesics,** including lidocaine injections into the spermatic cord to relieve severe pain.
4. **Antimicrobial drugs.** The choice of drug and route of administration depend on severity of symptoms, clinical setting, and results of urine culture. Ampicillin or cephalosporins are usually adequate. An aminoglycoside, with or without a cephalosporin, would be appropriate for severely ill patients, especially when this condition is acquired during hospitalization. Antimicrobial drugs are continued for 7–10 days.
5. **Epididymectomy.** This may be required for recurrent infections or for chronic infections that do not respond readily to medical measures. With acute epididymitis this procedure is technically difficult.

Follow-up studies after resolution of infection should include a complete urologic evaluation, intravenous pyelogram, cystourethrography, and cystoscopy.

C. "Idiopathic" epididymitis refers to cases in which bacteria such as gonococci and coliforms are not implicated. It is most commonly seen in young adults. The usual etiologic agent is *C. trachomatis,* but *Ureaplasma* is noted on occasion. Many patients concurrently have nongonococcal urethritis with a urethral discharge. The diagnosis is established by culturing the organism or showing a serologic response. Since these tests are not available in most clinical laboratories, a presumptive diagnosis is based on **negative cultures** for gonococci and urinary tract pathogens in a **susceptible host.** The preferred antibiotic is tetracycline (500 mg qid for 2 weeks). Differential features of epididymitis due to *C. trachomatis* and urinary tract pathogens are shown in Table 5-10.

D. Mumps epididymitis is usually associated with orchitis, but it may occur independently, (Diagnostic evaluation and therapy are noted under section **III**.)

E. Less common causes of epididymitis include tuberculosis, syphilis (secondary or tertiary), brucellosis, and fungi. The roles of *Ureaplasma urealyticum* and *T. vaginalis* are unclear.

Renal Abscess

Renal abscess can occur as multiple septic foci, a single abscess, or a large purulent collection (renal carbuncle). The symptomatology is variable; at times there is severe sepsis, but more commonly the course is indolent, with few localizing signs until late. The diagnosis is established preoperatively in only about 20% of cases. Once an abscess has formed, it may drain into the perinephric area or the renal pelvis, or it may encapsulate within the renal parenchyma.

I. Etiology

A. Hematogenous septic emboli to the renal cortex is the most frequent mechanism; usually *Staph. aureus* is the pathogen. Common sources of bacteremia are skin infections, endocarditis, and intravenous drug abuse.

Table 5-10. Causes of epididymitis

	Agent	
Etiologic factor	*Chlamydia trachomatis*	Urinary tract pathogens
Patient's age	18–45 years	Over 45 years
Concurrent genitourinary abnormality	Rare	Common
Inguinal pain	Common	Rare
Scrotal edema and erythema	Less severe	More severe
Recent sexual exposure	Common	Less common
Expressible urethral discharge	Common	Uncommon
Midstream urine culture for bacteria	Negative	Usually positive

B. Less frequently, lymphatic extension of ascending pyelonephritis can cause renal abscess. The pathogens are those associated with urinary tract infections, such as coliforms.

II. Diagnosis

A. Clinical findings are nonspecific—fever, chills, abdominal pain, muscle aches and pains, and leukocytosis. Localizing signs such as flank pain and tenderness, when present, appear late in the course. Lower urinary tract symptoms are infrequent, and urinalysis is generally of little value.

B. X-ray films during the early **acute phase** of infection tend to show diffuse and nonspecific changes, such as renal enlargement and a poorly defined renal outline. Intravenous pyelography reveals a localized area of impaired function. Retrograde pyelograms demonstrate nonfilling or displacement of a calyx. Arteriograms show delayed filling with little vascular displacement and no neovascularization.

In the **chronic phase** of infection x-rays show a more clearly defined mass, which must be differentiated from other space-occupying lesions. The mass is generally apparent on intravenous pyelography with nephrotomography. Arteriograms are useful for distinguishing abscess from neoplasm or cyst: With abscess there is focal decreased arterial flow, an avascular area with shaggy margins in the capillary phase, and little vascular displacement. CT scan with contrast is the best method of making the diagnosis. The presence of an enlarging renal mass, along with signs of sepsis, is strongly suggestive of renal abscess.

III. Treatment. Early lesions may respond to antimicrobial treatment alone. Drug selection is based on blood cultures and, in cases associated with pyelonephritis, urine cultures. Prior to culture results, an aminoglycoside in combination with nafcillin or a cephalosporin would be appropriate therapy. A well-encapsulated abscess should undergo percutaneous drainage with ultrasound guidance, surgical drainage, or nephrectomy. Which method to use depends on the size of the abscess, residual function in the kidney, and the status of the contralateral kidney.

Perinephric Abscess

Perinephric abscess refers to a suppurative collection between the kidney and the perirenal (Gerota's) fascia. This space is closed superiorly at the diaphragm; inferiorly it is open and communicates with the pelvic fat; laterally, the fascial layers fuse with the transversalis fascia; and medially they pass anterior to the aorta and vena cava. The infection is usually restricted to these anatomic boundaries. In rare instances there may be spontaneous drainage through the flank, intraperitoneal perforation, or transdiaphragmatic spread.

I. Etiology

A. Primary perinephric abscess results from hematogenous dissemination of bacteria, most often *Staph. aureus*.

B. Secondary perinephric abscess refers to direct extension from infection in the renal cortex, collecting system, or pelvic fat. The infecting organism is a urinary tract pathogen, *E. coli, Proteus, Klebsiella* or *Pseudomonas*. The common settings are pyelonephritis associated with renal calculi or an obstructing lesion. Less often, the infection arises from suppurative pyelonephritis, renal carbuncle, infected renal cysts, or an extrarenal focus such as the colon.

II. Diagnosis

A. Clinical findings are a tender flank mass, fever, and pain. Pain is variable in location; it is usually in the flank but may occur anywhere between the diaphragm and the inguinal ligament. When the infection abuts on the psoas or lumbar muscles, there is accentuation of pain with lateral flexion of the trunk away from the abscess or with hyperextension of the thigh.

B. Laboratory findings are leukocytosis and, in cases of secondary pyelonephritis, pyuria and bacteriuria. The diagnosis should be suspected in any patient with symptoms of pyelonephritis who fails to defervesce after 4–6 days of appropriate antimicrobial drugs.

C. X-ray findings are

1. Perinephric mass.
2. Renal fixation with upright or inspiration-expiration films.
3. Absence of psoas margin, loss of renal outline, curvature of the lumbar spine with concavity toward the lesion, and renal displacement.
4. On the intravenous pyelogram: nonvisualization, delayed excretory pattern, and renal displacement or extrinsic compression of the collecting system. Occasionally there is extravasation of contrast material into the perinephric space.
5. Chest x-ray films may show diaphragmatic elevation, diaphragmatic fixation, or pleural effusion.
6. The two most useful roentgenographic clues in terms of frequency and specificity are the appearance of a **perirenal mass** and **renal fixation.**
7. The diagnosis is best established by ultrasound or CT scan.

III. Treatment

A. Antimicrobial selection. Metastatic abscesses are usually caused by *Staph. aureus*, and the drug of choice is a penicillinase-resistant penicillin (nafcillin or oxacillin) or a cephalosporin. With secondary perinephric abscesses, urine culture yields the responsible organism, providing a useful guide for the initial selection of antibiotics. For seriously ill patients with no established bacterial etiology, an aminoglycoside and a cephalosporin would be a logical combination.

B. Surgical procedure. Incision and drainage is required in all cases. When the patient is seriously ill, this procedure can be performed under local anesthesia. Percutaneous drainage can be attempted under ultrasound guidance. A nephrectomy is performed in the presence of extensive renal involvement, provided the contralateral kidney functions well and the patient can tolerate the procedure.

Postprostatectomy Infections

I. Bacteremia. Routine blood cultures performed shortly after prostatectomy are positive in 20–50% of patients. The patients at greatest risk are those with preoperative bacteriuria. The blood culture isolate is usually the same as the preoperative urine culture. Most bacteremic episodes are transient and self-limited; only 1–3 percent of patients have sustained bacteremia with signs of sepsis and it is this group that requires antibiotic therapy. Treatment is based on the sensitivities of the pathogen, usually a gram-negative rod.

II. Urologic sepsis. Significant postoperative febrile reactions (temperature greater than 38.5°C) occur in 10–30% of patients following prostatectomy, usually in the first

2–3 postoperative days or when the catheter is removed. Leukocytosis and bacteriuria are often associated findings. Sepsis is most common with open resection surgical complications (postoperative obstruction or urinary dysfunction) and prolonged indwelling catheters. Treatment is based on urine and blood cultures. Therapeutic recommendations for the severely ill in the absence of culture data are an aminoglycoside along with a cephalosporin, ampicillin, or antipseudomonad penicillin.

III. Postoperative bacteriuria. Significant bacteriuria is noted in 30–60% of patients following prostatectomy. Possible complications are bacteremia (3%), pyelonephritis epididymitis, and urethral stricture. A 10- to 14-day course of antimicrobial therapy is recommended when asymptomatic bacteriuria persists after catheter removal.

IV. Prevention. The use of prophylactic antimicrobial drugs for prostatectomy is controversial and the data regarding efficacy are conflicting. It is recommended that an attempt be made preoperatively to render the urine bacteria-free. If this cannot be achieved, the drug used preoperatively (selected according to susceptibility tests) is continued through the operative period. Another approach is not to use an intraoperative antimicrobial drug, but rather to attempt clearing of bacteriuria after removal of the catheter. There is little evidence that intraoperative antibiotics reduce septic complications.

Antimicrobial Usage in Common Genitourinary Procedures

I. Instrumentation. Prophylactic antimicrobials are unnecessary for instrumentation when there is no urinary tract infection. Indeed, bacteriuria represents a relative contraindication to instrumentation, and there should be an attempt to clear the infection before genitourinary manipulation. If the infection proves refractory, an appropriate antimicrobial agent can be continued through the procedure and for at least 1–2 days thereafter. Drug administration should provide effective blood levels during manipulation to prevent bacteremia. Selection of drugs is optimally based on a **recent** urine culture, since urinary tract pathogens in the susceptible host often change during the course of treatment. This recommendation obviously does not apply when the procedure is intended for selective urethral cultures for localization purposes. In this instance antimicrobial treatment is delayed until specimens have been collected.

II. Catheter and tube drainage. Bacteriuria almost invariably accompanies prolonged usage of foreign bodies extending from external sites to the urinary tract. This includes suprapubic drainage, nephrostomy drainage, ureteral catheters and indwelling bladder catheters. Colonization or infection usually occurs within 7–10 days. Sequential cultures, even in the absence of treatment, show periodic changes in the organism involved. Prophylactic antimicrobial therapy predisposes to colonization of the urinary tract with resistant forms. Recommendations for use of antimicrobial drugs in this setting are

- **A. Signs of systemic infection.** Parenteral antimicrobials are given to control sepsis and bacteremia. Choice of drug is based on recent urine culture. If this information is not available, select a broad-spectrum agent such as gentamicin. Therapy can be modified if the culture subsequently shows an organism sensitive to a less toxic drug such as ampicillin or cefazolin. Therapy is continued for 3 to 5 days after fever and toxicity have subsided. However, bacteriuria is likely to persist as long as the foreign body is present.
- **B. Persistent bacteriuria,** after removal of the drainage tube. Therapy for 10–14 days with an appropriate oral agent is usually adequate, unless there is an underlying lesion.
- **C.** Some urologists instill 50 ml of polymyxin and neomycin solution when urinary drainage tubes are removed to clear bacteriuria. This procedure is also used after instrumentation or single catheterization in order to clear any bacteria introduced into a previously sterile bladder. Efficacy of this practice is not established.

III. **Genitourinary surgical procedure.** Prophylactic antimicrobial drugs are not indicated for genitourinary surgery in the absence of infection. Operations involving an infected urinary tract pose a threat of bacteremia or wound sepsis, however. If bacteriuria cannot be cleared preoperatively, a parenteral antimicrobial drug should be given according to results of urine cultures. Oral therapy can be substituted when the patient is able to take oral feedings. Treatment is continued for 7–10 days.

IV. **Urologic injuries.** Blunt or penetrating trauma may result in renal hemorrhage or urinary extravasation. These complications pose a minimal threat of infection, and antimicrobial drugs are generally not indicated. Exceptions are those cases in which a urinary tract infection is present at the time of injury, or bacteriuria develops during the posttraumatic period. Urine cultures should be followed and bacteriuria treated according to susceptibility tests. Extravasations of infected urine often require drainage to prevent retroperitoneal cicatrization and ureteral obstruction.

V. GU patients with **valvular heart disease**—see section on antimicrobial prophylaxis (pp. 295–296).

VI. **Foley catheter care** (see pp. 314–315).

Renal Tuberculosis

I. **General principles.** Tuberculosis of the genitourinary system represents blood-borne disseminated disease, almost invariably from a primary focus in the lung. The initial renal lesion consists of multiple, bilateral **miliary tubercles,** which generally remain dormant for many years. The usual mechanism of progression is entrapment of excreted bacilli in the loops of Henle, followed by the formation of medullary tubercles, which then coalesce and eventually slough into a calyx. The lesion progressively enlarges to involve the entire lobule, or it may extend to other calyces. At this stage urography shows characteristic large, ragged **caliceal cavities,** often with **infundibular contractures.** Eventually the entire kidney is destroyed, transformed into a calcified, caseous mass ("putty kidney").

II. **Types of infection.** Repeated shedding of tubercle bacilli into the urinary tract causes **secondary lesions** in the ureters, bladder, epididymis, or prostate. More than 90% of patients with lower genitourinary tract tuberculosis have involvement of the renal parenchyma, although it may not be readily apparent.

A. **Ureter.** The initial lesion is a **stricture** at the ureterovesical junction or, less commonly, at the ureteropelvic junction. With progression, the pyelogram shows ureteral ulcerations, which have a ragged, motheaten appearance. These eventually fibrose, causing stricture formation and a shortened ureter. Both ulceration and strictures can result from "nonspecific urethritis," but with tuberculosis these lesions tend to be more extensive and have a predilection for the distal ureter. Concurrent areas of healing and stricture produce a characteristic **beaded** or **corkscrew** appearance.

B. **Bladder.** Implantation of tubercle bacilli into the urinary bladder initially causes patchy mucosal inflammation or irregular, superficial ulcerations; there may be a greenish gray exudate, which is seldom seen with other conditions. These lesions generally clear within 1 month of chemotherapy. Persistent infection results in a thick, fibrotic **contracted bladder,** which is noted in approximately 10% of patients. Small, irregular nodules (tubercles) can be seen in the bladder wall by cystoscopy. Vesicoureteral junction involvement may cause ureteral reflux or stenosis, which threatens renal parenchyma on the affected side.

C. **Prostate.** The prostate is infected via the prostatic urethra, which is erythematous, thickened, and eventually dilated. Cavities within the prostate coalesce and slough, and the gland becomes small, firm, and irregular. (Large prostatic nodules are seldom caused by tuberculosis.) Retrograde or voiding cystourethrograms frequently show prostatic cavities and dilated prostatic ducts. Biopsy evidence of **granulomatous prostatitis** is a nonspecific finding—3% of patients with prostatitis have such changes due to extravasation of prostatic fluid alone. **Caseous necrosis** with palisading of histiocytes is highly suggestive of tuberculosis, however. Acid-fast stains and cultures of the biopsy specimen establish the diagnosis.

D. **Epididymis.** Infection of the epididymis follows tuberculous prostatitis with extension along the ductus deferens. The typical lesion is a small, firm nodule or beading of the epididymis. Occasionally the entire epididymis is destroyed and replaced by a large, often tender, cold abscess. If the ductus deferens is obstructed, sterility can occur. Tubercles may be difficult to visualize; acid-fast stains or cultures are required to establish the diagnosis.

III. **Diagnosis**

A. The most frequent **symptoms** reflect lower urinary tract involvement—chronic dysuria, frequency, nocturia and urgency, gross hematuria, bloody ejaculate, and chronic epididymitis. In the late stages, contraction of the bladder and stricture formation result in pain on urination and the need to void every 15–30 minutes. Back, suprapubic, or abdominal pain is also common. Constitutional symptoms (fever, fatigue, and weight loss) are noted in 20–40% of patients. Many patients receive repeated courses of antibiotics for bacterial urinary tract infection before the diagnosis of tuberculosis is appreciated.

B. An intermediate-strength **PPD skin test** is nearly always positive. Due to the frequency of positive reactions in older patients, the skin is more helpful in establishing the diagnosis in children and young adults.

C. **Laboratory tests. Pyuria, proteinuria,** and/or **microscopic hematuria** are noted in 70–90% of patients. Most urine specimens have an **acid pH.** Genitourinary tuberculosis is suspected in any patient with unexplained pyuria, especially if there is a history of pulmonary tuberculosis. CBC and sedimentation rates are variable and nonspecific; renal function tests are usually normal.

D. **X-rays.** Chest x-ray films are entirely normal in 25–50% of cases. When abnormal, they may show active or old, stable pulmonary tuberculosis (especially apical scars or calcified granulomas). Renal roentgenograms (KUB and excretory urograms) are abnormal in 60–90% of cases. **Tomography** is especially useful for detecting amorphous calcifications and small, papillary cavities. CT scan also shows these findings. Although the disease is bilateral, progression is asymmetric, and detectable lesions are often unilateral. X-ray changes that specifically suggest urinary tuberculosis are as follows.

1. **Renal parenchyma and pelvis.** Single or multiple medullary cavities communicating with the collecting system; cicatricial changes of the calyces or renal pelvis; "moth-eaten" papillary tips; localized or diffuse parenchymal calcifications
2. **Ureter.** Long segments of ulcerations; multiple strictures; beaded, corkscrew, pipestem, or calcified ureter
3. **Bladder.** Contracted and thick-walled; irregular scarring

IV. **Bacteriology.** The diagnosis is established by cultivation of *Mycobacterium tuberculosis* from a urinary tract source, usually the urine. Although 24-hour urine collections were previously recommended, most authorities now prefer at least **three first-morning, voided, clean-catch specimens.** Acid-fast examination of urine is of limited value due to contamination by the saprophyte *M. smegmatus*. The usual pathogen is *M. tuberculosis*. Rare cases involving *M. kansasii* and *M. avium intracellulare* ("Batty bacillus") have been reported.

The diagnosis of genitourinary tuberculosis is assumed in **culture-negative** cases if one of the following criteria is met:

A. Characteristic lesions on excretory urogram or cystoscopy, associated with a positive culture from a nonurinary source.

B. Caseating granulomas or positive AFB stain in biopsy from a genitourinary source, in association with a reactive PPD skin test.

V. **Treatment**

A. **Medical therapy** has supplanted surgical intervention as the treatment of choice for tuberculosis of the genitourinary system. The usual regimen is isoniazid (INH) (300 mg/day) and rifampin (600 mg/day PO) for at least 9 months. Some authorities also give streptomycin (1 gm IM twice weekly) for the 1st 3 months. Recent studies have indicated that prolonged treatment with two drugs such as

INH and rifampin is sufficient for sensitive organisms. Agents to be used for resistant strains are ethambutol, 15 mg/kg/day; cycloserine, 10–20 mg/kg/day up to 1 gm/day PO in 2 doses; ethionamide, 15–30 mg/kg/day up to 1 gm PO in 2 doses; and pyrazinamide, 15–30 mg/kg/day PO up to 2 gm/day in 2–4 divided doses.

B. Surgical procedures. In choosing between surgical and medical therapy, it must be noted that bilateral disease is the rule and that nearly all cases respond well to medical treatment. When surgery is required, it is desirable to administer antituberculous drugs for 3 weeks to 3 months preoperatively.

Indications for a surgical procedure are as follows:

1. **Ureteral strictures** may require dilatation. If this fails, the involved segment is resected and the ureter is reanastomosed. Ureteral stricture may occur during or several years after therapy. Therefore, periodic intravenous pyelogram or ureteral calibration is recommended. Nephroureterectomy is indicated when there is nontuberculous pyonephrosis with unilateral renal destruction proximal to a ureteral stricture.
2. **Severe bladder contracture** may improve with incorporation of an intestinal loop to increase capacity.
3. **Nephrectomy** may be required for intractable pain; drug-resistant organisms; intolerance to drugs with no available alternative agents; relapse after adequate therapy due to renal abscess; or autonephrectomy with intractable hypertension.

VI. Follow-up studies

A. Urinalysis and culture for tuberculosis are performed every 6 months for 3 years and then annually for 2 additional years. Antituberculous drugs should be discontinued for 3 days prior to urine culture. Previous studies indicate that 90–95% of patients under treatment have sterile urine at 6 months. Relapses are rare and nearly always occur within 2 years of the initial treatment course. Such patients should be retreated according to the previous guidelines, with due attention to the sensitivity of the organism. A search for renal abscess should be undertaken.

B. Urography should be done at the time of the initial evaluation and repeated at 3, 6, 12, 18, 24, and 36 months. Retrograde studies may be required when the collecting system fails to visualize with intravenous pyelography. The purpose of these studies is to detect urethral strictures that may occur during the healthy phase.

VII. Contagious aspects. Tuberculosis restricted to the urinary tract presents a minimal contagion hazard in a hospitalized patient who is continent. Such patients require isolation only when they have active pulmonary tuberculosis. Household contacts, however, should have skin tests and x-ray examinations. Young children in the family are particularly at risk, since they may crawl around the bathroom floor. Cystoscopes used in patients with urinary tuberculosis should be immersed in 10% formalin for 15–30 minutes. Other instruments can be autoclaved.

6 Pulmonary Infections

Pneumonia

I. General principles. Pneumonia is the 5th ranking cause of death in the United States and accounts for approximately 10% of all hospitalizations. A heterogeneous array of microorganisms can infect the lung, but bacteria are responsible for most of the serious cases of acute pneumonia.

II. Clinical features. Cardinal features of **bacterial pneumonia** are chills, fever, pleuritic chest pain, cough, and purulent sputum production. Involvement of the lower lobes may produce referred pain to the abdomen and simulate intraabdominal sepsis. All cases of pneumonia are accompanied by a pulmonary infiltrate on chest x-ray. Although usually evident when the patient initially seeks medical attention, on rare occasions the roentgenographic findings may not become apparent for 1–2 days, when the patient is seen early in the course.

III. Microbiology. The selection of antimicrobial agents in bacterial pneumonia is remarkably simplified when the responsible pathogen is known. The usual approach to an etiologic diagnosis is culture of expectorated sputum. In spite of the time-honored respect paid to sputum cultures, however, it should be noted that these specimens are invariably contaminated by orophayngeal flora and are notoriously misleading. **Gram's stain of expectorated sputum** is probably more accurate than culture, but even this approach is problematic due to difficulties of interpretation and variations among observers.

A. Cultures of expectorated sputum become even more difficult to interpret when the specimen has been obtained after antimicrobial drugs have been started. Depending on the dose, duration, and spectrum of activity of the antimicrobial agent, many patients have upper airway colonization by resistant microoganisms. This results in "sputum superinfection," which is not to be confused with patient superinfection. The point is that the physician should not redirect treatment at each new bacteria or fungus that emerges in the expectorated specimen during antimicrobial therapy of pulmonary infections. Indeed, even the pretreatment specimen should be cautiously interpreted; the clinical setting and the Gram's-stained slide of sputum are the most helpful guides to the etiologic agent (Table 6-1).

B. Reliable specimens for cultures in pulmonary infections are those devoid of oropharyngeal contamination. By this criterion, the usefulness of sputum is very low, but careful processing of such specimens, especially by Gram's stain, may prove helpful. (See Chap. 15 for details.) Blood specimens and pleural fluid, if present, should be obtained for culture in all cases of pneumonia prior to institution of antimicrobial treatment. Transtracheal aspiration provides reliable specimens in cases in which the infection is restricted to the pulmonary parenchyma. Being an invasive procedure with occasional serious complications, it should be reserved for selected patients. (See Chap. 15)

IV. Diagnosis. The pathogens can be predicted to some degree by age of the patient, history, clinical setting, and changes in x-ray films (see Table 6-1).

A. Community-acquired pneumonia in adults over 35 is usually due to *Streptococcus pneumoniae*. Aspiration pneumonia involving oral anaerobic bacteria is also

Table 6-1. Anticipated pulmonary pathogens according to type of infection and clinical setting

Type of infection	Clinical setting	Principal pathogens
Pneumonitis	Age	
	Infant	*Chlamydia trachomatis*, CMV *Escherichia coli*, *Staphylococcus aureus*, group B *Streptococcus*
	3 mos–5 yr	Viruses, *Streptococcus pneumoniae*, *Hemophilus influenzae*
	5–35 yr	*Mycoplasma pneumoniae*, *Staph. aureus*, viruses, *Strep. pneumoniae*
	>35 yr	*Strep. pneumoniae; H. influenzae; Legionella*
	Influenza—superinfection	*Strep. pneumoniae*, *Staph. aureus*
	Hospital-acquired	*Klebsiella* sp., other aerobic GNB,[a] *Staph. aureus*, *Strep. pneumoniae*, anaerobic bacteria, *Legionella*
	Aspiration	
	Community-acquired	Anaerobic bacteria[b]
	Hospital-acquired	Anaerobic bacteria,[b] aerobic GNB,[a] *Staph. aureus* (most cases involve combinations of the above bacteria)
	Tracheostomy	Aerobic GNB,[a] *Staph. aureus*
	Compromised host	*Strep. pneumoniae*, aerobic GNB,[a] *Staph. aureus;* opportunistic fungi—*Aspergillus*, Phycomycetes, *Candida albicans; Pneumocystis carinii; Toxoplasma; Nocardia;* viruses—CMV, herpes; Legionella
	Chronic	Pathogenic fungi,[c] tuberculosis, "organizing pneumonia," anaerobic bacteria[b]
Bronchitis	No chronic lung disease	Virus
	Exacerbation of chronic bronchitis	*H. influenzae*, *Strep. pneumoniae*
	Tracheostomy	Aerobic GNB[a], *Staph. aureus;* anaerobic bacteria
Lung abscess		Anaerobic bacteria[b] Other considerations: tuberculosis, atypical mycobacteria, pathogenic fungi;[c] *Pseudomonas aeruginosa*, *Klebsiella*, *Staph. aureus; E. histolytica*
Empyema	Associated with pneumonia	
	Children and young adults	*Staph. aureus*, less commonly *H. influenzae*, *Strep. pneumoniae*, *Strep. pyogenes*
	Adults	Anaerobes, *Strep. pneumoniae*
	Postthoracotomy	*Staph. aureus*, aerobic GNB[a]
	Penetrating chest wound	*Staph. aureus*, aerobic GNB[a]
	Subdiaphragmatic abscess	Anaerobes (including *B. fragilis*) plus aerobic GNB[a]

[a]Aerobic GNB (gram-negative bacteria) include *Klebsiella*, *E. coli*, *Proteus*, *Pseudomonas aeruginosa*, etc.
[b]Principal anaerobic bacteria in pulmonary infections are *Peptostreptococcus*, *Fusobacterium nucleatum*, and *Bacteroides melaninogenicus*.
[c]Pathogenic fungi include *Blastomyces*, *Coccidioides*, and *Histoplasma*.

common in this age group; but differentiation from pneumococcal pneumonia is generally not critical, since penicillin is the agent of choice for both conditions. Other bacteria, such as *Staphylococcus aureus, Legionella, Hemophilus influenzae,* and *Klebsiella,* account for 10–20% of cases of bacterial pneumonia in adults older than 35 with community-acquired disease. The most common treatable cause of pneumonia in persons aged 5–35 years is *Mycoplasma pneumoniae.* Erythromycin and tetracycline are the preferred agents; penicillins and cephalosporins are not effective against this organism. Neonates often have pneumonia involving group B streptococci, *Staph. aureus,* or *Escherichia coli.* Young children, 3 months to 4 years old, are vulnerable to pneumonia with *Strep. pneumoniae, Staph. aureus, H. influenzae,* and *Strep. pyogenes,* but most lower respiratory infections in this age group are viral.

B. Hospital-acquired* pneumonia occurs in 1–2% of all patients admitted to the hospital (see pp. 315–318). Surgical patients are at particular risk, especially those who have a thoracic surgical procedure, atelectasis, tracheostomy, endotracheal intubation, and compromised consciousness. The bacteriology of hospital-acquired pneumonia is quite different from that acquired in the community. The differences are best explained by the high rate of colonization of the oropharynx by gram-negative bacilli during hospitalization. The incidence of colonization by these organisms can be correlated with the severity of underlying diseases and prior antimicrobial treatment.

Major pathogens are aerobic gram-negative bacilli (especially *Pseudomonas* and *Klebsiella*) and *Staph. aureus*; less frequent are *Strep. pneumoniae* and anaerobic bacteria. Many cases involve multiple potential pathogens. Empiric treatment for the very ill patient should take into account this diverse pattern. If it is necessary to initiate antimicrobial therapy before the results of cultures are known, the combinations likely to be effective are an aminoglycoside (gentamicin, tobramycin, or amikacin) plus either a cephalosporin (cephalothin, cefazolin, cefamandole, or a third generation cephalosporin) or clindamycin.

C. An **immunocompromised host** can develop pneumonia related to a vast array of microbes, including bacteria (*Strep. pneumoniae, Staph. aureus,* aerobic gram-negative bacilli, anaerobic bacteria); opportunistic fungi (especially aspergillus, phycomyces, *Candida*); viruses (Cytomegalovirus [CMV], herpes); *Nocardia; Pneumocystis carinii; Toxoplasma;* and *Mycobacterium tuberculosis.* Noninfectious conditions, such as radiation pneumonitis, should be considered. In addition, patients with lymphoma or Hodgkin's disease often have pulmonary involvement, which may simulate pneumonitis by clinical findings and chest x-ray. Empiric treatment of pneumonia in the compromised host is extremely difficult due to the multiplicity of likely pathogens and the toxicity of therapeutic agents. Whenever possible, make a specific, etiologic diagnosis. The following plan is advised:

1. Obtain **expectorated sputum** for Gram's stain, acid-fast bacterial (AFB) staining, and potassium hydroxide (KOH) preparation for fungi. Specimens should be cultured for routine bacteria, fungi, and mycobacteria. **Note:** A positive AFB stain is considered diagnostic and means that treatment for *M. tuberculosis* should be initiated. Typical hyphae are seldom seen in pulmonary infections involving *Aspergillus* or Zygomycetes; when these forms are seen, and the clinical findings are consistent, amphotericin B treatment should be started. The recovery of *Candida* in expectorated sputum is of minimal diagnostic value, since this organism commonly colonizes the upper airways in sick patients.
2. A **transtracheal aspiration** should be performed, if the expectorated sputum is not diagnostic. Patients with a bleeding diathesis due to thrombocytopenia can have this corrected with packed platelet transfusions just prior to the procedure. Gram's stain, AFB stain, KOH preparation, and appropriate cul-

*An infection that is related to hospitalization. As a general rule, community-acquired pneumonia becomes clinically apparent within 72 hours of admission; all infections after 72 hours are considered to be acquired in the hospital.

tures are performed. **Note:** A transtracheal aspirate that yields no bacteria virtually eliminates the possibility of bacterial infection, provided there has been no antecedent antimicrobial treatment. Transtracheal aspirates infrequently yield *Aspergillus* or *Nocardia* even with documented pulmonary infections involving these organisms; and the recovery of *Candida* in transtracheal aspirates cannot be interpreted as diagnostic, since this organism may colonize the trachea and bronchi.

3. **Transthoracic needle aspiration** is advocated in cases in which the expectorated sputum and transtracheal aspirate are negative. Thrombocytopenia may be corrected with packed platelets to permit this procedure. The specimen should have a Gram's stain, methenamine silver stain (which detects *P. carinii* as well as fungi), and AFB stain, and should be cultured for aerobic and anaerobic bacteria, fungi, and mycobacteria.
4. **Lung biopsy** is generally reserved for cases that have been given a negative evaluation by the previous tests. An exception is in lymphoma or Hodgkins's disease, which frequently involves the pulmonary parenchyma; it may be prudent to bypass the transtracheal aspiration in order to obtain a tissue diagnosis in these cases. The method of biopsy varies at different centers depending on experience and expertise. Possibilities include fiberoptic bronchoscopy biopsy and open thoracotomy. The best yield for a specific diagnosis is achieved with open thoracotomy.

V. **Treatment.** Since many pathogens can cause pneumonia, the range of drugs for therapy is necessarily broad and diverse (Table 6-2). Initially, the pathogen is suspected from clues provided by the history, physical examination, age of the patient, and epidemiologic setting. Preliminary lab studies, such as a CBC with differential, sputum examination, and roentgenograms, give further information. The antimicrobial agent can now be selected with a high degree of confidence that the offending pathogen will be covered.

Aspiration Pneumonia

I. **General principles.** The tracheobronchial tree is normally protected from aspiration by glottic closure, cough reflex, and the gastrocardiac sphincter. Compromise of these defense mechanisms promotes abnormal entry of oropharyngeal secretions, gastric contents, or exogenous food and fluids into the lower respiratory passages. The consequences of aspiration depend on the composition and volume of the inoculum.

II. **Predisposing causes of aspiration**

A. Reduced levels of consciousness, e.g., anesthesia, central nervous system diseases, alcoholism, drug addiction, seizure disorder
B. Dysphagia from esophageal disease or neurologic disorders
C. Nasogastric feeding tubes
D. Protracted vomiting
E. Local anesthesia of upper airways
F. Tracheostomy or endotracheal intubation

III. **Preventive measures**

A. **Positioning** of susceptible patients
   1. Debilitated patients—elevate the head of the bed.
   2. Unconscious patients—elevate the foot of the bed.

B. **Nasogastric tubes.** Nasogastric tubes must function without coiling or obstruction. Feeding should be done slowly, without excessive volumes.

C. **Precautions** for patients undergoing **general anesthesia**
   1. Nothing by mouth for 24 hours or preoperative gastric aspiration
   2. Anesthesia given with a cuffed endotracheal tube
   3. For emergency procedures:
      a. Use wide-gauge gastric emptying tube before induction or after intubation, with cuff inflated

Table 6-2. Preferred antibiotics for pulmonary infections

Organism	Agent[a]	Alternatives (comments)
Bacteria		
Streptococcus pneumoniae	Penicillin	Cephalosporins Ampicillin Chloramphenicol Tetracycline Erythromycin Clindamycin
Staphylococcus aureus		
Meth-sensitive	Penicillinase-resistant penicillins	Cephalosporins (1st or 2nd generation) Clindamycin Vancomycin
Meth-resistant	Vancomycin	Vancomycin + rifampin, vancomycin + gentamicin
Klebsiella[b]	Aminoglycoside + cephalosporin	Cephalosporin
Pseudomonas[b]	Aminoglycoside + antipseudomonad penicillin	
GNB (other)[b]	Aminoglycoside + cephalosporin or broad spectrum penicillin	
Hemophilus influenzae[b]	Ampicillin or cefamandole	Tetracycline Chloramphenicol Third generation cephalosporin
Anaerobes	Penicillin or clindamycin	Tetracycline Cephalosporin Chloramphenicol
Nocardia	Sulfonamides	Sulfamethoxazole/trimethoprim Minocycline
Legionella	Erythromycin	Erythromycin + rifampin
Mycoplasma	Erythromycin or tetracycline	
Mycobacterium tuberculosis	INH + rifampin	INH + ethambutol or streptomycin
Fungi	Amphotericin B	Amphotericin B + 5FC for *Candida* or invasive aspergillosis (histoplasmosis and coccidioidomycosis confined to the lung is usually not treated)
Viruses		
Herpes simplex	Acyclovir	
Influenza A	Amantadine	
Pneumocystis carinii	Sulfamethoxazole/trimethoprim	Pentamadine

[a]Penicillin: Ampicillin and carbenicillin are considered equally effective. Carbenicillin: Ticarcillin, piperacillin, mezlocillin, and azlocillin are considered equally effective; in vitro testing facilitates choice. Cephalosporin: In vitro testing determines choice. Aminoglycoside: In vitro testing facilitates choice between tobramycin, gentamicin, and amikacin.
[b]GNB (gram-negative bacteria): In vitro testing required.

Table 6-3. Aspiration syndromes according to the composition of the inoculum

Inoculum	Pulmonary consequences	Therapy
Gastric acid	Chemical pneumonitis	Correction of hypoxia Tracheal suction IV fluids Corticosteroids
Pathogenic bacteria	Bacterial infection	Antimicrobials
Inert fluids (large volumes)	Mechanical obstruction	Tracheal suction
Foreign bodies	Early—mechanical obstruction	Extraction of foreign body
	Late—mechanical obstruction and bacterial infection	Extraction of foreign body and antimicrobials

b. Maintain patient in Trendelenburg or lateral recumbent position until gastric aspiration is performed
c. Induce anesthesia rapidly
d. Oral antacids before obstetric deliveries are advocated by some authorities

4. Extubation when patient is awake, after tracheal suction

IV. **Aspiration syndromes.** The pulmonary complications of aspiration may be classified according to the composition of the inoculum (Table 6-3). This classification delineates the pathophysiologic mechanism and the therapeutic approach.

A. **Gastric acid aspiration**

1. **Pathophysiology.** Experiments in animals have shown that **pH** and **volume** are the critical factors. Intratracheal instillation of sterile fluid with a pH of > 2.5 produces only transient hypoxia. A pH of < 2.5 at volumes of 1–4 ml/kg body weight causes massive accumulation of hemorrhagic fluid in alveolar spaces, intrapulmonary shunting, hypoxia, and reduced pulmonary compliance. This reaction is the equivalent of a **flash burn of the lung,** since it represents an immediate surface response to a chemical insult.
2. **Clinical features.** The aspiratory event, usually apparent because of the large volumes involved, is followed within 2 hours by acute dyspnea, which is invariably associated with a pulmonary infiltrate on chest x-ray. The most common changes seen on the x-ray film are mottled densities in one or both lower lobes. Patients frequently are wheezing, and most have frothy, hemorrhagic, nonpurulent sputum. About one-third are hypotensive, and 10% develop clinical shock. Fever is absent or low-grade. Blood gas determination shows hypoxia with abnormal or low PCO_2, indicating intrapulmonary shunting. Pulmonary function tests show reduced compliance or "stiff lungs." Bacteria play no role in the initial events; however, the patients are predisposed to infection during the subsequent course due to the respiratory supportive measures often required (e.g., endotracheal intubation and tracheostomy) and because the acid-injured lung is particularly susceptible to bacterial challenge.
3. **Treatment**
   a. **Ventilatory support** is the most important immediate therapeutic maneuver. Intubation or tracheostomy may be necessary. Monitoring of blood gases is crucial for optimal management.
   b. **Repeated tracheal suctioning** is often necessary to maintain a clear airway—initially to remove the aspirate and subsequently to clear edematous fluid.
   c. **IV fluids** in the form of colloid are necessary to support blood pressure in

hypotensive patients and may reduce vascular permeability changes. X-ray films showing pulmonary edema and frothy sputum may suggest congestive heart failure, but the patient is actually depleted of intravascular volume because of fluid aggregation in the lung. The amount of fluid to be infused depends on measurements of arterial and central venous pressures.

d. **Systemic corticosteroids** may have beneficial effects when administered within minutes or a few hours of aspiration; they are virtually useless if there is a delay of 12 hours or more. The purpose is to reduce capillary permeability and to reverse bronchospasm. Recommended doses are the equivalent of 600–1,600 mg cortisone daily for 2 days (prednisone, 25–60 mg/day, in 3 divided doses). We do not recommend corticosteroids unless there are initial signs of adverse effects, i.e., bronchospasm or wheezing. Vomiting and aspiration are common events, whereas only rare patients develop the clinical signs of chemical pneumonitis. Hence, it is not justifiable to expose all patients who aspirate to corticosteroids.

e. **Antimicrobial agents** are indicated at a later time only when there is subsequent evidence of infection, i.e., significant fever, progressive infiltrates on chest x-ray, and purulent sputum. Likely pathogens are *Staph. aureus*, gram-negative bacilli, and anaerobic bacteria.

f. Intratracheal instillation of alkaline agents is not advocated, since aspirated acid is quickly neutralized by the tracheobronchial secretions. For this reason tracheal aspiration for pH measurement also is futile. A gastric aspirate, vomitus, or fresh fluid in the mouth or oropharynx can be used for pH determinations.

g. Pulmonary lavage is not recommended, since the full extent of injury already has occurred by the time the diagnosis is recognized.

B. **Bacterial infection.** Infection may follow aspiration, since oropharyngeal secretions contain potentially pathogenic microorganisms as part of the normal flora.

1. **Clinical features.** Bacterial pneumonia following aspiration is a less fulminant process than acid pneumonitis, and the actual episode of aspiration is seldom observed. The diagnosis, however, is suspected when **typical symptoms** of fever and purulent sputum develop in a **susceptible host,** who has roentgenographic changes in a **dependent pulmonary segment.** The usual setting is in a patient with compromised consciousness or dysphagia. The involved pulmonary segments are the lower lobes, which are dependent in the upright position, and the superior segments of the lower lobes or posterior segments of the upper lobes, which are dependent in the supine position. Initially there is pneumonitis, but the infection may progress to abscess formation or empyema after 1–2 weeks. Thus, the presenting x-ray findings depend on the time in the natural history of the disease.

2. **Bacteriology.** The usual pathogens in community-acquired aspiration pneumonia are anaerobic bacteria, which are the major constituents of the oropharyngeal flora—principally, *Fusobacterium nucleatum, Bacteroides melaninogenicus,* and *Peptostreptococcus.* Hospitalized patients are likely to have colonization of the upper airway with enteric gram-negative bacilli, *Pseudomonas,* or *Staph. aureus.* These organisms assume pathogenic significance, along with the anaerobes, in hospital-acquired aspiration pneumonia.

3. **Treatment.** In the initial period before bacteriologic results are available, treatment is based on predicted pathogens. Establishment of the pathogens in such cases requires a specimen source devoid of oropharyngeal contaminants, i.e., blood culture, transtracheal aspirate, or empyema fluid. Expectorated sputum culture is not helpful in evaluating these cases.

   a. Predicted pathogens in community-acquired cases are penicillin-sensitive anaerobes that normally colonize the oropharynx. Suggested treatment is 500,000 to 1 million units of aqueous penicillin G q4–6h depending on the severity of the symptoms. When fever and toxicity subside, oral penicillin is continued to complete a 7–10-day course.

b. Predicted pathogens in hospital-acquired cases are gram-negative bacilli, *Staph. aureus*, and anaerobes. Recommended antibiotics are an aminoglycoside—gentamicin, tobramycin, or amikacin—in combination with a cephalosporin, clindamycin, or a penicillinase-resistant penicillin (nafcillin or oxacillin).

C. Aspiration of inert fluids. Patients may aspirate liquids that have no inherent toxic effect on the lung but can produce acute symptoms by airway obstruction. Examples include saline, water, gastric secretions (with a pH >2.5), nasogastric feedings, and barium. In most instances there is the combination of large volume aspiration and a host with a compromised cough reflex. Therapy consists of immediate tracheal suction. In the absence of a pulmonary infiltrate on chest x-ray, no further treatment is indicated.

D. Foreign body aspiration. Aspiration of particulate material causes variable degrees of respiratory obstruction depending on the relative size of the object and the caliber of the tracheobronchial tree. Most cases involve children 1–3 years old, and the usual foreign bodies are peanuts, other vegetable particles, inorganic material, and teeth. Adults are more likely to aspirate particles of meat.

1. **Clinical features.** Relatively large particles may lodge in the larynx or trachea causing sudden respiratory distress, aphonia, cyanosis, and rapid death. In adults this often follows aspiration of large chunks of meat at a restaurant, a syndrome sometimes referred to as the "café coronary." Smaller objects reach peripheral airways causing complete or partial obstruction. The initial symptom is cough due to bronchial irritation. When major bronchi are involved, there may be severe dyspnea, cyanosis, wheezing, chest pain, nausea and vomiting. Chest x-rays initially show atelectasis or obstructive emphysema. Expiration films are especially helpful in detecting the latter lesion. The objects most commonly aspirated are not radiopaque.

   Bacterial infection often follows, if the particulate matter is not removed from the tracheobronchial tree within 1–2 weeks. Types of infectious complications include pneumonitis (often recurrent), bronchiectasis, lung abscess and empyema. The usual pathogens are penicillin-sensitive oropharyngeal bacteria, which are probably aspirated and cleared by all persons, but which, in these cases, produce infection at a susceptible nidus.

2. **Treatment.** The usual method to remove retained particulate matter in the tracheobronchial tree is with the Jackson bronchoscope; occasional success has been reported with the fiberoptic bronchoscope. On rare occasions, a thoracotomy is required.

E. Approach to the patient who has been observed to aspirate

Aspiration is a relatively common event. Normal persons aspirate oropharyngeal secretions during sleep, and 10–15% of patients undergoing general anesthesia aspirate gastric contents. In most instances the inoculum is cleared by physiologic defense mechanisms of the lung, and there are no sequelae. On those occasions when a patient is observed to aspirate relatively large volumes, the following treatment measures should be instituted.

1. Patients who aspirate large volumes of liquids will develop respiratory distress if there is no effective cough reflex. This is most likely to occur with nasogastric feedings to unconscious patients and with oral or nasogastric feedings to those with neurologic deficits. Treatment consists of immediate tracheal suction. Subsequent x-ray films are generally clear, and no additional therapy is necessary except for precautions to avoid another episode.
2. Precipitous respiratory distress may be caused by aspiration of relatively small volumes of gastric acid. But with acid pneumonitis, symptoms are always associated with a pulmonary infiltrate on chest x-ray; wheezing and frothy sputum are additional suggestive features. The pH of the inoculum is a critical factor and may be tested by analysis of a gastric aspirate or vomitus. A pH of <2.5 is consistent with chemical pneumonitis. Patients who conform to this pattern should be suctioned and given ventilatory support, IV colloids, and corticosteroids.
3. Aspiration of oropharyngeal or gastric bacteria may eventually produce bac-

terial pneumonitis. However, routine use of antimicrobials represents **over-treatment** of a substantial portion of patients and predisposes to infection by resistant microorganisms. It is recommended that antibiotics be reserved for patients who subsequently develop clinical evidence of bacterial pneumonitis, including fever, increased sputum production, elevated WBC, and chest x-ray changes.

4. Patients with no respiratory distress nor any subsequent pulmonary infiltrate require no treatment other than measures directed at preventing future episodes.

Lung Abscess

I. **General principles.** Pyogenic lung abscesses are traditionally classified by three criteria and are
   A. **Acute** or **chronic** on the basis of the duration of symptoms preceding presentation, the usual dividing line being 4–6 weeks.
   B. **Primary** or **secondary** depending on the presence of an underlying pulmonary lesion.
   C. **Specific** or **nonspecific** according to cultivation of a likely pathogen with aerobic cultures of expectorated sputum.

   These distinctions are arbitrary and are not particularly helpful in the approach to individual patients.

II. **Pathophysiology.** Most lung abscesses result from the aspiration of oropharyngeal bacteria. Common features are an associated condition causing compromised consciousness or dysphagia, infection in a dependent pulmonary segment, and periodontal infection. Less common predisposing causes are bronchiectasis, bronchial obstruction, pulmonary malignancy, bland pulmonary infarction, and septic embolization. No underlying conditions are apparent in about 15% of cases.

III. **Clinical features.** Symptoms usually begin **insidiously** and are present for a period of several days or weeks before the patient seeks medical attention. Nearly all patients have **fever, leukocytosis,** and **purulent sputum** production. Additional findings are pleuritic chest pain, anemia, and weight loss. Approximately 50% of patients with anaerobic abscesses have foul-smelling expectorations. A less common presentation is acute pneumonitis followed by excavation and the appearance of an air-fluid level on chest x-ray.

IV. **Microbiology.** The bacteriology of lung abscess usually reflects the flora of the upper respiratory passages. Anaerobic bacteria such as *F. nucleatum*, *B. melaninogenicus*, and/or *Peptostreptococcus* are present in 90% of cases. These cases were previously classified as "nonspecific lung abscess" due to a failure to understand the etiologic mechanisms. Pathogens less frequently causing lung abscess are *Staph. aureus*, *Klebsiella*, *Strep. pyogenes*, *Nocardia*, *Pseudomonas pseudomallei*, *Pseudomonas aeruginosa*, other gram-negative bacteria (GNB), and *Entamoeba*.

V. **Diagnosis**
   A. **Bacteriology studies.** Culture of expectorated sputum is unacceptable as a means of determining the bacteriology of most lung abscesses. Bronchoscopy aspirates collected by the usual techniques are also of little value, since the bronchoscope introduces oral flora into the trachea during passage through the upper airways. An accurate bacteriologic diagnosis requires careful aerobic and anaerobic culture of a specimen that is devoid of oropharyngeal contamination, i.e., empyema fluid, transtracheal aspirate, or percutaneous lung aspirate. These specimens must be obtained before the institution of antimicrobial treatment. A **presumptive diagnosis of anaerobic lung abscess** may be made if there are **putrid expectorations** and other **typical clinical findings.** Aerobic pathogens are suspected if the course is acute and the sputum culture **and Gram's stain** reveal a specific pathogen in large numbers, e.g., staphylococci or *Klebsiella*.
   B. **Bronchoscopy.** Routine bronchoscopy in all cases of lung abscess had been recommended in the past to facilitate drainage and to detect underlying lesions such

as carcinoma or foreign body. More recently, bronchoscopy has been reserved for cases in which there is suboptimal response to antimicrobials or the likelihood of an underlying lesion.

C. Differential diagnosis. The differential diagnosis of an air-fluid level on chest x-ray is fungal infection, cavitating malignancy (with or without superimposed infection), Wegener's granulomatosis, tuberculosis, a thin-walled cyst or bulla that contains fluid, and loculated empyema. Nonpyogenic abscess or an underlying condition should be looked for when there are atypical findings: an edentulous patient, presence of hilar adenopathy, lack of fever or purulent sputum, or location of abscess in the apex or the anterior segment of an upper lobe. The diagnostic approach should include cytology studies, bronchoscopy, evaluation for tuberculosis and fungal infection, and review of previous chest x-rays.

VI. Treatment

A. Medical

1. Pulmonary abscesses involving anaerobes:

   Penicillin G in a total IV dose of 4–10 million units/day

   Alternative regimens for patients with penicillin allergy:

Clindamycin	300–600 mg IV q8h
Cefazolin	500 mg–1 gm IM or IV q8h

   Parenteral therapy is continued until the patient is afebrile and subjectively improved. Treatment should then be continued with an oral agent (penicillin G, penicillin V, clindamycin, or tetracycline), until the chest x-ray shows complete resolution or a small stable residual scar. In most cases this requires a total of 6–12 weeks. If treatment is discontinued before closure of the cavity, there is a high incidence of relapse.
2. Lung abscess due to other bacteria. Treat in a similar fashion using appropriate antimicrobials, e.g., for *Staph. aureus*, penicillinase-resistant penicillin or cephalosporin; for *Klebsiella*, cephalosporin with or without gentamicin, depending on susceptibility tests.
3. Empiric treatment for fulminant cases with no reliable specimens to document the bacterial etiology:

   Clindamycin **plus** gentamicin

   or

   Cefazolin **plus** gentamicin
4. **Postural drainage.** An important adjunctive measure (Table 6-4).

B. Surgical

Surgical treatment is seldom indicated for primary lung abscess, since nearly all patients respond to adequate medical treatment. Moreover, an operation may cause spillage of abscess contents into other bronchial segments, resulting in disseminated infection or acute bronchial obstruction.

Indications for surgical procedure:

1. Failure to respond to intensive antimicrobial therapy.
   a. Persistent sepsis. Most patients receiving appropriate antibiotics become afebrile within 7–14 days. By 5–7 days the temperature should at least be declining and the patient subjectively improved. If this is not achieved, the patient should undergo bronchoscopy. Possible explanations are inappropriate antimicrobial therapy, formation of empyema, nonbacterial disease, or an obstructing lesion. A surgical procedure (external drainage or resection) should be considered if there is no response following an attempt to drain by bronchoscopy.
   b. Failure of cavity closure by 4–6 weeks was once regarded as an indication for a surgical procedure. However, most cavities eventually close with extended courses of appropriate antibiotics. Occasional cases resolve clinically, leaving a thin-walled cavity. Resection would be indicated only if the cavity became the site of recurrent infection rather than true relapse.
2. Suspected underlying neoplasm. A surgical procedure generally can be de-

Table 6-4. Postural drainage positions

Pulmonary segment	Position
Upper Lobes	
Apical segments	Sitting position at 45°
Right, posterior segment	Prone, with right arm over pillow (one-quarter body turn)
Left, posterior segment	Prone, with left arm over pillow (one-quarter body turn) and shoulders slightly elevated.
Anterior segments	Supine
Lingula	Supine, with quarter turn to right and 12-inch elevation of hip (pillows under left hip)
Right Middle Lobe	Supine, with quarter turn to left and 12-inch elevation of hip (pillows under right hip)
Lower Lobes	
Superior segments	Prone, with pillow under abdomen
Anterior basal segments	Supine, with 18-inch elevation of hip
Posterior basal segments	Prone, with 18-inch elevation of hip
Left lateral basal segment	Right lateral decubitus with 18-inch elevation of hip
Right lateral basal segment	Left lateral decubitus with 18-inch elevation of hip

ferred until toxicity subsides, since the delay incurs minimal risk in terms of tumor progression. An exception to this approach is an abscess behind a totally obstructed bronchus.

3. Uncontrollable life-threatening hemoptysis.
4. An associated empyema (which should be drained).

Empyema

I. **General principles.** Empyema classically means "pleural pus," but a more practical definition is **infected pleural exudate.** There are three phases, which merge indistinguishably; variations in the time frame in this sequence of events account for variation in the findings and dictate the therapeutic approach. Initially there is the **exudative phase,** with thin fluid containing relatively few leukocytes. The lung at this stage is readily reexpanded. Next is the **fibropurulent stage,** with increasing polymorphonuclear cells and fibrin. During this phase there is a progressive tendency toward adhesions with loculation of fluid, a limiting membrane, and fixation of the lung. In the final, **organizing, stage** an inelastic membrane forms ("pleural peel"), and the lung becomes more completely fixed.

II. **Etiology**

A. **Pneumonic infection** is the most common precursor of empyema. Pleural involvement may result from direct extension through the alveolar spaces, bronchopleural fistula, or rupture of an abscess. In adults the infecting flora is usually complex, with multiple bacterial species.

1. **Seventy percent of cases** involve anaerobes (especially *F. nucleatum*, *B. melaninogenicus*, and *Peptostreptococcus*), and about one-half of these harbor aerobes as well (especially gram-negative bacilli and *Staph. aureus*). These conclusions are based on studies of empyema fluid cultured with optimal techniques prior to the initiation of antibiotic therapy. Once antibiotics are given, there may be rapid changes in the cultivable flora.

2. **Thirty percent of cases** are caused by a single bacterial species, usually pneumococci, *Staph. aureus*, *Strep. pyogenes*, or *Klebsiella*.
3. **In children** the most common pathogen is *Staph. aureus*, often following ruptured pneumatoceles and causing a pyopneumothorax.

B. **Postsurgical empyema** may complicate any thoracotomy procedure but is most likely to follow pulmonary resection in inflammatory conditions. The usual mechanism is (1) an infected or inadequately closed bronchial stump, followed by formation of a bronchopleural fistula; or (2) contaminated pleural space, with or without secondary rupture through the bronchus. The dominant pathogens are *Staph. aureus* and gram-negative bacilli. Preventive measures with thoracotomy procedures when the risk of infection appears high include
   1. Irrigation of the pleural space with antimicrobials before closure
   2. Pleural space drainage tube left in place (this is standard procedure with lobectomy but is not generally done with pneumonectomy unless the risk of empyema appears high)
   3. Postoperative systemic antibiotics

C. **Posttraumatic empyema** is associated with a hemothorax in which the infection develops within a susceptible nidus—the pleural clot. Reports of wartime injuries indicate that 10–25% of penetrating thoracic injuries are complicated by empyema. Infection may not become apparent for several days or even weeks; the bacteria are implanted with the original injury or with subsequent drainage procedures. Usual pathogens are *Staph. aureus* or aerobic gram-negative bacilli.

D. **Transdiaphragmatic spread** from intraabdominal suppuration, especially subphrenic abscesses. Most cases involve multiple bacteria derived from the intestinal tract, including both coliforms and anaerobes. Pyogenic or amebic liver abscesses also involve the pleural space, but usually in the form of a sterile effusion. Less commonly, a hepatic abscess ruptures through the diaphragm, resulting in an empyema.

E. **Tuberculosis.** (See Tuberculous pleural effusion, p. 148.)

F. **Miscellaneous causes** include ruptured esophagus, pleural seeding following septicemia, rupture of a paravertebral abscess, and extension from mediastinitis.

III. Diagnosis

A. The **x-ray picture** during the exudative phase generally shows pleural effusions in the posterior lateral gutter, which gravitate on lateral decubitus films. The appearance of a blunted costophrenic angle indicates the presence of at least 300–500 ml. In later stages empyema fluid tends to loculate and is less likely to gravitate on lateral decubitus films. Gas in the pleural space indicates a bronchopleural fistula, pneumothorax (spontaneous or after thoracentesis), or infection involving gas-producing bacteria.

B. **Thoracentesis** is indicated for all patients with undiagnosed pleural effusions. This procedure establishes the diagnosis, provides a guide to chemotherapy, and gives crucial information regarding the type of drainage procedure required. Occasionally, routine thoracentesis is unproductive, especially with small effusions or loculated pockets. Small effusions that gravitate can be tapped by needle aspiration from below, with the patient in the lateral decubitus position across two gurneys. Loculated effusions may require a #14 needle and roentgenographic markers, fluoroscopy, or ultrasound.

C. The **diagnosis of pleural effusions** is based on fluid analysis and associated clinical findings (see Table 6-5).

D. **Bronchopleural fistula formation** is indicated by bubbling of suction drainage tubes, bronchography, or a sonogram with contrast material or with methylene blue injected into the pleural space, followed by sputum analysis.

IV. Management

A. **Medical.** Systemic antimicrobials are given to treat the associated parenchymal infections, to facilitate healing of a bronchopleural fistula, to eliminate bacteria from the pleural space (pleural penetration for most agents is good), and to prevent cellulitis or rib osteomyelitis at drainage sites. The efficacy of local instillations of antimicrobials or enzymes has not been convincingly demonstrated.

B. Surgical drainage

1. Empyema in the **exudative phase** with thin free-flowing pleural fluid can usually be managed with repeated **needle aspiration.** If the fluid reaccumulates rapidly, it is necessary to institute continuous drainage with an intercostal catheter under water-seal suction. Open drainage in this stage is contraindicated due to the potential complication of pneumothorax.
2. During the **fibropurulent phase,** the fluid is purulent and cannot be adequately drained by needle aspiration. Delay in establishing adequate thoracotomy drainage is the most important cause of morbidity from empyema.
   a. **Closed drainage** is used initially. It should be under water-seal suction if loculation is not well established. Tubes are used rather than collapsible drains. The tubes are secured to the chest wall and are not removed until the cavity is obliterated by complete lung expansion. Cavity size is evaluated by soundings or a sonogram.
   b. **Open drainage** is necessary when the closed procedure fails. Indications are persistent sepsis, failure to demonstrate progressive reduction in cavity size, or inadequate removal of the infected material despite rearranging of tubes. Open drainage with rib resection permits breaking up of adhesions and provides a large outlet for dependent egress of purulent collections.
3. **Decortication** is required for thick-walled chronic empyema with entrapped lung. This procedure should be deferred until after the acute inflammatory reaction subsides. The goal is removal of the infected membrane and obliteration of the pleural space. Decortication combined with pulmonary resection is indicated when the lung is severely diseased, especially in the presence of a bronchopleural fistula.
4. **Thoracoplasty** is used when there is insufficient remaining lung to obliterate the pleural space. (This procedure is seldom required.)

V. Postoperative bronchopleural fistula. This is a major complication of pulmonary resections.

A. Fistulas during the early postoperative period (at 1–2 days) generally result from inadequate closure of the bronchial stump. The patient develops massive subcutaneous emphysema and varying degrees of respiratory insufficiency. Treatment consists of pleural drainage, sometimes followed by reoperation to close the defect.

B. Fistulas developing at 1–2 weeks indicate inadequate tissue coverage of the stump or rupture of an empyema through the stump suture line. The patient coughs up serosanguineous fluid, and prompt drainage is necessary to prevent aspiration into the healthy lung.

C. Fistulas developing after 2 weeks usually represent frank empyemas, which rupture through the bronchial stump. The patient is febrile, and the sputum is purulent.

D. Closure of infected bronchopleural fistulas may be attempted after the pleural space has been divested of any infected membrane. The bronchial stoma is denuded, sutured, and buried. A pedicle flap of skeletal muscle may be used to reduce the pleural pocket.

Bronchiectasis

I. General principles. Bronchiectasis is an irreversible dilation of proximal and medium-sized bronchi caused by obstruction and infection. Resected segments show a dilated lumen filled with suppurative material, and inflamed, often necrotic, mucosal surfaces. Bacterial infection of the lung is the most common precursor, particularly when associated with bronchial obstruction, delayed treatment, delayed resolution, or parenchymal necrosis. In the past, tuberculosis was an important cause of bronchiectasis, with several mechanisms involved: enlarged, obstructing, perihilar lymph nodes; distortion of bronchial architecture by contracting parenchymal lesions; and direct destruction from endobronchial tuberculosis. Other causes are

Table 6-5. Differential diagnosis of pleural effusions

Effusion	Patient characteristics	Gross fluid appearance	Exudate*	RBC >10,000/mm	Glucose <40 mg/100 ml	WBC >2,500/mm	Dominant cell type	Culture	Adjunctive tests
Bacterial empyema	Symptoms of pneumonitis infiltrate on x-ray film	Turbid or purulent	+	–	+	+ +	Nearly all PMNs	+	Gram's stain Pleural fluid pH ≤ 7.0
Pneumonitic	Symptoms of pneumonitis infiltrate on x-ray film	Serous	+	–	–	±	Nearly all PMNs	–	Pleural fluid pH > 7.0
Tuberculous effusion	Young adult +PPD	Serous or sanguineous	+	5%	+	75%	Lymphocytes	25%	Pleural biopsy
Congestive heart failure or anasarca	Signs and symptoms of CHF	Serous	<10%	–	–	–	Lymphocytes, PMNs, or eosinophils	–	
Pulmonary embolism	Susceptible host	Serous or sanguineous	+	+	–	–	Lymphocytes, PMNs, or eosinophils	–	Lung scan Angiogram

Rheumatoid arthritis (collagen-vascular disease)	History of arthritis, subcutaneous nodules	Turbid	+	–	+	+	Lymphocytes or PMNs	–	Rheumatoid factor
Malignancy	Older patient	Serous or sanguineous	±	65%	±	±	Lymphocytes or eosinophils	–	Pleural fluid cytology + in 50%
Trauma	History of trauma	Sanguineous	+	+ + (Hct >1–2 gm/100 ml)	– –	– –	Lymphocytes or eosinophils	–	
Chylothorax	Trauma or malignancy	Milky (chylous)	+	–	–	–	–	–	Fat droplets on Sudan stain
Pancreatitis	Susceptible host serum amylase	Sanguineous or serous	+	±	–	+	Lymphocytes, PMNs, or eosinophils	–	Pleural fluid-serum amylase ratio >1

*Specific gravity >1.016, protein >3 gm/100 ml, pleural fluid-serum LDH ratio >0.6.

obstruction (foreign body, tumor, and congenital); viral infections (particularly pertussis, measles, and influenza); and certain associated disease states (agammaglobulinemia, Kartagener's syndrome, cystic fibrosis, and sinusitis).

II. Clinical features. The classic form of the disease was described in the preantibiotic era. The disease usually developed in young adults and was characterized by copious amounts of putrid sputum, emaciation, severe secondary parenchymal infections, clubbing, and reduced life expectancy. This presentation is now seldom seen, and with improved diagnostic techniques, less severe forms of bronchiectasis are more readily detected. Symptoms in the present era are chronic cough, purulent sputum production, hemoptysis, and recurrent bouts of pneumonia. Secondary pulmonary infections tend to recur in the same location and respond well to antibiotic therapy.

III. Diagnosis

A. Routine chest x-rays are often normal or show only nonspecific increased bronchial markings extending from the hilar region.

B. Bronchography establishes the diagnosis and is useful in evaluating the extent and distribution of disease. It should not be performed until at least 3 months after any parenchymal pulmonary infection, since reversible bronchiectatic changes are expected during this period. Bronchiectatic changes are classified into three forms—**cylindric, fusiform,** and **saccular.** The most common sites of disease are the **posterior basilar segments of the lower lobes,** presumably due to their lack of gravitational drainage. The middle lobe is also predisposed to this disease due to angulation of the bronchus at the take-off and peribronchial lymph nodes at the origin. Upper lobe disease is more common with previous tuberculosis or lung abscess.

C. Bronchoscopy is useful for detecting underlying conditions such as tumor, stricture, or foreign body.

D. X-rays of nasal sinuses show sinusitis in up to 40% of patients.

E. Sputum cultures are of little value except in rare cases associated with active tuberculosis.

IV. Treatment

A. Medical. Since the anatomic defects are irreversible, medical treatment is directed at controlling symptoms and preventing progression. Principles of medical treatment are

1. Postural drainage to mobilize secretions, with positioning appropriate to the segment involved (Table 6-4).
2. Hydration—systemic and local—to facilitate expectoration. Bedside nebulizers and cold vapor humidifiers are relatively ineffective. Heated humidified air or a nebulizer that produces small particles (such as a deVilbiss #40 or a bronchodilator for intermittent positive pressure breathing [IPPB]) are preferred.
3. Bronchodilators are useful prior to postural drainage for patients with bronchospasm.
4. Antibiotics are indicated for
   a. Exacerbations, as manifested by increased purulent sputum, progressive dyspnea and fever. Ampicillin or tetracycline usually is effective.
   b. Complicating pulmonary infections, usually respond to penicillin G.
   c. Prolonged use of antibiotics to prevent exacerbations is controversial.
5. Discontinuation of smoking and treatment of associated sinusitis are important adjunctive measures.

B. Surgical. Surgical intervention has a limited role. Patients with mild symptoms generally respond to medical measures; those with severe symptoms usually have extensive involvement of multiple segments, which precludes complete resection. Factors to consider when surgical intervention is contemplated are response to optimal medical treatment, age of the patient, extent and distribution of disease, associated bronchitis, and pulmonary reserve. Indications for surgery are

1. **Disease restricted to a single lobe,** which does not respond adequately to medical therapy. This particularly applies to younger patients and those with recurrent bouts of pneumonia in the same pulmonary segment or lobe.

In such cases segmental resection or lobectomy is generally curative. Surgery is sometimes advocated when there is involvement of more than one lobe, and if there is a marked difference in the extent of disease. Preoperative pulmonary function tests are important in determining whether the patient will tolerate general anesthesia and how much resection can be undertaken. Differential pulmonary function studies may be helpful when findings of the usual ones are not definitive.

2. **Serious hemoptysis.** This usually results from aneurysmal vascular deformity in the bronchiectactic cavity.
3. **Bronchiectasis secondary to a resectable carcinoma.**
4. **Bronchiectasis related to a foreign body** that cannot be removed by bronchoscopy.
5. Rare cases that are complicated by **amyloidosis.**

Postoperative Atelectasis

I. **General principles.** Atelectasis is the most common cause of fever in the early postoperative period. The precipitating events are **inspiratory insufficiency** or **retained secretions** due to impaired cough reflex and dehydration. Patients at greatest risk are those with chronic obstructive pulmonary disease. Additional predisposing factors are obesity, debility and the duration of anesthesia. The most common preceding operations are laparotomy (especially upper abdominal incisions) and thoracotomy.

II. **Diagnosis**

A. **Low-grade fever, tachycardia,** and **tachypnea** during the 1st 3 postoperative days commonly indicate atelectasis. There may also be mild chest discomfort, dyspnea, and cyanosis.

B. **Careful auscultation** for rales and decreased breath sounds often is more revealing than chest x-rays. The physical examination is optimally performed with the patient breathing deeply in the sitting position.

C. **Blood gases** typically show low PO_2 with normal or low PCO_2. This pattern indicates ventilation-perfusion abnormalities; it is also noted with pulmonary embolism, bronchospasm, congestive failure, and pneumonitis.

D. **Chest x-ray** films reveal linear shadows ("discoid atelectasis"), segmental or lobar atelectasis, or simply an increased pulmonary density.

E. **Major complications** are arrhythmias, hypoxia, and pneumonitis. Pneumonitis commonly supervenes with atelectasis and may be the presenting finding.

F. **Lobar or total lung collapse** causes severe agitation, acute dyspnea, cyanosis, substernal oppression, hypertension, and deviation of the trachea toward the involved side. Chest x-ray shows mediastinal shift, narrowing of the intercostal spaces, diaphragmatic elevation, and a dense lobe or lung. This represents an extreme (and unusual) form of atelectasis.

G. The **differential diagnosis** of dyspnea in the early postoperative period includes pneumonitis, pulmonary edema, aspiration pneumonia, and pulmonary embolism.

III. **Preventive measures**

A. **Preoperative preparation** of patients with chronic pulmonary disease undergoing elective surgery:

1. Discontinuation of smoking for 2–4 weeks.
2. Bronchodilators for wheezing, either systemic (i.e., Tedral, ephedrine, or aminophylline) or local (Isuprel nebulizer; IPPB with Bronkosol, 0.5 ml added to 2–4 ml of half-isotonic saline; or IPPB with Isuprel, 0.6 ml of 1:200 isoproterenol added to 2–4 ml of half-isotonic saline).
3. Postural drainage two to four times daily for patients with excessive sputum production. A useful regimen is IPPB with a bronchodilator for 5 minutes, then a mist humidifier for 15–20 minutes, followed by percussion postural drainage.

4. A 7–10-day course of preoperative tetracycline or ampicillin (250 mg PO qid) as an effort to decrease purulent sputum production.
5. Coughing and diaphragmatic breathing exercises.

B. Postoperative measures

1. Adequate hydration.
2. Humidification of inspired air, preferably with a heated mist humidifier or ultrasonic nebulizer.
3. "Stir-up" routines, such as frequent turning, forced deep breathing (e.g., "blow bottles"), and forced coughing. Patients who are unable to cough may benefit from IPPB with saline or periodic intratracheal injections of 1–2 ml of saline. If the latter procedure is to be repeated, a transtracheal aspiration may be performed and the polyethylene catheter left in the trachea for intermittent saline instillation.
4. Analgesia sufficient to permit cough without suppressing respiration.

IV. Treatment

A. Recommendations are similar to those for postoperative prevention.

B. Nasotracheal suction aspiration is indicated for patients who fail to improve with forced breathing and coughing. If symptoms persist, the patient is bronchoscoped to remove impacted plugs. Endotracheal intubation or tracheostomy is considered if repeated bronchoscopy is required.

C. Antimicrobial treatment is controversial. Most patients with atelectasis respond to mechanical measures alone. Pneumonitis often supervenes, however, if atelectasis persists for extended periods.

Clues to a superimposed infection are fever >38°C; leukocytosis, which is not present with uncomplicated atlectasis; purulent, rather than mucoid, sputum production; and pulmonary infiltrate, rather than collapse, on chest x-ray. Likely pathogens in this setting are anaerobic bacteria, aerobic gram-negative bacilli, and *Staph. aureus*. Optimal treatment is based on Gram's stain and culture of a transtracheal aspirate. Empiric treatment of seriously ill patients should be directed against all likely pathogens—an aminoglycoside in combination with nafcillin, cefazolin, or clindamycin.

Infectious Complications of Tracheostomy

I. General principles. The normal trachea is sterile under usual conditions, but it becomes colonized 24–48 hours following tracheostomy. Common isolates from tracheostomies include *Klebsiella*, *E. coli*, *Pseudomonas*, *Enterobacter*, *Proteus*, *Staph. aureus*, and *Candida*. Usually multiple microbial species colonize simultaneously. Some degree of inflammation is also inevitable—most commonly at the stoma, tip of the tube, and around the cuff. Autopsy studies show that nearly all patients with tracheostomy have tracheitis and ulceration. Antimicrobials have no effect on the incidence of colonization or on local inflammation. Major infections requiring antimicrobial treatment are serious wound sepsis, febrile tracheobronchitis, and pneumonitis. Less common complications of tracheostomy are mediastinitis, tracheoesophageal fistulae, persistent stoma, and tracheal stenosis. For these reasons, the decision to perform a tracheostomy should be given considerable thought, with due accord paid to the positive and negative aspects of the procedure.

II. Predisposing factors. Factors predisposing to colonization and infection are

A. Obliteration of upper airway defense mechanisms.

B. Foreign body.

C. Pressure necrosis from inflated cuffs.

D. Atelectasis due to loss of humidification from upper airways, inadequate suctioning, excessive secretions, administration of dry gases, and aspiration of solid particles.

E. Excessive exposure to pathogens through frequent use of contaminated inhalation therapy equipment and failure to employ aseptic cleansing techniques.

F. Aspiration of oropharyngeal secretions. This event is common and may be demonstrated by tracheal suction after oral administration of methylene blue. Inflated cuffs dᵒ not provide complete protection, since they are seldom "watertight," and if they impinge on the esophagus, actually predispose to aspiration.

III. Prevention of serious sepsis

1. Elective rather than emergency procedures significantly lessen possible complications.
2. Irrigation and suction procedures are performed with sterile gloves, sterile catheters, and sterile fluids for instillation. Inhalation therapy equipment is cleaned daily. The inner cannula is removed and cleaned at least four times daily.
3. Patients who aspirate significant volumes of oral feedings should be given nothing by mouth and possibly fed through a nasogastric tube.
4. Prophylactic antibiotics have no established value in preventing major complications, and predispose to infection with resistant organisms

IV. Treatment of septic complications

A. Wound sepsis with significant cellulitis, fever, lymphadenopathy, or mediastinitis is treated with systemic antimicrobials as well as local wound care. Antimicrobial selection is based on Gram's stain and culture of purulent drainage. Less serious wound infections can be managed with local measures.

B. Tracheobronchitis and pneumonitis are characterized by fever and purulent tracheal secretions. These conditions are distinguished by the presence or absence of an acute infiltrate on chest x-ray. The bacteriology in both is similar to that of tracheostomy aspirates without systemic signs of sepsis—principally gram-negative bacilli and *Staph. aureus*. A logical initial choice of antimicrobials for severely ill patients pending culture results is an aminoglycoside and a cephalosporin.

Pulmonary Tuberculosis

I. General principles. Tuberculosis most commonly involves the lung, probably because the respiratory tract is the usual portal of entry. The disease may occur as a **primary** form, involving hilar lymph nodes and an adjacent area of lung as well as pleural effusion, miliary spread, or meningitis. **Recrudescent** tuberculosis follows a primary event (which may not have been recognized) by several months to years. This recurrent form usually involves the upper lobes of the lung; other sites include liver, urinary tract, genital tract, intestine, and miliary spread.

II. Clinical features

A. Symptoms. Cough, hemoptysis, weight loss, fever, night sweats, and pleuritic chest pain are the most frequent complaints. Symptoms are usually indolent over several weeks or months.

B. Chest x-ray. Most common findings in adults are infiltrates, nodules, or cavities in the apex or in the posterior segments of the upper lobes.

III. Skin test. Intermediate-strength PPD is positive (>10 mm induration) in over 85% of patients with active disease. False-negatives are most common in patients who are elderly, debilitated, receiving corticosteroids, and overwhelmed by infections. Approximately 50% of patients over 50 yrs old have a positive skin test indicating previous infection but usually inactive disease. Thus, the PPD is of greatest value in establishing the diagnosis in young patients and for excluding the disease in older persons.

IV. Microbiology

A. AFB smears of expectorated sputum are positive in one-half to two-thirds of all patients with active pulmonary tuberculosis and in nearly all with cavitary tuberculosis.

B. Culture of *M. tuberculosis* establishes the diagnosis of active disease. Three specimens of early morning coughed sputum should be collected in all suspected cases. Patients without sputum production should have three induced sputum and/or bronchoscopic or gastric aspirates. Therapy does not interfere with cultivation of the organism for several days or even weeks.

V. Tuberculous pleural effusions. Tuberculin-positive young adults with pleural effusions have a high incidence of developing active pulmonary tuberculosis within three years. Cultures of pleural fluid in only about 25% of these individuals yield acid-fast bacilli. Closed pleural biopsies are diagnostic in about 80% of patients with tuberculous effusions. Remaining cases can be detected with open pleural biopsy. Long-term follow-up studies of patients with "nonspecific pleuritis" demonstrated by **open** biopsy show that, when tuberculosis is excluded by this procedure, it is not necessary to treat with antituberculous drugs. On the basis of these observations the following diagnostic evaluation is recommended:

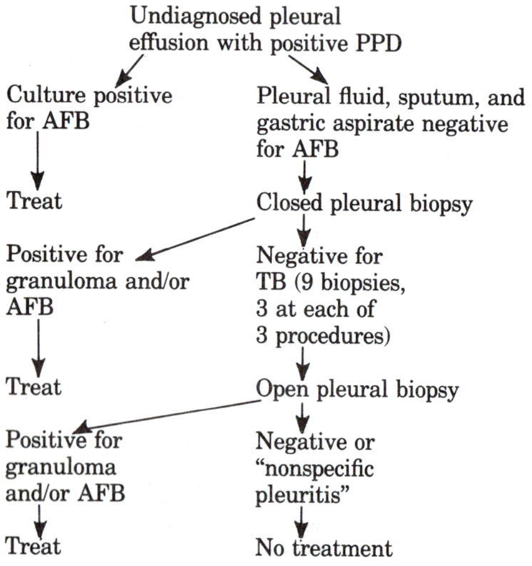

VI. Medical treatment

A. All patients with **active pulmonary tuberculosis** (positive culture, symptoms, or progressive changes in chest x-rays ascribed to tuberculosis) should receive two antituberculous drugs for 9–12 months.

B. Preferred treatment in a newly diagnosed uncomplicated adult case is:

1. INH, 300 mg PO daily, plus rifampin, 600 mg PO daily. Pyridoxine, 15–50 mg daily, is often given concurrently to minimize the risk of polyneuritis due to isoniazid-induced pyroxidine deficiency.
2. Alternative "first-line" drugs to be combined with INH are ethambutol, 15 mg/kg/day, or streptomycin, 1 gm daily for 2–4 weeks, then 1 gm 2–3 times weekly for up to 6 months.
3. Intermittent treatment under supervision may be preferred for noncompliant patients. The usual regimen is isoniazid 15 mg/kg twice weekly combined with rifampin, 600 mg twice weekly.
4. Abbreviated courses utilizing multiple bactericidal drugs are sometimes advocated for noncompliant patients and to reduce the duration of treatment. These regimens utilize isoniazid and rifampin combined with streptomycin and/or pyrazinamide for 2 months followed by isoniazid and rifampin for 4–7 months.

C. Treatment with three antituberculous drugs has not proved superior to treatment with two, for any form of tuberculosis, provided that both agents are active against the organism involved. Therapy with three or more agents is advocated for patients exposed to drug-resistant organisms and emigrants from areas where drug resistance rates are high, such as Southeast Asia. Some authorities routinely advocate triple therapy against selected forms of tuberculosis, e.g., advanced cavitary tuberculosis, miliary tuberculosis, tuberculous pericarditis, or tuberculous meningitis: the third drug given with isoniazid and rifampin is usually ethambutol or streptomycin. Patients previously treated with antituberculous drugs should receive at least two drugs not previously used, usually in combination with isoniazid.

D. Second-line agents to be considered in cases involving resistant mycobacteria are cycloserine, 15 mg/kg PO daily in divided doses; ethionamide, 250 mg PO tid or qid; pyrazinamide, 20–35 mg/kg PO daily in 2–4 divided doses; viomycin, 15 mg/kg IM 3–5 times weekly; and kanamycin, 15 mg/kg IM 5 times weekly.

E. Primary drug resistance is unusual in previously untreated adults. More than 90% of strains are sensitive to isoniazid, ethambutol, streptomycin, and rifampin. Drug resistance is most common in (1) previously treated reactivated cases, (2) inadequately treated cases (premature discontinuation of drugs or use of a single agent for active disease), (3) atypical mycobacteria, (4) children with tuberculosis, (5) Asians or Hispanics, (6) persistent positive cultures (3 mo.).

VII. Surgical treatment—indications

A. Suspected pulmonary neoplasm

1. There is a disproportionate incidence of carcinoma in patients with active or inactive tuberculosis ("scar carcinoma"). Clues suggesting carcinoma are
   a. Atypical x-ray appearance for tuberculosis
   b. Suboptimal x-ray or clinical response to antituberculosis treatment
   c. Negative PPD skin test, since bronchogenic carcinoma patients are often anergic
2. A mass or cavitary lesion in which noninvasive procedures fail to yield a diagnosis (see solitary pulmonary nodule, p. 152).

B. Inability to control tuberculosis or its residual effects

1. Persistent active disease (positive sputum) despite 4–6 months of at least two drugs that prove active in repeated in vitro tests. Surgical intervention may be considered if there are progressively enlarging infiltrates, continued open cavities, or resistant organisms that make medical treatment unfeasible.
2. Open cavitary disease with negative sputum cultures ("open negative"). This condition often can be managed with indefinite continuation of chemotherapy. Surgical intervention may be considered when an individual is unreliable and continued therapy is judged unfeasible.
3. Irreversible destructive lesions that cause disability or recurrent pyogenic infections or represent foci for tuberculosis extension. Examples are bronchostenosis, bronchiectasis (hemorrhage or positive sputum), and large areas of destroyed lung (providing there is satisfactory pulmonary reserve).
4. Persistent or recurrent hemoptysis, usually from persistent cavities or bronchiectasis.
5. Tuberculous bronchopleural fistula arising spontaneously or following surgery or trauma. This is a serious complication because
   a. The fistula provides a pleural reservoir for the development of resistant organisms.
   b. Communication with the pleural space provides ready access for the development of bacterial as well as tuberculous empyema.
   c. Periodic drainage of pleural collection may result in disseminated infection to other areas of the lung or result in massive aspiration with death from drowning. Tuberculous bronchopleural fistulae do not heal with antituberculous drugs or surgical intervention alone. Optimal results are obtained when an operation is performed after 3–4 months of antituberculous treatment. Immediate drainage is indicated when there is a superimposed pyogenic empyema or threat of massive aspiration.

C. Pleural tuberculosis. This usually follows extension of parenchymal tuberculosis at a subpleural location.

1. Serous effusions in tuberculin-positive young adults with no x-ray evidence of parenchymal disease generally clear within 2–3 months. Treatment consists of thoracentesis and two antituberculous drugs for 1½ years. Decortica-

tion is considered only if x-ray pictures (especially lateral views) at 2–3 months show encapsulated collections (see **2**).

2. In encapsulated pleural tuberculosis, decortication should be undertaken when pleural involvement is significant (occupies one-fourth to one-third of the hemithorax), collections are thick and loculated (especially with lateral x-rays showing a clearly defined mass), and thoracentesis fails to yield fluid or to alter the roentgenographic appearance.

D. Atypical mycobacterial disease. Indications for surgical intervention are similar to those in *M. tuberculosis*, except that resection is more frequently required due to greater drug resistance and generally poor response to medical treatment. Initial treatment consists of multiple agents such as isoniazid, rifampin, ethambutol, and streptomycin. The regimen is tailored to the in vitro susceptibility profile. Localized lesions should be excised when there is failure to respond to optimal medical treatment, or drug toxicity precludes continued use of active agents. *Mycobacterium kansasii* infections often can be controlled with drugs. *Mycobacterium intracellulare* is resistant to most antituberculous agents and usually requires combined medical and surgical treatment.

VIII. Surgical considerations

A. Antituberculous drugs should be given to patients 3–6 months prior to surgery. Optimal candidates are those who have negative sputum cultures preoperatively. Patients with resistant strains should receive several weeks of second-line drugs before operation.

B. Type of procedure

1. A resectional surgical procedure generally is preferred. This includes wedge resection, subsegmental and segmental resection, lobectomy, and pneumonectomy. The goals are extirpation of all lesions and preservation of normal lung. Preoperative tomograms or bronchography assist in determining the extent of involvement. Contraindications to resection are
   - **a.** Inadequate pulmonary reserve according to pulmonary function tests. In all cases a minimum of two normal lobes should be preserved.
   - **b.** Extensive bilateral disease, unless the contralateral side is stable.
   - **c.** Involvement of the entire lung, so that active foci must be entered.
   - **d.** Endobronchial tuberculosis. This should be excluded with bronchoscopy if the patient has persistently positive sputum cultures.
   - **e.** Advanced age, cardiac disease, and other serious underlying conditions (relative contraindications).
2. Extraperiosteal plombage thoracoplasty is occasionally indicated for cases in which resectional surgery is contraindicated. Anticipated functional loss is 8–12% of the preoperative maximum breathing capacity.
3. Pleural tuberculosis. When there is significant parenchymal disease, the patient is treated medically. If the parenchymal lesion responds, pleural involvement is considered an independent process. Decortication is combined with resection (or pleuropneumonectomy) only when criteria for resection apply. Long-standing empyema with a thick calcified peel and entrapped lung often requires a staged thoracoplasty.

C. Complications of surgery are correlated with the extent of involvement and the presence of positive preoperative sputum cultures. (The latter applies to *M. tuberculosis* but not atypical mycobacteria.) The most common complication is bronchopleural fistula with either a large pleural air space or empyema.

Surgical Intervention in Pulmonary Mycotic Infection

I. Coccidioidomycosis

A. Indications for surgical intervention

1. In **acute** pulmonary coccidioidomycosis a surgical procedure is generally contraindicated, except when there is **empyema** or severe persistent **hemoptysis.**

2. **Chronic solitary nodules** do not require operation (or chemotherapy), except to exclude carcinoma when the etiology is unknown.
3. **Stable asymptomatic cavities** represent a controversial group. Many authorities adopt a "wait-and-see" attitude. Those that persist for 6–12 months will seldom close spontaneously or with amphotericin B therapy. Compelling indications for resecting such cavities are
   a. Location near the visceral surface, since they pose a threat of pneumothorax, bronchopleural fistula, and empyema
   b. Large size (>4 cm in diameter)
   c. Continued enlargement despite amphotericin B treatment
   d. Hemoptysis and secondary infections
4. **Coccidioidomycosis empyema** may result from a bronchopleural fistula, rupture of a peripheral cavity, or after resectional surgery. Immediate drainage and amphotericin B treatment (at least 300–500 mg) are indicated. Decortication and resection (usually lobectomy) often are required.

B. **Resection.** Segmental resection may be adequate when the cavity or granuloma is confined to the segment, without satellite nodules. Lobectomy is preferred for more extensive involvement. This decision is made by consulting preoperative tomograms and by careful inspection during the operative procedure.

C. **Major postoperative complications** are pleural space problems, empyema, and recurrent cavities. They are more common following operation for cavitary disease (rather than granulomas) and when the disease has been incompletely resected (segmental resection rather than lobectomy). Hematogenous dissemination of coccidioidomycosis following a surgical procedure is rare.

D. **Amphotericin B treatment**
1. **Preoperative.** Some authorities suggest preoperative amphotericin B in a total dose of at least 400–600 mg for all patients undergoing operations for coccidioidomycosis. Others restrict preoperative use of this drug to certain high-risk groups: those with extensive pulmonary disease; susceptible (dark-skinned) races, especially blacks and Filipinos; pregnant females; and patients with high complement-fixation titers (>1:32).
2. **Postoperative.** Amphotericin (in the range of 300–500 mg) continues to be given postoperatively to all patients who have received it preoperatively. Treatment with amphotericin B is also advocated for patients who develop postoperative space problems, empyema, or a rising complement-fixation titer.

II. Histoplasmosis

A. Indications for surgical intervention
1. Right middle lobe syndrome or bronchiectasis, especially when complicated by severe hemoptysis.
2. Chronic progressive cavitary histoplasmosis. Experience has taught that these lesions, although indolent, are associated with significant morbidity and mortality. Most cases can be treated with amphotericin B in a total dose of 2–2.5 gm. Surgical intervention is reserved for patients who fail to respond to medical therapy. (Concurrent pulmonary tuberculosis must be excluded in these cases.)
3. Granulomatous nodules do not require surgical intervention (or chemotherapy) except to exclude carcinoma.

B. Amphotericin B treatment
1. Amphotericin B is unnecessary for solitary histoplasmosis nodules that have been excised for diagnostic purposes.
2. When resection of chronic cavitary histoplasmosis is planned, it is most prudent to give amphotericin B preoperatively, in a dose of at least 500 mg–1 gm, in an attempt to control the disease and to convert positive sputum cultures. The drug is continued postoperatively to provide a total dose of 2–3 gm.
3. When the diagnosis of chronic cavitary histoplasmosis is initially established at surgery, the total dose of 2–3 gm of amphotericin B is given postoperatively.

4. These recommendations are controversial; some authorities would reserve amphotericin B for patients with incomplete resections or postoperative recurrences.

III. Blastomycosis

A. Surgical excision is indicated for chronic pulmonary blastomycosis that fails to respond to a complete course of medical therapy. The preferred regimen is amphotericin B (1.5–2.5 gm); others are hydroxystilbamidine, miconazole, and ketoconazole.

B. Following surgical excision, either in previously undiagnosed cases or in those who fail to respond to chemotherapy, drug therapy consists of either amphotericin B (1 gm) or hydroxystilbamidine (8 gm). This recommendation is based on the risk of local extension or hematogenous dissemination after excisional surgery.

IV. Aspergillosis. The principle form of aspergillosis requiring surgical intervention is **intercavitary mycetoma,** a condition of colonization, without invasion, of preexisting cavities or diseased bronchi. The fungal ball per se is usually asymptomatic and may disappear spontaneously. The natural history of most cases of aspergilloma is relatively benign. The usual indication for a surgical procedure is hemoptysis with severe episodes of hemorrhage or chronic, persistent bleeding despite antibiotics. Another approach to treating a fungal ball is local administration of amphotericin B by means of a thin, plastic catheter running directly into the cavity via the tracheobronchial route (this technique has been advocated by only a few physicians).

V. Cryptococcosis

A. Therapeutic indications. The course of pulmonary cryptococcosis is variable, but whenever the diagnosis is established, there should be a careful search for extrapulmonary involvement—especially skin, bone, and meninges. If the lesion is believed to be confined to the lung, some authorities recommend careful follow-up and advocate surgical resection or amphotericin B treatment, in a total dose of 2 gm, only for patients who fail to show spontaneous clinical and roentgenographic improvement within 1–2 months. A contrary recommendation is that all patients with pulmonary cryptococcosis receive treatment in order to prevent meningeal dissemination. Results with medical and surgical treatment of these localized lesions are equivalent.

B. There are numerous reports of **cryptococcal meningitis** following surgical resection of pulmonary cryptococcomas. Meningitis antedating the procedure has seldom been excluded in such reports, however. The actual incidence of postoperative dissemination is only about 3%. Thus, the danger of amphotericin B must be weighed against its potential benefits. Many authorities now prefer to avoid the drug and, to detect this complication, simply follow patients postoperatively with periodic cerebrospinal fluid examination.

Solitary Pulmonary Nodule

I. General principles. Patients with solitary pulmonary nodules are commonly referred to a surgeon for a definitive diagnosis. The principal differential is between malignancy, granuloma, and hamartoma. Results from operative procedures indicate that 40–60% of solitary nodules are malignant. Since these reports are based on referred patients, however, they are considerably biased. X-ray surveys of solitary nodules among unselected patients indicate the incidence of malignancy is less than 20%; the majority of nodules are granulomas due to tuberculosis, histoplasmosis, coccidioidomycosis, or cryptococcosis.

II. Diagnosis

A. X-ray. The most useful guidelines are previous x-rays for comparison of size and tomograms to detect calcification. Lesions showing concentric and regular or central calcification are nearly always benign. Malignant tumors generally show doubling times of 1 month to 1 year. Previous films showing no progression in size over 2 years nearly exclude malignancy.

Other roentgenographic features are less useful. The following suggest malignancy but must be considered nonspecific: large size (>4 cm in diameter); serrated or irregular margin; and lack of satellite lesions.

B. Skin tests are nonspecific. About 50% of all patients over 50 years of age in the United States have positive intermediate-strength PPD tests. Most persons who have lived in areas endemic for histoplasmosis and coccidioidomycosis have positive skin tests for these fungi. The incidence of false-negative skin tests with granulomas is about 5–10% for tuberculosis, 20% for histoplasmosis, and 30% for coccidioidomycosis.

C. Serologic tests for coccidioidomycosis and histoplasmosis are usually negative or nondiagnostic when these fungi are responsible for solitary granulomas. There are no other serologic tests that can be used in this situation.

D. Cultures of sputum or bronchoscopy aspirates for tuberculosis and fungi are generally negative when the primary disease is a solitary nodule.

E. Cytology studies of three or more specimens are positive in 20–50% of patients with nodular carcinomas.

F. Bronchoscopy with bronchial brushing is seldom diagnostic with granulomatous nodules; results are variable with malignant lesions and depend on the location of the lesion.

G. Percutaneous needle biopsy can usually be directed successfully into even small nodules under fluoroscopic guidance in the hands of an experienced operator. Unfortunately, the quantity of aspirate may be scanty, and the histologic appearances often are considered nonspecific.

H. Scalene node biopsy in the absence of a palpable supraclavicular node is seldom diagnostic.

I. Mediastinoscopy or parasternal mediastinotomy is particularly useful when there is paratracheal or hilar node enlargement. As many as 50% of patients with malignant nodules have positive mediastinal nodes, indicating nonresectability.

III. Diagnostic approach. On the basis of the above observations it is concluded that many of the routine preoperative tests are of limited value. Noninvasive tests such as sputum cytology and cultures for AFB and fungi can be justified on the basis of safety, simplicity, and occasional diagnostic yield. With invasive procedures, the anticipated yield must be balanced against the risk and expense. Unless the procedure yields a specific diagnosis, a thoracotomy will still be required for a definitive result. There are occasions, however, when the invasive tests are employed to establish a diagnosis in a patient who is not a surgical candidate. Factors that generally militate against thoracotomy are

A. Strong clinical and roentgenographic evidence against malignancy, especially

1. Age under 35 years (fewer than 1% of nodules are malignant)
2. Lack of smoking history
3. Previous x-rays showing no increase in size over 2 years
4. Calcifications that are central, laminated, or diffusely punctate

B. Evidence of metastatic spread

C. Compromised pulmonary or cardiac status or other physical conditions that contraindicate surgery

IV. Diagnostic thoracotomy must be considered when these criteria do not apply. To detect agents responsible for granulomas, a portion of the operative specimen should be submitted to the laboratory without fixation and cultured for fungi and tuberculosis. The yield of positive cultures is good for tuberculosis, fair for coccidioidomycosis, and poor for histoplasmosis. An additional portion of the specimen should be fixed and submitted for the mycobacterial and fungal stains (periodic acid–Schiff [PAS] and Giemsa stains are suggested). These specialized stains are particularly important, since the routine hematoxylin-eosin stain frequently fails to demonstrate the responsible organism.

Patients with resected granulomas that prove to be tuberculous should receive a drug regimen advocated for active disease (see pp. 147–149) or should receive INH for 1 year with careful follow-up. When the resected granuloma is caused by fungi, no medical treatment is indicated.

7 Cardiovascular Infections

Endocarditis

I. General principles. There are two forms of endocarditis, distinguished by clinical presentation and bacteriologic patterns.

A. Subacute bacterial endocarditis (SBE) usually occurs on previously damaged valves and involves relatively nonpathogenic bacteria, such as *Streptococcus viridans*. The disease begins insidiously, and the patient typically presents with symptoms of more than 6 weeks' duration. Common complaints are weakness, weight loss, fever, night sweats, and arthralgias. The usual findings are low-grade fever (seldom over 38.5°C), murmur, splenomegaly, and anemia. Leukocytosis is unusual.

B. Acute bacterial endocarditis (ABE) tends to involve previously normal heart valves and is caused by more pathogenic bacteria, such as *Staphylococcus aureus*. In comparison with SBE, the onset is more abrupt and the fever is higher, while anemia and splenomegaly are less common. The course tends to be fulminant, with rapid valve destruction and early congestive failure.

C. Despite this traditional separation, there is considerable overlap in clinical findings and bacteria involved. For practical purposes, cases with an acute onset require rapid diagnosis and early institution of therapy, regardless of the bacterial etiology.

II. Pathophysiology. Certain underlying conditions predispose to endocarditis.

A. Valvular heart disease. Damaged valves cause turbulence of blood flow. This results in thrombus deposition, which then serves as a nidus for bacterial implantation. The pressure gradient is an important determinant of turbulence. Thus, left-sided lesions (damaged aortic or mitral valve, ventricular septal defect, patent ductus arteriosus, and tetralogy of Fallot) are more common underlying conditions than right-sided lesions (damaged pulmonic or tricuspid valve and atrial septal defect). The infection usually occurs on the distal or downstream side of the lesion. Several types of valvular disease have been implicated (Table 7-1).

B. Degenerative heart disease, acquired with aging. The major causes are calcification of the mitral anulus, atheromatous deposits on the aortic valve, mural infarction, and papillary muscle dysfunction.

C. Cardiac surgical procedure. At great risk are those cases in which endothelial surfaces are sutured. The infection typically involves suture lines.

D. Intravenous drug abuse. Heroin addicts and occasional drug users are subjected to frequent, often high-level, bacteremia as well as possible valvular damage from inoculated particulate matter. Three unique features of endocarditis are found in these patients:

1. Frequent tricuspid valve involvement. The common presentations are acute symptomatology, bacteremia, low-grade or absent murmur, and septic pulmonary emboli.
2. *Staph. aureus* is the most common pathogen.
3. Probable return to a drug habit by addicts, despite reassurances to the contrary, is an important consideration when a cardiac operation is indicated.

Table 7-1. Valvular lesions in endocarditis

Underlying heart disease	Frequency in endocarditis cases (%)	Comment
Rheumatic valve disease	40–60	Mitral valve most commonly affected, aortic valve next most commonly
Congenital heart disease	6–20	Patent ductus arteriosus, IV septal defect, tetralogy of Fallot, pulmonary stenosis, coarctation, bicuspid aortic valve
Degenerative heart disease	5	Incidence is 5% of all patients, but 20–50% in those over 60 years of age; most common lesions are calcified mitral anulus, calcified or nodular valve lesions, and thrombus following myocardial infarct
Artificial devices	5–20	Includes prosthetic valves (hetero- and homografts) and septal patches
Miscellaneous	1	Includes cardiomyopathies and syphilitic aortic valve disease
No history of valvular disease	20–40	Many patients have undetected lesions, including rheumatic valve disease, congenital heart disease (especially bicuspid aortic valve), degenerative heart disease, Marfan's syndrome, and mitral valve prolapse (systolic click syndrome)

This poses a serious threat to prosthetic valves. An alternative approach with tricuspid endocarditis refractory to medical treatment is to excise the valve, leaving wide-open tricuspid insufficiency. Initial results with this procedure have been good, although long-term follow-ups are not available.

III. Diagnosis. Diagnostic hallmarks of endocarditis are fever, murmur, "embolic" phenomena, hematuria, and persistent bacteremia.

A. Fever is present in nearly all cases. Occasional exceptions are noted with uremia, old age, complicating cerebrovascular accident, severe congestive heart failure, and previous antimicrobial therapy.

B. Murmur is present in 95% of all cases. Absence of murmur is most likely early in the course of acute endocarditis and with involvement of the tricuspid valve or mural endocardium. Changing murmurs are considered particularly suggestive but are relatively infrequent in subacute cases; even when present, a changing murmur must be interpreted with caution, since it may represent flow changes due to anemia or fever. Marked changes or the appearance of a new diastolic murmur are more significant.

C. Mucocutaneous lesions

1. Petechiae. Nonblanching, nontender, hemorrhagic lesions on the skin, mucous membranes of the mouth, palate, or conjunctivae. Such lesions may appear in showers and tend to fade in a few days. They are noted in 20–40% of cases but are not specific for endocarditis. About 50% of patients undergong cardiopulmonary bypass develop conjunctival petechiae in the immediate postoperative period. These are probably due to fat emboli and do not occur following thoracic surgical procedures without cardiopulmonary bypass.

2. **Osler's nodes.** Tender, discolored nodules of the fingers, palms, or soles, which may ulcerate. These lesions are sterile. Histologic study indicates vasculitis, and they are often considered diagnostic of endocarditis. **Janeway lesions** are nodular, painless lesions on the palms, soles, fingers, or toes. They usually represent septic emboli, and cultures may yield the pathogen.
3. **Splinter hemorrhages.** Subungual linear hemorrhages, usually parallel to the nail edge, found in the distal third of nail beds. They are strongly suggestive of endocarditis if they occur without trauma.
4. **Eye lesions.** Petechial hemorrhages on conjunctivae or retinas; small retinal flame-shaped hemorrhages with pale centers; and **Roth spots** which are cotton-wool exudates caused by infarction of the nerve fiber layer.
5. **Clubbing.** Occasionally noted late in the course of SBE.

D. **Microemboli or macroemboli** involve the **kidney** (flank pain and hematuria); **spleen** (right upper quadrant pain, sometimes with a splenic friction rub); **bone** (osteomyelitis); **joint** (septic joint); **coronary vessels** (acute myocardial infarction or congestive failure, most commonly with aortic valve endocarditis); **lung** (especially with right-sided endocarditis); **cerebrum** (cerebrovascular accident or mycotic aneurysm); and **skin** (see **III.C.1–4**). Emboli to other nonmucocutaneous sites, such as the liver and myocardium, are commonly noted at autopsy but are infrequently documented ante mortem. In some cases, however, they represent the presenting complaint, and may account for atypical presentation. Embolic occlusions of large vessels are uncommon except with fungal endocarditis.

E. **Splenomegaly** occurs in 30–60% of SBE cases.

F. **CNS lesions** include aseptic meningitis, purulent meningitis, cerebritis, cerebral abscess, and mycotic aneurysms. The most frequently seen form is aseptic meningitis, with a sterile cerebrospinal fluid that shows pleocytosis, elevated protein, and normal glucose.

G. **Metastatic abscesses** usually occur in the skin, brain, lung, bone, joint, or myocardium. These are most common with endocarditis cases involving virulent bacteria, especially *Staph. aureus.*

H. **Mycotic aneurysms** of peripheral vessels tend to occur late and may appear months or even years after the valvular infection has been eliminated. The most common sites of involvement are at bifurcations of cerebral vessels; abdominal aorta; ligated ductus arteriosus; superior mesenteric, coronary, or pulmonary arteries; and sinus of Valsalva. Causative organisms usually are relatively nonpathogenic bacteria, such as *Strep. viridans.* With CNS vessel involvement, the patient may present with a cerebrovascular accident; such cases can be managed with medical treatment and usually do not require neurosurgical intervention.

I. **Renal involvement** is rather common, occurring in three forms:
1. Infarction due to sterile or septic emboli. An abscess can be formed by virulent bacteria such as *Staph. aureus.*
2. Diffuse glomerulonephritis due to immune-complex disease. Histology shows membranoproliferative changes comparable to renal lesions of lupus, syphilis, and malaria. Deposits of immunoglobulin and complement are noted along the basement membrane and in the mesangium. Renal failure may result and is usually reversible with treatment, unless scarring has occurred.
3. Focal embolic glomerulonephritis—a misnomer, since the usual mechanism is immune-complex disease. Only a few glomeruli are involved, and renal failure is rare.

J. **Laboratory findings of anemia, hypergammaglobulinemia,** and **positive latex fixation** (rheumatoid factor) are noted in 50% or more of patients who have had symptoms of endocarditis for more than 6 weeks (SBE). **WBC** is usually normal or only mildly elevated; a high WBC suggests emboli with infarction or metastatic abscess. **Hematuria,** usually microscopic, is a helpful sign. Two-dimensional and M-mode **echocardiography** may detect vegetations, a finding that generally indicates an unfavorable prognosis.

Table 7-2. Causes of bacterial endocarditis

Organism	Incidence in endocarditis (%)
Streptococcus viridans	25–50
Enterococci	8–12
Streptococci (anaerobes and other)	10–20
Staphylococcus aureus	15–20
Staph. epidermidis	1–3
Gram-negative bacilli	1–3
Fungi	1–2
Miscellaneous (pneumococci, *Neisseria*, diphtheroids, *Bacteroides, Salmonella, Listeria, Hemophilus, Brucella*, Q fever, etc.)	5–10

K. **Blood cultures** are the most important diagnostic tool in endocarditis. Since a distinctive feature of endocarditis is **continuous bacteremia,** blood cultures are likely to be positive on repeated occasions. A major cause of negative blood cultures is previous antimicrobial treatment, and this emphasizes the need for multiple cultures prior to the initiation of therapy. Nevertheless, 5–10% of well-established endocarditis cases are associated with negative blood cultures, and this held true even in the preantibiotic era.

Five blood cultures should be obtained prior to initiation of antimicrobial therapy. The first culture yields the responsible pathogens in over 90% of culture-positive cases. In the absence of previous therapy, additional cultures seldom yield an organism when the first three are negative. The advantage of multiple cultures is clarification of the role of possible contaminants, such as *Staph. epidermidis* or diphtheroids. Additionally, multiple positive cultures can distinguish the continuous bacteremia associated with endothelial infections from the intermittent bacteremia seen with an extravascular portal of entry such as an abscess.

With acute infections requiring emergency antimicrobial therapy, blood cultures can be collected in rapid succession (every 10 minutes) from different veins. In less fulminant cases the cultures should be obtained at spaced intervals over 48 hours, preferably during periods when the fever begins to rise. The strategy regarding patients who have received previous antimicrobial therapy is to discontinue treatment and collect multiple blood cultures over several days if the clinical situation permits. Bone marrow and arterial blood cultures offer no advantage over venous blood samplings.

IV. **Bacteriology.** Virtually any bacterium recovered from humans has been incriminated in endocarditis. Many are considered nonpathogens and seldom cause infections at other sites. Gram-positive cocci are responsible for more than 90% of all endocarditis cases. Gram-negative bacilli, despite their prevalence in bacteremia, seldom invade heart valves, even damaged ones. This remarkable difference between gram-positive and gram-negative bacteria is presumably related to certain inherent properties of the organisms (i.e., adherence factors) and to the protective effect of humoral antibody to gram-negative bacteria.

The organisms most often responsible for endocarditis, according to recent studies, are shown in Table 7-2.

A. ***Strep. viridans*** ("green strep") causes 70–80% of SBE cases and is less common in ABE cases. It almost always involves previously damaged valves. An oral portal of entry was traditionally suspected, although this association has been less frequent in recent years; indeed, some cases of SBE have occurred in edentulous patients. However, it is still recommended that penicillin prophylaxis be used in susceptible hosts undergoing dental manipulation or an oral surgical procedure (see pp. 295–296).

B. **Enterococcal** (*Strep. faecalis,* group D *Streptococcus,* "fecal strep") endocarditis accounts for 20% of SBE cases and usually affects previously damaged valves. Enterococci cause a more virulent disease with a higher mortality than *Strep. viridans*. The genitourinary tract is a common portal of entry; antecedent events are childbirth, a gynecologic surgical procedure, abortion, genitourinary instrumentation, and a urologic surgical procedure. This has led to the recommended prophylactic regimen of penicillin plus streptomycin for patients with valvular disease who undergo these procedures (see pp. 295–296).

C. **Anaerobic and microaerophilic streptococci** amount for 8–15% of endocarditis cases. For this reason, anaerobic blood cultures (thioglycolate medium) as well as aerobic blood cultures should be obtained. The presentation, treatment, and prognosis are similar to those of *Strep. viridans* endocarditis.

D. ***Strep. bovis*** causes a small portion of endocarditis cases, although precise incidence figures are not known. This organism is easily confused with the enterococcus, since both grow on bile-esculin, the medium generally used to identify group D streptococci. The two may be distinguished by testing growth in 6.5% salt—*Strep. bovis* is salt-sensitive, and enterococci are salt-tolerant. This differentiation has important clinical significance, since *Strep. bovis* is more sensitive to penicillin, and endocarditis caused by *Strep. bovis* carries a better prognosis.

An association has been observed between *Strep. bovis* bacteremia and intestinal tumors, especially colon cancer. Some authorities recommend a full gastrointestinal workup when this organism is discovered in the bloodstream, including x-rays of the upper and lower bowel and colonoscopy. Enough negative workups have been performed, however, to make the universal application of this suggestion questionable. A careful history and several stool guaiac tests should suffice in many cases.

E. ***Staph. aureus*** causes over 50% of cases of acute endocarditis (75% in heroin addicts), and previously normal heart valves are particularly vulnerable to it. As many as 65% of patients with fatal *Staph. aureus* bacteremia prove to have endocarditis at autopsy. Consequently, **treatment for endocarditis** is suggested for patients with repeatedly positive blood cultures for *Staph. aureus* and no extracardiac focus, even in the absence of corroborating clinical findings.

The prognosis for *Staph. aureus* endocarditis depends largely on host factors, especially age. The mortality of elderly patients is approximately 75%, while younger patients generally survive. *Staph. aureus* endocarditis is also associated with a relatively high rate of central nervous system complications, annular abscesses, and myocardial abscess.

F. **Pneumococci, *Strep. pyogenes*** (group A), and **gonococci** were responsible for 20–25 of endocarditis cases in the preantibiotic era. These organisms now account for only 1–5% of cases; the change is presumably related to early antibiotic treatment of infections with these organisms at the primary infection sites. When they do invade the heart valves, these organisms cause rapidly destructive lesions and a high mortality.

G. ***Staph. epidermidis*** (*Staph. albus* or coagulase-negative staphylococci), micrococci, diphtheroids, and propionibacteria occasionally cause endocarditis. False interpretations are also possible, since these organisms are frequent contaminants in blood cultures, either from the skin during blood sampling or from manipulations of cultures in the laboratory. Corroborating clinical findings and multiple positive blood cultures are necessary to implicate these organisms in endocarditis.

Staph. epidermidis has become a major cause of endocarditis following open-heart surgery. This organism is usually resistant to penicillin G and occasionally to penicillinase-resistant penicillins (methicillin, nafcillin, and oxacillin). Vancomycin is effective in resistant cases.

H. **Enteric gram-negative bacilli, *Pseudomonas aeruginosa, Ps. cepacia,*** and ***Serratia marcescens*** seldom cause endocarditis except in intravenous drug abusers, postcardiotomy patients, or immunocompromised hosts. Prognosis with medical therapy is poor, even with antimicrobial combinations in high dosage for extended periods. Some patients have persistent bacteremia; others improve clinically and have negative blood cultures, only to relapse either during or after therapy. Antimicrobial resistance often develops during the course of treatment. This necessitates repeated cultures and in vitro susceptibility tests during treatment, as well as careful follow-up to detect relapse.

I. Fungi. The most common cause of fungal endocarditis is *Candida,* followed by *Aspergillus* and *Histoplasma.* Although *Candida albicans* is responsible for nearly all other forms of candidiasis (e.g., skin and vagina), 25–50% of endocarditis cases involve other species, such as *Candida tropicalis, Candida parapsilosis,* and *Candida guilliermondi.* Open-heart surgery is the most common underlying condition. Contributing factors are contamination during the procedure, indwelling polyethylene intravenous catheters, and the use of broad-spectrum antibiotics. Distinctive clinical features are

1. Indolent course with low-grade or intermittent fever for extended periods.
2. Organisms difficult to recover in blood cultures. Optimal yield is with a biphasic media (brain-heart infusion agar and broth) incubated at 30°C and held for 4 weeks.
3. Failure of a susceptible host to respond to empiric antibiotic treatment.
4. Large vegetations that often cause embolic occlusion of major vessels or obstruct the valve orifice.
5. Endophthalmitis. This finding is highly suggestive of candidiasis. Funduscopic examination should be performed regularly on postcardiotomy patients with unexplained fever.
6. Poor outcome with medical treatment. Candidemia may clear with amphotericin B, but viable fungi often persist in vegetations. Overall survival rates are less than 10%. Many authorities advocate early surgical intervention, since antifungal treatment seldom sterilizes vegetations and major embolic complications can occur at any time. Cures have been recorded with valve replacement following institution of full doses of amphotericin B alone or combined with 5-fluorocytosine or rifampin.

V. Medical treatment. Endocarditis is universally fatal if untreated. With appropriate antimicrobial agents, 50–70% of patients are cured of infection, although survivors are often left with serious cardiac disease. The best results are seen with *Strep. viridans* infections (>90% cured) and the worst results with gram-negative bacilli and fungi (<10% cured). The major causes of medical failure are intractable congestive failure, resistant organisms, embolic complications, and renal failure. Factors associated with a poor prognosis are summarized in Table 7-3.

A. Certain principles of **antimicrobial therapy** are unique to endocarditis:

1. **Bactericidal agents are preferred.** These include penicillins, cephalosporins, and vancomycin.
2. Antimicrobial **combinations** are used under certain circumstances (to treat enterococci, gram-negative bacteria, and fungi), either to accomplish synergy or to prevent emergence of antimicrobial resistance.
3. Antimicrobial drugs should be administered **parenterally** (usually intravenously) in **large doses.**
4. **Extended courses** are advocated, at least 4–6 weeks.

B. Suggested **drug regimens** are summarized in Table 7-4. Antimicrobial susceptibility patterns, however, should be confirmed with laboratory testing of the blood culture isolate in all cases. The standard disk diffusion antibiotic test is inadequate, since it determines bacterial inhibition rather than bactericidal activity. Furthermore, the disk test does not measure precise end points of susceptibility and does not permit evaluation of antimicrobial combinations. The preferred method is to measure the minimum inhibitory concentration (MIC) and the minimum bactericidal concentration (MBC), using serial dilutions of antibiotics against a standardized inoculum of the organism. Antibiotics can be tested alone and in various combinations.

Therapeutic decisions are remarkably simplified when the responsible organism has been recovered. This emphasizes the importance of obtaining cultures prior to initiation of treatment. A recommendation for culture-negative cases consists of therapy for enterococci as well as for other common organisms. A special

Table 7-3. Risk factors in endocarditis

Risk factor	Favorable Prognosis	Unfavorable prognosis
Onset	Subacute	Acute
Infecting microorganism	*Streptococcus viridans*	*Staphylococcus aureus*
	Strep. bovis	Enterococci
	Microaerophilic or anaerobic streptococci	Gram-negative bacilli (esp. *Pseudomonas*) Pneumococci Gonococci Fungi
Valve	Mitral, tricuspid, pulmonic	Aortic, prosthetic
Cardiac status	Compensated	Heart failure
CNS status	—	Coma
Age	—	> 60 years
Associated diseases	—	Cirrhosis, malignancy, uremia

problem exists when *Staph. aureus* is particularly suspect, i.e., in a patient with a fulminant course or in a heroin addict.

C. Response to medical therapy

1. **Follow-up blood cultures** should be obtained daily for the initial 5 days; weekly for the duration of therapy; and monthly for 2 months after therapy. More frequent cultures are indicated when the response is suboptimal or when symptoms recur. In most cases the cultures will be negative 1–2 days after institution of antimicrobial treatment.
2. The expected clinical response during the first 2–7 days of antibiotics is defervescence and subjective improvement. The differential diagnosis of persistent or recurrent fever includes inadequate antibiotic therapy (insufficient dosage or inappropriate agent); superinfection with a resistant organism; drug fever; metastatic abscess; embolic infarction; complications at injection sites (e.g., thrombophlebitis and myositis); or an unrelated febrile illness. Splenomegaly, glomerulonephritis, and anemia respond slowly. Changing murmurs generally mean little in regard to adequacy of antimicrobial treatment.
3. A number of adverse factors lead to a poor prognosis in endocarditis (see Table 7-3). The unfavorable factors are acute onset, virulent pathogen, aortic or prosthetic valve involvement, heart failure, coma, advanced age, and serious associated diseases.
4. **Long-term follow-up** is crucial in the management of endocarditis. Up to one-third of patients expire from late complications after bacteriologic cure. This is usually due to hemodynamic changes that occur during the healing process, progressive valve stenosis or insufficiency, mitral valve aneurysm, valve perforation, valve distortion, or myocardial fibrosis. Patients with these complications should be evaluated for an elective cardiac surgical procedure on the same basis as other patients with valvular heart disease. Additional late sequelae are mycotic aneurysm, chronic renal failure, embolization of sterile thrombi, and recurrence of endocarditis.

VI. Surgical intervention during active infection

A. Despite the risks of operating in an infected field, cardiotomy and valve replacement are justified for certain complications. Mortality is high (25–40%) when cardiotomy is performed on an emergency basis. The most important factor in surgical mortality is the hemodynamic status of the patient at the time of the

Table 7-4. Recommended therapy for endocarditis

Organism	Preferred regimen	Alternatives	Comment
Nonenterococcal streptococci	Penicillin G, 6–10 million units daily for 4 wk, ± streptomycin, 1 gm/day for 2 wk	Cephalothin, 8–12 gm/day for 4 wk Vancomycin, 2 gm IV daily for 4 wk	For relatively resistant strains (minimum bacteriocidal concentration [MBC] penicillin >0.3 μg/ml), add streptomycin
Enterococci	Penicillin G, 20 million units daily for 4 wk **plus** streptomycin, 2 gm IM daily for 2 wk, then 1 gm IM daily for 1 wk **or** gentamicin, 3 mg/kg/day for 4 wk	Vancomycin, 2 gm IV daily for 4 wk, **plus** streptomycin or gentamicin for 4 wk	Gentamicin is preferred to streptomycin for strains with minimum inhibitory concentration > 2,000 μg/ml; ampicillin is alternative to penicillin; cephalosporins are unacceptable
Staphylococcus aureus	Nafcillin, 9–12 gm IV daily for 4–6 wk	Cephalothin, 8–12 gm IV daily for 4–6 wk Vancomycin, 2 gm IV daily for 4–6 wk	Vancomycin is preferred for methicillin-resistant strains. 4-week regimen may be adequate for those with good prognosis, e.g., addicts
Staph. epidermidis	Penicillin, 20 million units IV daily for 6 wk **or** cephalothin, 8–12 gm IV daily for 6 wk **or** nafcillin, 9–12 gm IV daily for 6 wk **or** vancomycin, 2 gm IV daily for 6 wk **plus** gentamicin, 3 mg/kg/day for 1 wk **plus** rifampin, 600 mg PO daily for 6 wk	Preferred regimen **followed by** rifampin, 600 mg PO daily, **plus** cloxacillin or cephalexin, 2 gm PO daily for 6 mo	Preferred initial treatment is vancomycin **plus** gentamicin **plus** rifampin. Preference for penicillin, cephalosporin, nafcillin, or vancomycin is determined by sensitivity tests
Coliforms, *Pseudomonas*	Ampicillin, 12–20 gm IV daily for 6 wk **or** cephalothin, 8–12 gm IV daily for 6 wk **or** carbenicillin, 30–36 gm IV daily for 6 wk **plus** gentamicin, 4–5 mg/kg/day for 4–6 wk		Preferred regimen depends on sensitivity tests; other aminoglycosides may be substituted for gentamicin, depending on these results
Candida	Amphotericin B, 0.8–1 mg/kg IV 3 days weekly		Poor prognosis; usually requires an operation for cure

procedure. The major cause of operative mortality is cardiac insufficiency, especially inability to come off cardiopulmonary bypass. Other postoperative complications include valve dehiscence, peripheral emboli, and reinfection, usually with a different organism. Whenever possible, sepsis and hemodynamic complications should be vigorously managed to permit elective surgical intervention 3–6 months after a complete course of antibiotics. Medical management alone, when a surgical procedure is indicated, is associated with mortality rates of 80% or more. An early operation is advocated for some high-risk patients with deteriorating hemodynamic status, even in the face of persistent bacteremia.

B. If a surgical procedure is required during the course of antibiotic therapy, the entire nidus of infection should be removed. This can be accomplished when only the leaflets are involved, but it may prove difficult or impossible in extensive infection of the valve and its supporting structures or the myocardium. Excised vegetations should always be Gram's-stained, cultured, and studied histologically. The entire recommended course of antimicrobials for the original pathogen should be completed postoperatively. The duration of postoperative drug treatment is based on the histologic appearance of the resected valve; the presence of active infection indicates that antibiotics should be given for 4 additional weeks.

C. Valvectomy without valve replacement is often adequate for endocarditis involving the tricuspid or pulmonic valves. A valve prosthesis may be inserted at a later time if this results in serious right heart failure. Pulmonary hypertension or significant mitral disease interdict valvectomy alone.

D. Indications for surgical intervention:

1. **Irreversible cardiac failure,** the most common indication for emergency cardiac surgery, is caused by valve perforation, progressive valve damage, valve prolapse, ruptured chordae tendineae, myocarditis, myocardial abscess, or myocardial infarction due to coronary emboli.
   - **a.** Surgical intervention can only reverse complications resulting from **damage to the valve** or its supporting structures. It has no effect on myocardial failure. Valvular damage is most frequent with aortic valve endocarditis, less common with mitral valve involvement, and uncommon with right-sided endocarditis.
   - **b.** When **heart failure** due to valvular insufficiency is severe, a surgical procedure should be performed immediately. For less severe congestive failure, operation is indicated for patients who fail to improve or who deteriorate despite aggressive medical therapy.
   - **c.** The most common cause of intractable heart failure is **aortic insufficiency** due to extensive vegetations with leaflet destruction, perforation, or valve detachment with flail cusps. Patients with slowly evolving aortic insufficiency show the classic signs, which include ventricular dilatation and hypertrophy, a large stroke volume, and a wide pulse pressure. These are not found with acute aortic regurgitation, in which compensation is not accomplished by ventricular dilatation and hypertrophy. Tachycardia becomes an important mechanism in maintaining cardiac output. Chest x-ray films show only mild-to-moderate cardiomegaly with pulmonary vascular insufficiency. Physical examination typically uncovers a soft and brief diastolic decrescendo murmur and a first heart sound that is soft or absent. The severity of ventricular volume overload has a correlation with the degree of premature mitral valve closure; this can be determined by echocardiogram.
   - **d.** With **mitral insufficiency,** angiographic studies are often recommended to distinguish valve damage from myocardial disease as the cause of heart failure. The role of myocardial disease in congestive failure can be clarified with echocardiography and blood pool imaging.
2. **Resistant infection** is the indication for surgical intervention in 10–20% of cases. The responsible organism may be relatively resistant to antimicrobials, or become resistant during treatment, or never be identified. Gram-negative bacilli, such as *Pseudomonas* and *Serratia,* and fungi are notorious in this regard. In such instances patients may respond initially to treatment,

but the relapse rate is high, and medical cures are accomplished in only 10–20% of cases. Nevertheless, antimicrobial drugs are employed on a trial basis and to improve the postoperative condition. The usual indications for surgical intervention are persistent bacteremia after 10–14 days of appropriate antimicrobial treatment or relapse after a course of treatment. A highly resistant organism is an added argument for early operation. Some authorities consider fungal endocarditis an absolute indication for a surgical procedure. Before proceeding, however, it is important to be certain that optimal antibiotic therapy has been given, based on sensitivities of the pathogen, and that there is no extracardiac focus to explain persistent sepsis.

3. **Multiple systemic emboli** occurring during the course of medical treatment are the reason for surgical intervention in 5–10% of endocarditis cases. Anticoagulants do not prevent continued embolization and are not indicated for such emboli. This complication generally occurs during the first few weeks of treatment, when vegetations are friable. Embolization to the coronary or cerebral arteries is the principal concern.
4. **Septal or anular abscess** requires surgical intervention, and an early procedure reduces the extent of tissue destruction. These are most common with aortic valve endocarditis. The usual finding is persistent fever despite appropriate antibiotic treatment, especially when associated with typical ECG changes. Extension of infection into the conduction system of the septum is to be suspected from cardiograms that show progressive prolongation of P–R and Q–T intervals, bundle branch block, or complete heart block. Atrioventricular dissociation and multifocal premature ventricular contractions are less common. Rupture through the membranous septum results in a left-to-right shunt; this is an uncommon complication, but it is surgically correctable.

Endocarditis of Prosthetic Valves

I. General principles

A. The **incidence** is generally 0.2–1% during the early postoperative period and 2% during the 36 months following the surgical procedure.

B. The **prognosis** is poor, since invasion of myocardial tissue and serious valve dysfunction are common. Reported mortality rates for early-occurring cases are 70–90%, and for late cases, 35–50%.

II. Risk factors. Factors associated with an increased risk of postoperative endocarditis include

A. Use of cardiopulmonry bypass. The increased risk with a bypass pump may be related to a reduction in humoral defense mechanisms, which correlates with the duration of pump perfusion.

B. Amount of prosthetic material implanted

C. Operation on the aortic valve

D. Quality of aseptic technique, duration of procedure, and number of persons in the operating room

E. Porcine heterografts and mechanical valves—approximately equal risk with each

III. Measures that decrease risk

A. Treat extracardiac foci of infection. Any infection, such as those involving the skin, urinary tract, or teeth, should be eliminated prior to an elective cardiac surgical procedure. Dental procedures, cystoscopy, prostatectomy, and other procedures associated with an endocarditis risk should also be performed before elective cardiac surgery.

B. Extracardiac infections that occur in the postoperative period should be aggressively treated. Metal needles are preferred over polyethylene catheters for postoperative intravenous infusions. Urinary catheters, intraarterial or intravenous lines, and tracheostomies should be used sparingly and eliminated as soon as possible.

C. **Prophylactic antimicrobials** are used for nearly all cardiotomy procedures, although their efficacy is occasionally disputed. Most commonly, penicillinase-resistant penicillins (nafcillin or oxacillin) or cephalosporins are employed. Some surgeons also add ampicillin, penicillin G, or an aminoglycoside, but this is not generally recommended. Prophylactic antimicrobials should be initiated no more than 24 hours preoperatively, administered to provide effective levels throughout the intraoperative period, and continued for 2–3 days after the surgical procedure.
Suggested regimens are

Nafcillin	1 gm IV or IM **or**
Cefazolin	0.5 gm IV or IM

given the night before operation (optional), ½–1 hour preoperatively, repeated within 4 hours during the operative procedure, and continued every 6 hours thereafter for 48–72 hours.
More extensive use of prophylactic antimicrobials is discouraged, as it appears to be unnecessary and may select out resistant organisms.

IV. **Early postoperative endocarditis** (within 2 months of cardiotomy)

A. **Source of Infection.** Infection can be introduced during the operation from an exogenous source, e.g., operating room air, personnel, donor blood, or the pump reservoir. Cultures of the perioperative site just prior to closure have yielded *Staph. epidermidis* or diphtheroids in up to 60% of cases. Intravenous catheters, arterial lines, and urinary catheters may also be important sources of valve seeding.

B. **Bacteriology.** In order of frequency, the following organisms cause early endocarditis: *Staph. epidermidis,* gram-negative bacilli, *Staph. aureus,* and miscellaneous organisms including streptococci and fungi. Types of pathogens vary among institutions and with different prophylactic regimens.

C. **Clinical features**

1. Fever, chills, and positive blood cultures are common.
2. Petechiae, splenomegaly, and urine sediment changes are highly suggestive but are **relatively infrequent.**
3. **Valve dysfunction** is evidenced by auscultatory, hemodynamic, or roentgenographic changes. Infected **patches** following septal defect repair may tear loose, resulting in recurrence of shunts. With **prosthetic valves** there may be impaired closure or detachment from the anulus, causing an insufficiency murmur. Thrombi may partially occlude the valve, with disappearance of the valve click. These changes must be differentiated from those of ball variance or valve detachment due to nonseptic processes. Phonocardiograms can detect alterations in prosthetic valve sounds, indicating valve dysfunction, which are not heard with auscultation.
4. Prolonged exposure roentgenograms of valves with extensive suture line disruption show an abnormal tilting of the prosthesis (**double exposure sign**). Aortic prosthetic valves should have little movement; even minor degrees of tilt are considered abnormal. On the other hand, mitral prostheses have a normal to-and-fro movement, and greater angulation is required for diagnostic significance. Cinefluorography should be performed to detect these changes when endocarditis involves a prosthesis with a radiopaque base. The echocardiographic demonstration of vegetations on prosthetic valves has proved difficult; however, this procedure can be helpful in assessing poppet mobility.

D. **Treatment.** Mortality for early postoperative endocarditis **exceeds** 70%. The role of antimicrobial drugs in treating this complication is debated. Some feel that an antibiotic trial is indicated since medical cures have been reported and there is a reluctance to reoperate. Others argue that this approach is mere temporizing and that relapse is predictable. The two different approaches commonly advocated are as follows:

1. A trial of medical treatment, with systemic antibiotics for up to 8–12 weeks. Prolonged administration of oral agents for an additional 6–12 months has

also been suggested. The choice of drugs depends on the sensitivities of the specific pathogen. The general recommendations for bactericidal drugs in high dosage apply in this setting as well (see Table 7-4).

2. Surgical intervention in all cases—advocated by some authorities because of the high rate of failure with medical treatment and the frequency of severe valve dysfunction or perivalvular tissue involvement. The timing of surgical intervention is dictated by the clinical circumstances. Valve dysfunction with severe congestive failure requires an emergency procedure. Additional findings that indicate high risk are evidence of annular or myocardial tissue involvement (perivascular leak, persistent fever, or conduction disturbances), valve dysfunction with leaflet destruction, poppet entrapment, and obstructing vegetations. Unfortunately, many patients with early prosthetic valve endocarditis are not surgical candidates due to other medical complications.

V. **Late prosthetic valve endocarditis** (more than 2 months after cardiotomy)

A. **Source of infection.** The pathogen is introduced from an endogenous source, related to inapparent bacteremia, toothbrushing, or dental manipulation. Thus, valve seeding in this situation is analogous to that in patients with rheumatic valvular disease.

B. **Bacteriology.** The pathogens in late cases are reminiscent of infections on natural valves, with streptococci (*viridans* and enterococci) causing the majority of cases. Even in these cases, however, there remains a disproportionately high frequency of *Staph. epidermidis,* gram-negative bacilli, and fungi.

C. **Clinical features.** Fever, chills, malaise, and anorexia usually take a more indolent course, with less likelihood of early congestive failure than in the early postoperative cases.

D. **Treatment.** Medical therapy has a better chance of success with uncomplicated endocarditis caused by streptococci, although the overall mortality is 45%. The specific antibiotics are selected by sensitivity patterns (see Table 7-4), and the approach is the same as to other forms of endocarditis. Surgical intervention is usually required for infections involving resistant organisms and for late prosthetic valve endocarditis complicated by heart failure, persistent bacteremia during antibiotic therapy, frequent embolization, or bacteriologic relapse. Loss of the prosthetic valve click, appearance of insufficiency murmurs, or roentgenographic evidence of disrupted suture lines are ominous signs that dictate early surgical intervention. Relapse after a single extended course of appropriate antibiotics usually necessitates reoperation.

Infected Pacemakers

I. **General principles.** Infection is usually localized to the electrode or generator site, often necessitating removal of the entire foreign body. Despite direct continuity with and impingement on the endocardium, endocarditis is rare.

II. **Pathophysiology.** The infection may occur at any time following implantation. Early postoperative infections (within 6 weeks) result from breaks in aseptic surgical techniques. Late infections may be associated with skin erosions over superficial implants, especially in thin patients. More commonly there is no antecedent event, and the organism has probably settled in the foreign body during a transient bacteremia. In either early or late cases, the pathogen is nearly always *Staph. aureus.* Many surgeons use antibiotic prophylaxis when inserting pacemakers, but its efficacy has not been demonstrated. If used, the prophylactic agent should be a penicillinase-resistant penicillin (oxacillin or nafcillin) or a cephalosporin.

III. **Clinical findings.** Erythema and tenderness, wound drainage, wound dehiscence, and skin necrosis are found at the electrode or pulse generator site. In most cases there is a minimal systemic reaction—the temperature and WBC are normal or only mildly elevated.

IV. **Management**

A. Traditional treatment is **removal** of the generator and electrode with local debridement of the infected area. Another pacemaker can be inserted at a distant site, or a temporary transvenous pacemaker can be utilized and a permanent pacemaker inserted at a later time.

B. Alternatively, there may be an **attempt to salvage** the original pacemaker with local antibiotic irrigations. While this approach has its adherents, it is not widely practiced. The infected site is widely debrided, including excision of a margin of viable tissue. The generator and electrodes may be removed, chemically sterilized, and reinserted either at the original site or below the pectoral muscle. A polyethylene catheter is inserted through a stab wound for infusions, and drainage is accomplished with a rubber drain placed in the dependent portion of the pocket. Irrigation consists of bacitracin alone (for *Staph. aureus* infections) or a combination of bacitracin (50,000 units/L) and neomycin (200 mg/L). Long-term oral antimicrobials should be given according to susceptibility tests.

C. Parenteral antibiotics are given during removal and replacement of another pacemaker and for 48–72 hours thereafter. Longer durations of therapy are indicated only for severe local infections and those associated with a systemic reaction (fever and leukocytosis). Selection of agents is based on Gram's stain and culture of drainage, needle aspirates, or debrided tissue. Empiric treatment should always include an agent active against *Staph. aureus*—a penicillinase-resistant penicillin (nafcillin or oxacillin) or a cephalosporin.

D. Bacteremia in association with infection of the pacemaker site often means superinfection of the cardiac valves or of the endocardial implantation site of the wire, especially when staphylococci are the isolates. The approach for bacteremic infection is more aggressive: immediate removal of the pacemaker and its wire, and 4 weeks of appropriate antibiotic therapy.

Fever Following Cardiac Surgical Procedure

I. General principles. Fever and leukocytosis, unrelated to infection, are common following cardiac surgical procedure. The fever is noted within hours of extracorporeal circulation, usually peaks to 38–39°C, and then subsides within 2–4 days. The WBC is often elevated to 10–20,000/mm^3 on the first postoperative day and returns to normal within 2–4 days. High fevers and those extending beyond 4–7 postoperative days should be regarded as abnormal, and require workup for several potential causes (Table 7-5).

II. Endocarditis may occur at any time during the postoperative period. Corroborative findings are positive blood cultures and evidence of valve dysfunction.

III. Extracardiac infections occur at the sternal incision, in intravascular catheters, and in the lung and urinary tract. These infections are generally noted within 3 weeks of operation and tend to involve bacteria resistant to the prophylactic antimicrobial regimen.

IV. Bacteremia in most cases following cardiac surgery originates from extracardiac sources. Bacteremia that is not obviously due to endocarditis should be investigated by the following:

A. Chest x-ray, urinalysis, inspection of intravascular catheter sites, and examination of the wound.

B. Removal of all dispensable predisposing factors, such as intraarterial lines, intravenous lines, and urinary catheter.

C. Culture of blood (5 times), urine, intravascular catheters, and any purulent drainage.

D. Treatment for the blood culture isolate with a 7–10-day course of systemic antimicrobials.

E. Presumption of endocarditis if bacteremia recurs after antibiotics are discontinued.

V. Postpericardiotomy syndrome may follow any type of cardiac surgical procedure. An analogous syndrome has been noted with myocardial infarction, viral pericar-

Table 7-5. Differential diagnosis of fever following cardiac surgery

Factor	Endocarditis	Postpericardiotomy syndrome	Postperfusion syndrome	Hepatitis
Onset after surgery	Any time	1–12 wk (usually 2–4 wk)	1–12 wk (usually 2–6 wk)	2–20 wk (usually 3–8 wk)
Fever	Variable, often spiking	Variable	Low-grade	Low-grade or normal
Chest pain	Usually absent	Common	Not present	Not present
Principal physical finding	Valve dysfunction	Pericardial friction rub or effusion	Splenomegaly	Tender hepatomegaly
WBC	Normal or leukocytosis	Normal or leukocytosis	Lymphocytosis with atypical lymphs	Normal or lymphocytosis with atypical lymphs
Principal lab test	Blood culture	ECG Chest x-ray	CBC Urine or serology for CMV (usually present but nonspecific)	Liver function tests, especially SGOT and SGPT HAA Blood for HBsAg
Treatment	Antimicrobial; reoperation, if required	Salicylates Corticosteroids, if severe	No specific treatment	No specific treatment

ditis, and chest trauma. The illness usually begins in the second or third postoperative week with the onset of fever and chest pain. Less commonly, the fever merges imperceptibly into the usual postoperative temperature elevation. The pain is retrosternal, intensified with respirations or swallowing, and alleviated in the upright position. Approximately 30–50% of patients have a pericardial friction rub. X-rays and physical examination often show evidence of a pericardial and/or pleural effusion. ECG shows generalized S–T segment elevation, indicating pericarditis, or nonspecific S–T and T wave changes that simulate ischemia or the effects of digitalis. The complete blood count (CBC) is normal or shows neutrophilic leukocytosis without atypical lymphocytes.

This illness is self-limited, usually lasting 2–4 weeks. Therapy is directed toward making the patient more comfortable with antipyretics, analgesics, and antiinflammatory agents. Aspirin is particularly effective. Pericardiocentesis is occasionally required to prevent cardiac constriction. Severe cases should be treated with corticosteroids, which relieve pain and fever dramatically within 1–2 days.

VI. **Postperfusion syndrome** affects 3–8% of patients undergoing a cardiac surgical procedure. The onset of fever is usually 2–6 weeks after operation but may blend with the expected postoperative fever or may be delayed for several months. Hallmarks of this syndrome are low-grade **fever, splenomegaly,** and **lymphocytosis** with **atypical lymphocytes.** There may be peripheral adenopathy, a generalized maculopapular rash, or mild abnormalities in liver function tests. The syndrome appears to be related to the use of large amounts of **fresh blood** rather than to cardiopulmonary bypass per se. Serology and viral cultures suggest that **cytomegalovirus** (CMV) is usually responsible. However, positive findings of CMV infection are sometimes noted after cardiopulmonary bypass without postoperative complications. Epstein-Barr virus (infectious mononucleosis) has also been implicated in this syndrome. The prognosis is excellent, and symptoms clear spontaneously in 1–4 weeks. No therapy other than salicylates is required.

VII. **Hepatitis.** The incidence is related to the amount and source of blood used. Hepatitis risk is greater with blood from paid donors than from volunteer donors. The onset usually occurs 3–8 weeks postoperatively but may be as early as 1 week or as late as 20 weeks following operation. Characteristic features are abnormal findings of liver function, especially the (1) serum glutamic-oxalacetic transaminase (SGOT) and (2) serum glutamic-pyruvic transaminase (SGPT), which are universally elevated. Additional findings are tender hepatomegaly, low-grade fever, anorexia, and malaise. Arthritis, urticaria, or glomerulonephritis are occasionally noted. CBC may show lymphocytosis with atypical lymphocytes. The test for hepatitis B antigen (HBsAg) is considered diagnostic. However, most cases are non-A, non-B hepatitis, for which no specific test is available (p. 56). Hepatitis may bear strong resemblance to the postperfusion syndrome. Principal features favoring a diagnosis of hepatitis are jaundice, tender hepatomegaly, marked elevations in SGOT, and positive serology for hepatitis B. No specific therapy for hepatitis is available.

Mediastinitis Following Cardiac Surgical Procedure

I. **General principles.** The incidence of wound infections is 0.5–5% following median sternotomy incisions for cardiac surgical procedures. They are a major complication because they present a threat to the cardiotomy incision and prosthetic implants. Furthermore, chronic infections of the costal cartilages may continue for months or even years, requiring repeated operative procedures. The incidence is higher among patients who have prolonged procedures, infected tracheostomy stomas, postoperative closed-chest massage, low cardiac output postoperatively, reoperation in the early postoperative period, and wound hematoma.

II. **Clinical features.** Usual findings are local tenderness, erythema, purulent wound drainage, sternal wound dehiscence, persistent or recurrent postoperative fever, and leukocytosis. Less commonly, there is sternal instability with a rocking motion.

Patients with early infections (< 4 weeks after operation), representing 70% of such cases, have higher fever, toxicity, and bacteremia. The late cases (> 4 wk after operation) are often afebrile, and drainage from the operative site is the hallmark of infection. X-rays show no characteristic changes until late in the course of infection.

III. Bacteriology. Patients with early infections usually have pathogens resistant to the antibiotics used as prophylaxis. The most common organisms are coliforms, *Pseudomonas,* and *Staph. epidermidis. Candida* and *Aspergillus* are occasionally seen. Late cases are caused by staphylococci (either *Staph. aureus* or *Staph. epidermidis*), gram-negative bacilli, or *Mycobacterium chelonei.* The marked variations in pathogens emphasize the need for careful culturing to guide selection of antimicrobials.

IV. Treatment.

- **A.** The wound should be reopened, debrided, and irrigated. Exudate and excised tissue should be Gram's-stained and cultured.
- **B.** Sternal bone is rongeured away to the point of fresh bleeding. It is important to remove all infected bone, since chronic osteomyelitis of the sternum and costal cartilages may continue to simmer for months or even years. Steel wire sutures at the site of infected bone should be removed.
- **C.** The wound is packed and allowed to heal secondarily. The use of topical antibiotics and irrigation tubes in this setting is arbitrary and may cause superinfection with resistant organisms, particularly *Pseudomonas* and *Candida.*
- **D.** Systemic antibiotics should be administered for 4–6 weeks according to results of antibiotic susceptibility tests. Infections with *M. chelonei* are usually treated with amikacin ± cefoxitin.

V. Prevention.

- **A.** Adequate aseptic technique and careful wound hemostatis are mandatory.
- **B.** The use of orotracheal or nasotracheal tubes is favored for postoperative ventilation in deference to tracheostomy. If necessary, a cricothyroid tracheostomy is preferred to isolate the stoma from the sternal wound.
- **C.** Sternal closure with sutures through intercostal spaces rather than costal cartilages tends to prevent chronic osteomyelitis.
- **D.** Extended courses of prophylactic antibiotics have failed to prevent sternal wound infections and appear to encourage emergence of resistant microorganisms.

Purulent Pericarditis

I. General principles. Purulent pericarditis is a highly lethal infection that requires prompt drainage and intensive antimicrobial treatment. Formerly, nearly all cases were caused by direct extension of pulmonary infections or seeding from septicemia. Recent studies indicate that up to 20–30% of cases are postoperative complications of thoracic surgical procedures. There has also been a shift in bacteriologic patterns. *Staph. aureus* remains the most common pathogen, but there has been a decline in pneumococcal pericarditis accompanied by a rising incidence of cases caused by gram-negative bacilli. One factor that has not changed is the high mortality rate, still 50–75% according to recent reports. The diagnosis is established by pericardiocentesis with analysis of fluid and culture. Many cases are not diagnosed until late in the course or are detected only at autopsy.

II. Etiology

- **A.** Direct extension from primary infections of the **lung, pleura, or mediastinum.** Pneumococcal pneumonia in a pulmonary segment adjacent to the pericardium is the most frequent underlying condition in this group. Most instances involve an excessive delay in initiation of treatment, and pericarditis represents a late complication.
- **B.** Direct extension from **postoperative infections,** especially cardiotomy procedures or esophageal surgery. Usually there is antecedent infection of the sternal wound. The most common pathogens are *Staph. aureus,* gram-negative bacilli, and fungi (*Candida* or *Aspergillus*).
- **C. Bacteremia** with seeding of the pericardium. The most frequent pathogen is *Staph. aureus.*

D. Direct extension of **cardiac infections,** either endocarditis or myocardial abscess. The bacteria that usually cause endocarditis are implicated, but there is a disproportionate incidence of *Staph. aureus* in this group.

E. Underlying **systemic conditions,** such as burns and debilitating disease, are two of many additional factors predisposing to purulent pericarditis. Occasional cases occur in patients with pericarditis due to nonbacterial causes, such as uremia and viral infections.

III. Bacteriology. The most frequently encountered pathogens are *Staph. aureus, Strep. pneumoniae,* and gram-negative bacilli. Less common are *Neisseria meningitis, H. influenzae,* anaerobic bacteria, and *Candida.* As already noted (**II**), there are substantial differences in the distribution of pathogens according to the underlying cause.

IV. Diagnosis

A. Signs and symptoms. The infection is fulminant, with prominent systemic signs of sepsis. The main problem in clinical diagnosis is to localize the process to the pericardium. Two factors tend to interfere with early diagnosis: First, there is usually an associated infection, such as pneumonia, to account for the systemic toxicity. Second, the classic signs of pericarditis—especially typical pain, diagnostic ECG changes, "water-bottle" heart on x-ray, and pericardial friction rub—are often absent because of the gluelike exudate, which may not necessarily be abundant in volume. Thus, it may be necessary to proceed with echocardiography followed by pericardiocentesis on the basis of minimal direct evidence and adroit clinical judgment.

B. Clinical clues to pericarditis.

1. Precordial pain—often pleuritic or related to position
2. Evidence of tamponade—elevated central venous pressure, hypotension, narrowed pulse pressure, or paradoxic pulse (fall of $>$ 10 mm Hg in blood pressure on inspiration)
3. Precordial dullness, distant heart tones, or pericardial friction rub
4. X-ray films showing diffuse cardiomegaly—especially rapid increases in cardiac silhouette without pulmonary congestion
5. ECG changes—especially generalized S–T elevations with a "coving" pattern or T wave inversions

C. Techniques that demonstrate pericardial effusions or thickening are echocardiography, radioisotope scanning, and CO_2 infusion studies. Echocardiography has proved especially useful in distinguishing pericardial disease from chamber dilatation. Cardiac catheterization shows a typical pressure curve and pericardial thickening, but noninvasive techniques often give sufficient information to establish the diagnosis.

D. Differential diagnosis of pericardial effusions includes other causes of pericarditis: idiopathic, viral, tuberculous, fungal (especially histoplasmosis and coccidioidomycosis), traumatic, lymphomatous, carcinomatous (especially lung and breast), uremic causes; as well as toxoplasmosis, rupture of a left lobe amebic liver abscess, collagen vascular disease and irradiation. Purulent pericarditis is distinguished by a more rampant clinical course and one of the predisposing disease states just listed, but the definitive test is analysis and culture of pericardial fluid.

E. Pericardiocentesis should be performed whenever purulent pericarditis is suspected. Routine tests to be performed on the aspirate include (1) stains and cultures for bacteria (aerobes and anaerobes), fungi, and AFB; (2) cell count and differential, and (3) glucose concentration. The diagnosis is based on the recovery of a pathogen and/or purulent fluid (WBC $>$30,000/mm^3 with a predominance of polymorphonuclear cells). Gram's stain provides an immediate clue to the etiologic agent and is occasionally positive when cultures fail to yield growth. Glucose concentration is usually low in bacterial infections but may be normal early in the course.

1. **Technique of pericardiocentesis.** An 18–21-gauge spinal needle is inserted 1 cm below the costal margin to the left of the xiphoid process. Electrocardiogram monitoring is accomplished by attaching a chest lead to the needle

hub with the machine set at the V position. The needle is angled toward the left shoulder and advanced until fluid is obtained. If the epicardium is contacted, the ECG shows a large S–T segment elevation (injury pattern) or ventricular ectopic beats. Bloody aspirates must be tested to assure that the myocardium has not been entered. Blood in pericardial aspirates fails to clot and has a lower hematocrit than peripheral blood. Failure to obtain fluid may indicate that the fluid is organized or loculated.

V. **Treatment**

A. **Parenteral antimicrobials** are given in high dosage and continued for 4–6 weeks. Selection of agents is based on Gram's stain and culture of pericardial fluid. When empiric decisions are necessary, an intravenous cephalosporin is appropriate for likely bacterial pathogens in cases unrelated to a thoracic surgical procedure. For postoperative infections, a penicillinase-resistant penicillin (nafcillin or oxacillin) or a cephalosporin should be combined with an aminoglycoside. The regimen can be modified as soon as culture results become available. Direct inoculation of antibiotics is unnecessary, since pericardial penetration with systemic administration is good.

B. Careful observation of the patient should be made for signs of **tamponade**—hypotension, narrowed pulse pressure, increasing tachycardia, elevated venous pressure, and hepatomegaly. Tamponade may occur precipitously and requires immediate pericardiocentesis. Intravenous fluids and isoproterenol are adjunctive and temporizing measures to use while preparing for emergency needle aspiration. A large-bore needle (14-gauge or 16-gauge) may be necessary to permit free flow of purulent or blood pericardial effusions. Removal of 50–100 ml often promptly relieves tamponade due to rapid changes in pressure when critical volumes are reached. As much pericardial fluid as is obtainable should be aspirated when possible.

C. **Surgical drainage** is almost always necessary. Although some authorities advocate repeated cardiocentesis, it should be recognized that the fluid may quickly reaccumulate to dangerous levels; in addition, the procedure itself is not without risk. Similarly, indwelling polyethylene catheters inserted into the pericardium through large-bore needles are generally inadequate. These tend to become plugged, thereby providing incomplete drainage.

1. **Pericardiostomy** to provide continuous drainage of the pericardium is the preferred technique in dealing with impending tamponade. Loculations are removed at the time of surgical procedure, and drains are generally left in place for several days. The pericardium may be irrigated with antibiotic solutions, but this is unnecessary, since adequate levels of antibiotics are easily achieved in the pericardium with systemic administration. The route of drainage may be through (1) a simple intercostal incision after excision of one or more costal cartilages (usually the left 5th and/or 6th; (2) the subxiphoid route, which provides the advantage of pericardial drainage at its most dependent site; or (3) the posterolateral route, which it may be necessary to take if the anterior pericardial layers are fused precluding anterior drainage.
2. **Pericardiectomy** is preferred for chronic infections that have resulted in thick pus and dense adherent membranes. It is usually performed through a left anterior thoracotomy incision. Drainage of the left pleural space is accomplished with a chest tube.

Mycotic Aneurysms

I. **General principles.** Mycotic aneurysm refers to infection in the wall of an artery. Since most cases are caused by bacteria rather than fungi, and aneurysmal dilatation is not invariably present, the term is a misnomer.

II. **Pathophysiology**

A. **Primary mycotic aneurysm** results from hematogenous seeding directly through the intima or via the vasa vasorum. The vessel usually has a damaged endothelial surface from atherosclerosis, which provides a nidus for circulating bacteria. Additional predisposing conditions are preformed aneurysms and arteriovenous fistulas. The bacteremic episode may be overt, with an obvious extravascular focus, or it may be transient and occult. Arteries most frequently involved are the aorta and its major branches. Usual pathogens are salmonellae, especially *Salmonella typhimurium* and *S. choleraesuis*. Less common culprits are staphylococci, streptococci, and gram-negative bacilli.

B. **Bacterial endocarditis** causes mycotic aneurysms by septic embolic occlusion. This mechanism accounted for 80% of mycotic aneurysms in the preantibiotic era, but accounts for only 10% now. The bacteriology reflects that of endocarditis, with streptococci and staphylococci predominating. Previously normal peripheral vessels are usually involved, especially at bifurcations.

C. **Direct invasion** of arteries can be associated with adjacent suppurative foci, such as wound infection, paravertebral abscess, intraabdominal sepsis, or osteomyelitis. The aneurysm results from external erosion when the supporting structure (arterial intima) is destroyed. Virtually any pathogen, including *Mycobacterium tuberculosis,* may be involved.

D. **Vascular trauma** is assuming greater importance in recent years. It may result from a vascular surgical procedure, mainline drug addiction, penetrating or blunt trauma, cardiac catheterization, arteriography, or hemodialysis shunts. Often there is an initial pseudoaneurysm due to a periarterial hematoma. Bacteria are introduced, either from the injury or from another septicemic source, and localize at the susceptible focus. The most common pathogens are *Staph. aureus,* coliforms, *Pseudomonas,* and anaerobes.

III. Clinical features

A. **Pain** at the infected site and **fever** are almost invariably present.

B. A **pulsatile** or **enlarging mass** is generally present when peripheral arteries are involved. Mycotic aneurysms at less accessible sites, such as the visceral arteries, are difficult to detect and usually require arteriography.

C. **Blood cultures** are positive for the offending organism in 60–80% of cases. As with endocarditis, bacteremia is continuous rather than intermittent.

D. **Stool cultures** and **agglutination titers** are generally positive when *Salmonella* is responsible.

E. **Persistent** or **recurrent sepsis** despite antimicrobial therapy suggests mycotic aneurysm, since these infections are notoriously refractory to medical treatment.

IV. Treatment

A. **Medical.** Systemic antimicrobials are given according to susceptibility tests and continued for 6 weeks. However, antibiotic therapy of a primary mycotic aneurysm caused by *Salmonella* almost invariably leads to failure. The only cures reported in recent years have been achieved by a combined medical and surgical approach.

B. **Surgical**

1. The artery should be ligated, oversewn, or bypassed at proximal sites that are not infected.
2. All infected tissue should be excised.
3. A vein graft may be used in preference to bypass for true aneurysms associated with minimal purulence.
4. Immediate bypass is preferably avoided due to probable contamination. This approach is sometimes mandatory, however, as with aortic mycotic aneurysm. For peripheral arteries, it is usually possible to ligate the vessel; bypass is delayed until the infection has subsided. Vascular insufficiency provides the indication for subsequent surgical procedures.

V. Major complications are hemorrhage, disseminated infection, and overwhelming septicemia.

The initial hemorrhage usually signals more extensive subsequent bleeding. The ultimate prognosis depends largely on the vessel infected. Aortic mycotic aneurysms usually terminate fatally with exsanguination, often before the diagnosis is appreciated. The outlook is much better for peripheral vessels. In either situation, prompt diagnosis and surgical intervention are considered crucial.

Infected Arterial Graft

I. **General principles.** The incidence of arterial graft sepsis is only 1–6%, but it represents a potentially catastrophic complication that can cause massive hemorrhage from a suture line, graft thrombosis with distal ischemia, and overwhelming septicemia. The mortality of graft sepsis in recent years is 25–40%, and surviving patients often require amputation.

II. **Pathophysiology.** Several factors predispose to vascular graft infection.

A. Vascular reconstruction in the **inguinal area.** Over 75% of infected grafts occur at this site, due to the difficulty of controlling contamination from the perineum, groin, and local lymph nodes. Abdominal aortic grafts are also at risk, whereas grafts in the head and neck, thorax, and upper extremities are relatively free of infection.

B. **Perioperative contamination** of the graft. This is the route of organisms causing early infections (within 8 weeks of surgery).

C. **Transient bacteremia** during the operation or in the postoperative period. Experimental studies demonstrate the vulnerability of vascular graft sutures, particularly silk sutures, to circulating bacteria. This risk is reduced when a pseudointima is formed over junctional sites after 1–2 weeks. Endothelialization of the graft itself, however, requires several weeks and may never be complete. This persistent foreign body in continuity with the circulatory system represents a susceptible focus, analogous to a prosthetic cardiac valve.

D. **Perigraft hematoma,** by providing a nidus for infection.

E. **Placement** in an **infected** or **contaminated field.** Although such sites are at particular risk, they are not absolutely destined for infection. Autogenous graft material has the best chance to heal and function in a contaminated field.

III. **Diagnosis.**

A. Graft sepsis may become apparent from 1 week to several years after the operative procedure. The usual interval is 3–8 months. **Early cases** (within 2 months) are generally associated with **wound sepsis.** It is uncertain whether **late cases** represent contamination during the procedure, with symptoms being delayed due to prophylactic antimicrobials, or involvement with relatively nonpathogenic bacteria. The late cases may also be caused by inapparent bacteremia, normally well tolerated, but in these patients the circulating organisms localize to the susceptible nidus.

B. **Clinical findings** depend largely on the site of the infection. Graft sepsis near skin surfaces generally shows erythema, tenderness, false aneurysm, and sinus tracts. Graft sepsis in less accessible sites, such as the retroperitoneal space, is more likely to present with systemic signs and few localizing findings. For example, infected aortoiliac grafts commonly present with hemorrhage into the peritoneal cavity or gastrointestinal tract, even in the absence of other signs of infection. Aortofemoral or iliofemoral graft infections are most often recognized by skin drainage or cellulitis in the area of the inguinal wound.

1. **Hemorrhage or false aneurysm.** This indicates suture line involvement and imminent massive bleeding. Arteriography may prove useful in defining false aneurysms.
2. **Graft thrombosis.** The clot may propagate to involve the entire graft, suture lines, and contiguous proximal vessels.
3. **Wound infection with draining sinus.** A sinogram will assist in determining the extent of a sinus tract.
4. **Septicemia** or distal **septic embolization.**
5. **Gastrointestinal hemorrhage** in a patient with an aortic graft suggests an intestinal erosion with arterial-enteric fistula formation.
6. **Fever, leukocytosis,** and **local pain** and **tenderness** are common. These may be the only findings prior to massive hemorrhage, especially with intraabdominal grafts.

IV. **Bacteriology**

A. **Culture sources.** These include peripheral blood and local collections, spontaneous wound drainage, careful needle aspirates, incised wounds, and operative specimens. Gram's stain provides an immediate clue to the type of organism involved.

B. Pathogens. In older studies most graft infections were caused by *Staph. aureus* and *Strep. pyogenes.* More recently about one-third involve *Staph. aureus,* and two-thirds yield coliforms, *Pseudomonas, Serratia* or *Staph. epidermidis.* Mixed infections are frequent. The bacteriology is also related to the operative site. In aortofemoral and femoral-popliteal bypasses, staphylococci, both *Staph. aureus* and *Staph. epidermidis,* are most common. In aortoiliac bypasses, gram-negative bacilli are most common.

V. Treatment

A. Medical. Antimicrobial agents are administered parenterally in large doses to control sepsis. Drug selection is based on blood cultures and cultures of any local drainage. Empiric therapy, when necessary, should be directed against likely pathogens: for most grafts, *Staph. aureus* (nafcillin, cephalosporin, etc.); for grafts associated with inguinal incisions, *Staph. aureus* and enteric flora (clindamycin plus gentamicin or cephalosporin plus gentamicin). Systemic antimicrobials are administered for at least 6 weeks.

B. Surgical. A trial of medical treatment is often attempted initially, especially for patients with mild sepsis and for those who are considered unsuitable for reoperation. The goals of surgical treatment, if it is required, are to remove all foreign material and reestablish circulation with a new bypass through clean tissue.

1. **Suture line involvement** is a harbinger of impending hemorrhage, if it has not already occurred. The host artery must be ligated, oversewn, or resected immediately. Resuturing at the site of sepsis is destined to failure.
2. **Thrombosed grafts** should be excised.
3. **Bypass procedures.** Graft removal generally necessitates an alternative circulatory route or amputation. If distal ischemia is inevitable, there should be immediate bypass grafting followed by removal of the original graft. In some situations a two-stage procedure is used: immediate placement of an alternative bypass, away from the infected site, followed subsequently by removal of the infected prosthesis. Potential alternative routes for infected aortic grafts are thoracic aortofemoral or axillary-femoral bypass. With infected femoral-popliteal grafts, the obturator foramen may be used to reestablish circulation from the iliac to the lower popliteal artery. If the infection involves only the midportion of the graft, the original anastomotic sites may be used for regrafting.

   When graft exclusion does not threaten distal viability, reconstruction surgery should be delayed until several months after the original debridement. This approach can be employed even with aortofemoral or aortoiliac bypass by removing the graft and observing the limb for signs of ischemia. With aortofemoral grafts, a portion of the original graft may be salvaged if the infection is restricted to one femoral limb. This is accomplished by a staged partial excision. The iliac portion of the involved side is examined and, if not infected, this segment is removed. As long as distal viability is retained, removal of the infected distal segment can be delayed for 1–2 weeks. This staged approach permits removal of the infected portion of the graft without contaminating the proximal segment.
4. **Antimicrobial irrigations.** There may be an attempt to salvage the original infected vascular graft with antimicrobial irrigations when thrombosis has not occurred and suture lines are not involved. The infected bed is debrided, catheters are inserted, and skin is closed secondarily. This technique is most successful when the infection is localized to the midportion of the graft and there are no purulent collections. Parenteral antibiotics, followed by a prolonged course of an oral agent, should also be given. This approach may be attempted when graft excision is not feasible.

VI. Preventive measures

A. When elective procedures are planned, any extravascular infection should be controlled preoperatively. **Skin infections,** in particular, represent a major contraindication to elective vascular surgical intervention. **Ischemic foot ulcers** pose a special problem, in part due to lymphatic drainage to the inguinal and femoral nodes. Foot lesions should be vigorously treated preoperatively with local dressings and systemic antimicrobials. These may prove refractory to healing without revascularization, however.

B. **Inguinal incisions should be avoided** whenever possible. Thus, aorta–external iliac bypass is preferred over aortofemoral bypass.

C. Clinical trials and experimental animal data have demonstrated the value of **antimicrobial prophylaxis.** The usual regimen is an antistaphylococcal drug, such as penicillinase-resistant penicillin (oxacillin or nafcillin), or a cephalosporin.

D. Some authorities prefer prosthetic grafts that have **soaked in antimicrobials.** The value of this maneuver has not been established.

E. Meticulous **aseptic technique** is crucial. This includes careful skin preparation, care to avoid contact of the graft with skin or dermal edges, use of plastic drapes to exclude the skin from the operative field, and copious irrigation (with or without antimicrobials) prior to wound closure. Laminar flow systems are sometimes used, but their efficacy has not been documented.

F. Careful **hemostasis** and prompt evacuation of hematomas is essential.

G. Wound **drains** should be **avoided.**

H. **Wound infections** without graft involvement should be treated aggressively by drainage and systemic antimicrobials.

I. Many authorities believe vascular grafts are as susceptible to transient episodes of bacteremia as damaged heart valves. Thus, **prophylactic antimicrobials** are sometimes advocated for dental procedures, oral surgical procedures, or genitourinary manipulation. Guidelines are the same as those outlined for patients with rheumatic valvular disease.

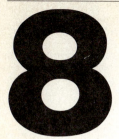

8 Bacteremia and Septic Shock

I. Definitions

Sepsis refers to a systemic disease caused by microorganisms or their products in the bloodstream.

Bacteremia implies viable bacteria in the blood as indicated by positive blood cultures. It may be transient, intermittent, or sustained.

Septic shock is a clinical syndrome characterized by sepsis with evidence of circulatory insufficiency and inadequate tissue perfusion.

II. Bacteriology of bacteremia.

Bacteria most commonly recovered in blood cultures can be divided into four categories:

A. **Aerobic gram-positive cocci** account for 30–50% of all bacteremias. The predominant isolates are *Streptococcus pneumoniae, Staphylococcus aureus*, and enterococci.

B. **Aerobic gram-negative bacilli** account for 40–60% of all bacteremias. The incidence of gram-negative bacteremia is generally estimated at 2–10/1,000 patients, depending on the patient population and hospital surveyed. The predominant gram-negative isolates are shown in Table 8-1.

C. **Anaerobic bacteria** account for 8–12% of all bacteremias. *Bacteroides fragilis* is the most common organism in this group and is responsible for 70–80% of all anaerobic bacteremias; most of the balance consists of *Clostridium, Fusobacterium*, anaerobic streptococci (*Peptostreptococcus*), and *Bacteroides* species other than *B. fragilis*.

D. *Staph. epidermidis, Propionibacterium*, and diphtheroids are common blood culture isolates but usually represent contaminants. In certain clinical settings, however, such as infections associated with prosthetic devices, these organisms are repeatedly recovered.

III. Pathophysiology of gram-negative sepsis and septic shock.

Septic shock results from several interrelated factors, including the direct effect of bacterial products on the cardiovascular system, activation of the complement cascade system, the volume status at the onset of sepsis, and the nature of associated diseases. Endotoxin is the most readily identifiable microbial component responsible for septic shock; it is the lipopolysaccharide component of the cell wall found in all gram-negative bacteria, including Enterobacteriaceae, *Pseudomonas*, and *Neisseria* sp. Although a form of lipopolysaccharide is present in *B. fragilis*, this material is not a biologically active endotoxin. However, other anaerobic gram-negative bacteria, such as *Fusobacterium*, do possess typical endotoxin with full biologic activity.

A. **Endotoxin** causes vasoconstriction of arterioles and venules in the renal, mesenteric, and pulmonary circulation, causing hypoperfusion and stagnant anoxia. Lactic acidosis develops locally and induces arteriolar dilatation while the venules remain vasoconstricted. This sequence perpetuates stagnant anoxia and acidosis, increases hydrostatic pressure in the vascular bed, and promotes leakage of plasma into the interstitial space. The circulating volume decreases, further causing reflex vasoconstriction and arteriovenous shunting. Eventually, local anoxia and acidosis cause tissue damage, leading to widespread capillary leakage, systemic acidosis, and death.

B. There is also direct tissue damage caused by endotoxin through a mechanism

Table 8-1. Predominant gram-negative isolates in bacteremia

Organism	Percent of all gram-negative bacteremia cases
E. coli	30–40
Klebsiella	15–20
Pseudomonas	10–15
Proteus sp.	5–10
Enterobacter	5–10
Serratia	3–5
Others*	5–10

*Includes *Neisseria* (gonococci and meningococci), *Hemophilus influenzae*, and *Salmonella*. These compose a relatively small portion of all bacteremias, but they are common in certain susceptible hosts.

similar to the generalized Shwartzman reaction. This results in **venous microthrombosis,** with pulmonary hemorrhage, cortical necrosis of the kidney, and widespread tissue damage to other organ systems.

C. **Polypeptides** play a role in septic shock due to release of vasoactive peptides and coagulation peptides. Endotoxin causes endothelial damage, resulting in activation of factor XII, which converts kallikreinogen to kallikrein, bradykinin, and other vasoactive peptides. These kinins cause vasodilatation and increased capillary permeability. The early hypotension and vasodilatation seen in gram-negative sepsis may result from the action of these vasoactive peptides. Activation of factor XII also initiates the clotting cascade. Fibrin thrombi are deposited in the vascular system, causing ischemia and tissue necrosis. Eventually the blood is depleted of fibrinogen, platelets, and other clotting factors. The fibrinolytic system is also activated, resulting in a breakdown of fibrin and fibrinogen with the formation of noncoagulable **fibrin split products.** Hemorrhagic diathesis results from the combined effects of depleted clotting factors, activation of the fibrinolytic system, and the presence of fibrin split products. The final picture in severe cases is that of disseminated intravascular coagulation (DIC) with elevated prothrombin time, decreased platelets, elevated fibrin split products, falling hematocrit, and low sedimentation rate.

D. Endotoxin also **activates the alternative complement pathway** and, to a lesser extent, the classic pathway. Complement consumption activates peptides that enhance the inflammatory process, promotes tissue damage, and increases capillary permeability. A marked decrease in serum complement during sepsis is regarded as a poor prognostic sign and is often associated with shock.

IV. Bacteriology of septic shock

A. The common association of gram-negative bacteremia and the shock syndrome has led some to use the terms **septic shock, gram-negative shock,** and **endotoxin shock** synonymously. This is unfortunate, because infections due to gram-positive bacteria, fungi, and viruses can also cause the shock syndrome. Hemodynamic studies of patients with shock due to gram-positive bacteremia give results identical to those in studies of patients with gram-negative bacteremia with respect to aortic root pressure, central venous pressure, heart rate, stroke volume, vascular resistance, left ventricular end-diastolic pressure, and left ventricular stroke work. The only significant difference is that the cardiac index is lower with shock due to gram-negative bacteremia. The point to emphasize is that the clinician confronted with a septic patient in shock cannot accurately categorize the responsible pathogen without culture results. Certain differentiating points deserve emphasis, however.

1. The incidence of septic shock is 30–40% in gram-negative bacteremia, compared to 3–5% in gram-positive bacteremia. Statistically, the most likely pathogen in a patient with septic shock is a gram-negative rod.
2. Patients with gram-negative bacteremia are likely to develop shock within

2–8 hours, whereas shock is generally delayed in patients with infections due to other microbes.

3. Thrombocytopenia and disseminated intravascular coagulation are more common in patients with gram-negative bacteremia.

B. Virtually all clinically significant gram-negative bacteria can cause septic shock. The incidence of this complication is approximately equal with the various coliform bacteria and pseudomonads. It is of interest that about 35% of patients with *B. fragilis* bacteremia develop shock, despite the fact that this organism does not possess biologically active endotoxin. However, disseminated intravascular coagulation is rarely observed with *B. fragilis* bacteremia.

V. Signs and symptoms of bacteremia

A. **The classic presentation** is sudden onset of shaking chills, high fever, and prostration followed by hypotension within 2–8 hours. However, 40–60% of patients with gram-negative bacteremia do not have this classic presentation, exhibiting some or none of these findings.

B. **Fever** is noted in the vast majority of patients and may be the only finding. A small percentage of patients lack fever or are even hypothermic; this exception is most commonly associated with advanced age, uremia, or corticosteroid therapy.

C. Hyperpnea with a **respiratory alkalosis** is common in gram-negative bacteremia. It may be so prominent as to suggest pneumonia, atelectasis, or pulmonary embolism.

D. **Hypotension** is noted in 30–40% of patients with gram-negative bacteremia. Findings of decreased peripheral perfusion can dominate the clinical presentation: changes in mentation, oliguria or anuria, and cold skin with diaphoresis.

E. Unexplained **acidosis** suggests bacteremia.

F. **Thrombocytopenia** is found in 50–60% of patients with gram-negative bacteremia, although the complete syndrome of disseminated intravascular coagulation (DIC) is seen in fewer than 5%.

VI. Portal of entry in bacteremia. It is possible to define a primary focus of infection that serves as the portal of entry in the majority of patients with bacteremia. An exception is immunocompromised patients with leukopenia, lymphoma, or cancer chemotherapy. The predominant identifiable portals of entry are shown in Table 8-2.

VII. Prognosis. A number of factors have been identified as prognostic in gram-negative bacteremia.

A. **Underlying condition.** The clinical status of the patient is critical to outcome (Table 8-3).

B. **Septic shock.** This condition, as previously defined, is associated with a mortality of 40–80% as compared to 20–35% in cases without the shock syndrome.

C. **Appropriate antimicrobial selection.** Initial selection of an antimicrobial regimen that proves active against the blood culture isolate reduces mortality to 20–30% vs. 50–60% with inappropriate antibiotics. The proper choice of antibiotics also decreases the incidence of septic shock.

D. **Portal of entry.** The prognosis is relatively good for patients with gram-negative bacteremia associated with urinary tract infection, septic thrombophlebitis, a surgical wound, and intraabdominal sepsis. The prognosis is poor for pneumonia, burn wound sepsis, and the immunocompromised host with no defined portal of entry.

VIII. Management of septic shock

A. Clinical evaluation

1. Establish septicemia as a likely diagnosis. Major alternative considerations in the differential diagnosis of hypotension are acute myocardial infarction, cardiac arrhythmias, dehydration, and pulmonary embolism.

2. Identify a likely portal of entry in order to support this diagnosis, guide initial antimicrobial selection, facilitate appropriate consultations, and plan surgical intervention. The severity of the infection necessitates expeditious assessment, with attention focused on those clinical findings that are immediately available. Important considerations in the history are recent surgical procedures, invasive diagnostic studies or instrumentation, recent or current use of antimicrobials, and previous infections. The physical examina-

Table 8-2. Common portals of entry in bacteremia

Focus of infection	Approximate frequency (%) in gram-negative bacteremia	Comment
Urinary tract	30–40	Most common in virtually all studies
Respiratory tract	15–20	Especially common in hospital-acquired pneumonia and pneumonia in the compromised host
Intraabdominal or pelvic sepsis	10–15	
Phlebitis	5	Usually associated with IV catheters
Burn wound	5	
Surgical wound	5–10	

Table 8-3. Mortality associated with clinical status in gram-negative bacteremia

Underlying disease	Percent mortality in gram-negative bacteremia
No ultimately fatal underlying disease	15–25
Ultimately fatal disease, but anticipated survival > 1 yr	45–65
Fatal disease with anticipated survival < 1 yr	75–95

tion should concentrate on areas likely to be rewarding, especially the chest, abdomen, wounds, and indwelling lines.

3. Evaluate severity with measurements of temperature, blood pressure, cardiac rate, central venous pressure, and urinary output.

B. Laboratory evaluation

1. **General studies:** CBC, urinalysis, liver function tests, electrolytes, and creatinine. When feasible, it is appropriate to obtain pertinent roentgenograms (chest, plain films of the abdomen, etc.) and an electrocardiogram.
2. Preferred tests for evaluating the **hematologic changes** associated with septic shock: platelet count, total hemolytic complement, fibrin split products, and prothrombin time.
3. **Cultures.** In all cases, at least two blood cultures should be obtained before antimicrobial therapy is started. These may be drawn in rapid sequence but should be done with separate venipunctures. Urine should also be cultured in all cases, since the urinary tract is the most common portal of entry. The appropriateness of other cultures is dictated by the clinical setting, e.g., cultures of the wound, intravenous catheter site, aspiration of potentially infected body fluids, or sputum.

IX. Therapy

A. Volume replacement. Aggressive volume replacement is the initial therapeutic imperative in cases of hypotension due to sepsis. This approach is necessary to prevent stagnant anoxia and lactic acidosis, which, if progressive, can end in irreversible shock. Fluid (15–20 ml/min) should be administered in the form of colloid (plasma, albumin, or blood) or crystalloid (electrolyte solutions such as saline). The question of crystalloid vs. colloid is controversial, but many authorities prefer large amounts of crystalloid with judicious use of colloid.

B. Corticosteroids. Corticosteroids stabilize lysosomes, improve microcirculation, and inhibit the interaction of complement with endotoxin. Reports of corticosteroid therapy for patients with septic shock suggest efficacy, although virtually all studies are fraught with problems in interpretation due to inadequate design. Nevertheless, corticosteroids are advocated here with an attitude of cautious skepticism, with an overriding impression that they may work and that short-term steroid therapy is relatively benign.

Suggested regimens are

Methylprednisolone, 30 mg/kg **or**
Dexamethasone, 3 mg/kg

The drug should be given in a single dose IV over 10–15 minutes. The treatment should be repeated once at 4–6 hours if hypotension persists. When steroids are used, it is important to note that these agents may alter some parameters that are useful in monitoring the clinical course. Nonspecific effects of steroids are leukocytosis with lymphopenia, decrease in fever, and alterations in mental status ranging from euphoria to psychosis.

C. Vasoactive drugs. Vasoactive drugs are used when hypotension persists, despite adequate fluid replacement as determined by central venous pressure or pulmonary wedge pressure. Vasoconstrictor agents such as levarterenol (Levophed) and metaraminol (Aramine) are not generally recommended, since septic patients already have intense sympathetic stimulation.

1. **Dopamine** is the preferred agent. It is an endogenous catecholamine that increases myocardial contractility and causes nonadrenergic vasodilatation of the renal and mesenteric vasculature. The expected effect is a slight increase in blood pressure, decreased or unchanged heart rate, increased cardiac output, and increased renal and mesenteric blood flow. Suggested dosage is 2–10 μg/kg/min, with adjustments based on response.
2. **Isoproterenol** may also be useful. It increases cardiac output and improves microcirculation by vasodilatation of the arteriolar and venous systems. Suggested dosage is 2–8 μg/min, with adjustments based on response.

D. Heparin. The use of heparin has been suggested to reverse the clotting abnormalities associated with septicemia and disseminated intravascular coagulation. Experimental animal studies and clinical trials show, however, that anticoagulation potentiates the bleeding diathesis and does not improve survival. Therefore this treatment is not recommended.

E. Antimicrobial treatment. Early use of antimicrobials that subsequently prove to be active against the blood culture isolate has been shown to improve survival rates and reduce the incidence of shock syndrome in patients with gram-negative bacteremia. No specific regimen can be suggested that would be appropriate for all patients. Instead, the choice should be tailored to the clinical setting according to predicted pathogens for the suspected portal of entry. Table 8-4 summarizes the recommendations for the most common sources of bacteremia in critically ill patients. The following points are emphasized:

1. Aminoglycosides are included in all regimens in which gram-negative bacteremia is suspected. This recommendation is based on the high rates of resistance to alternative choices. Aminoglycosides considered adequate are gentamicin, tobramycin, and amikacin. The choice between these agents depends on the individual physician's preference and on resistance profiles in the particular hospital.
2. Large doses of antibiotics are recommended in the initial period for the seriously ill patient (see Chap. 12).
3. The intravenous route should be used for all hypotension patients.
4. All regimens include two agents, the purpose being to expand the spectrum.

Table 8-4. Antibiotic selection for severely ill patients with suspected gram-negative bacteremia

Portal of entry	Anticipated pathogens	Antimicrobials
Urinary tract	Coliforms Pseudomonads Enterococci	Aminoglycoside + ampicillin
Lower respiratory tract	Coliforms Pseudomonads *Streptococcus pneumoniae* *Staphylococcus aureus*	Aminoglycoside + 1. Cephalosporin 2. Carbenicillin, ticarcillin
Biliary tract	Coliforms Enterococci	Aminoglycoside + 1. Ampicillin 2. Cephalosporin
Intraabdominal sepsis	Coliforms Anaerobes	Aminoglycoside + 1. Clindamycin 2. Cefoxitin 3. Chloramphenicol 4. Metronidazole
Female genital tract	Coliforms Anaerobes	Aminoglycoside + 1. Clindamycin 2. Cefoxitin 3. Chloramphenicol 4. Metronidazole
IV catheter	Coliforms Pseudomonads *Staph. aureus*	Aminoglycoside + 1. Cephalosporin 2. Oxacillin
Site unknown		Aminoglycoside + 1. Cephalosporin 2. Carbenicillin, ticarcillin 3. Oxacillin

It is necessary to provide activity against anaerobes or aerobic gram-positive bacteria that may also cause shock syndrome.

5. After culture results are available, the initial antimicrobial regimen should be modified to one that is less toxic and narrower in spectrum.

F. Surgical drainage. Areas of localized infection must be searched for and drained. Failure to drain localized infection will cause continuous or relapsing septic shock despite medical therapy.

G. Monitoring. Parameters that should be monitored to evaluate response to therapy and to dictate subsequent courses of action are as follows:

1. Temperature, blood pressure, pulse, creatinine, and mental status are watched; more seriously ill patients may require regular monitoring of blood gases, clotting parameters, serum electrolytes, and urine electrolytes.
2. Urinary output is measured by voided volumes, spot catheterization with a thin catheter, or an indwelling catheter.
3. Volumes of fluid replacement and decisions regarding vasopressors can be determined by central venous pressure measurements made by using a large-bore needle. For improved accuracy, however, the preferred method is pulmonary wedge measurements using a Swan-Ganz line.

9 Skin and Soft-Tissue Infections

Staphylococcal infections

I. Definitions

A. *Staphylococcus aureus* is a gram-positive coccus with individual cells that tend to form clumps, appearing like a bunch of berries in a Gram's stain of infected material. These organisms are distinguished from the less virulent *Staph. epidermidis* by being hemolytic on blood agar, coagulase-positive, and able to ferment mannitol.

B. There is a high prevalence of **carriers** of *Staph. aureus,* approximately 20–30% of normal individuals, and double that incidence among hospital personnel. The anterior nares is the most common site of carriage, although some individuals also harbor these organisms in their mouth, skin, and perianal region. Chronic skin diseases such as psoriasis can be colonized by large numbers of staphylococci.

C. The **spread** of staphylococci to patients is by direct contact or by air-borne inoculation of infected particles over distances of less than 6 feet. Hospital personnel with staphylococcal boils are a major source of transmission of the organism. There may also be autoinfection in patients carrying the organism in their nares or on the skin.

D. Certain **conditions** are particularly disposed to staphylococcal infections: diabetes, cystic fibrosis (lung infections), influenza, and certain immunodeficiency diseases, especially those that entail decreased leukocyte function.

II. Staphylococcal pyoderma

A. Definitions. Perhaps the commonest bacterial infection in humans, pyoderma involves the hair follicles, usually on the face or extensor surfaces of the extremities. The mildest form, **folliculitis,** has an uncomplicated evolution from a vesicle that points to the outside, to drainage, encrustment, and finally spontaneous healing. Trauma or irritation by scratching can lead to deeper local infection, spreading cellulitis, inoculation of other skin sites, and even septicemia. A **furuncle** (boil) is a follicular infection that has spread to the subcutaneous layers of the skin. There is a firm, discrete nodule with purulent drainage. Systemic manifestations are not seen. A **carbuncle** is a deeper and more extensive lesion, containing multiple loculated pockets of purulent material. There is abundant pus and spreading erythema. This lesion tends to occur in skin which is thick and less elastic such as found on the back of the neck. It is painful, indurated, and often associated with systemic signs of fever, headache, and malaise.

B. Differential diagnosis. It is important to distinguish these staphylococcal infections from *acne vulgaris,* which involves the sebaceous follicles: the comedone of acne is **rarely** infected with *Staph. aureus,* more often being colonized by *Staph. epidermidis* and *Propionibacterium acnes.* Another disease to be differentiated is *hidradenitis suppurativa,* an inflammation of the apocrine glands of the axilla or of the perianal or inguinal area.

C. Treatment. Treatment of staphylococcal pyoderma depends on the appearance of the lesion, the location, and the presence of systemic manifestations.

1. Mild forms of **folliculitis** are managed with warm, moist packs. No medical or surgical therapy is necessary.
2. More severe forms, such as **furuncles,** require judicious incision and drainage. In the case of a **carbuncle** with loculated pockets, it is necessary to use a small wick drain in order to encourage drainage and to prevent closure of the incision. Drainage of such lesions, while often necessary, also carries some risk of spreading infection to distant sites. Such lesions are well demarcated by pyogenic membranes. Incising these natural boundaries can lead to local dissemination and even septicemia.
3. **Antibiotic treatment** is indicated for furuncles and carbuncles, especially when surgical incision is performed. The preferred treatment is a penicillinase-resistant penicillin (oxacillin or nafcillin) or a cephalosporin. Penicillin-allergic patients can be treated with erythromycin or clindamycin. Most patients are treated on an ambulatory basis, and oral therapy is indicated.
   a. **Resistance to penicillin G** (and related compounds, such as ampicillin, amoxicillin, and carbenicillin) is extremely common among strains of *Staph. aureus*. This resistance is mediated by an enzyme, penicillinase, so that increased doses of antibiotic induce more enzyme, thereby destroying all the drug. The incidence of penicillin-resistant *Staph. aureus* among hospitalized patients is approximately 95%. In community-acquired staphylococcal infections, the incidence is also high, ranging from 50 to 90% in various areas. Hence, **all** staphylococcal infections should be considered resistant to penicillin until appropriate sensitivity tests can be performed. The correct treatment, pending the laboratory results, includes one of the following antibiotics:

Cephalosporins (cephalexin, cefaclor)	250 mg 4 times daily
Erythromycin	250 mg 4 times daily
Clindamycin	150 mg 4 times daily
Penicillinase-resistant penicillins (nafcillin, oxacillin, or dicloxacillin)	250 mg 4 times daily

   b. **Methicillin-resistant staphylococci** have caused sporadic infections and occasionally hospital-based epidemics. These organisms are invariably resistant to all the penicillins, including oxacillin, nafcillin, and dicloxacillin. In addition, the majority are resistant to clindamycin and erythromycin, and approximately 50% are resistant to cephalosporins. The most reliable treatment is vancomycin, administered intravenously in doses of 500–750 mg q6h.
4. Indications for hospitalization and parenteral antibiotic administration are
   a. Significant local spread with cellulitis
   b. Metastatic staphylococcal lesions, suggesting bacteremic spread
   c. Systemic manifestations, such as chills and fever
5. Staphylococci infections involving the **muzzle area of the face** require special consideration, since the organism can be spread by venous drainage to the **cavernous sinus,** with subsequent suppurative thrombophlebitis. In general, staphylococcal skin lesions in this area of the face should not be drained in an aggressive manner, since the organism may be spread to deeper structures. If there is only simple folliculitis, the lesion can be treated with hot, moist packs and observed for any spread or signs of toxicity. For more extensive involvement, such as furuncles, oral antibiotics should be administered. Hospitalization for parenteral antibiotics and close observation should be considered for more extensive lesions or for those that fail to respond to oral antibiotic therapy. (See p. 224 for discussion of cavernous sinus thrombosis.)

III. Staphylococcal cellulitis

A. Staphylococci tend to spread through the subcutaneous tissues of the skin in a circumferential, slowly progressive fashion. As distinguished from streptococcal erysipelas, **cellulitis** is characterized by tender, diffusely erythematous skin without a distinct border. Cellulitis progresses rather slowly, over a period of days, compared to erysipelas, which can move forward in a matter of hours. To be sure, these two organisms can imitate one another, so that cellulitis can be caused by *Staph. aureus* as well as by *Streptococcus pyogenes.*

B. Treatment consists of appropriate oral antibiotics, employing a penicillinase-resistant penicillin (oxacillin, nafcillin, or dicloxacillin) or a cephalosporin. Severe cases require parenteral antibiotic therapy, so that hospitalization is mandatory. When a limb is involved, it should be elevated in order to relieve the edema fluid. Warm soaks are advisable when there is a wound or skin abrasion. Since the infection is confined to the superficial layers of skin, there is no need for incision and drainage.

IV. Staphylococcal wound infections

A. Clean surgical wounds can be infected by this organism, usually through contact with medical personnel in attendance. The route of transmission is direct contact, e.g., from contaminated hands, soiled dressings, or dirty instruments. Clinically, a staphylococcal wound infection usually becomes obvious 3–4 days after the surgical procedure. The suture line becomes reddened, tender, and somewhat tense. A slow ooze of odorless, yellow pus can be discerned at the edges and on the dressing. Gram's stain of the discharge reveals multiple polymorphonuclear leukocytes (PMNs) with gram-positive cocci in clumps.

B. Treatment of a local wound infection is achieved by simply opening the involved sutures and allowing the subcutaneous tissues to drain. If abundant pus is present, a small wick drain should be inserted to prevent closure. Warm soaks should be applied to the area. Antibiotics are not indicated for these superficial wound infections.

Indications for parenteral antibiotic therapy are

1. Local extension with surrounding cellulitis. The adjacent subcutaneous tissue is firm and tender, often displaying a blush of erythema
2. Systemic signs, such as fever and toxicity
3. An underlying prosthetic device or graft that should be protected from a superficial infection by this organism

Streptococcal Infections

I. Definitions

Streptococci are classified by the Lancefield system, based on cell wall polysaccharide, which divides the organisms into 18 groups. Clinically, group A *Strep. pyogenes* is the most important in skin infections; group B organisms cause pneumonia and meningitis in infants; and group D (enterococcus) organisms produce endocarditis, urinary tract infections, biliary tract infections, and intraabdominal sepsis. There are also nongroupable strains, known as *Strep. viridans,* which cause endocarditis. The infections described here are caused mostly by group A *Strep. pyogenes,* although a few are caused by groups C and G streptococci.

II. Streptococcal pyoderma (impetigo)

A. Impetigo is characterized by a cluster of vesicular lesions in the horny layer of the skin, usually on the legs, arms, face, and scalp. It is seen most commonly in young children, especially during hot seasons, and can be initiated by insect bites. Impetigo follows an indolent course: The vesicles progress to pustules, and are then covered by a thick yellow crust with very few systemic signs. Local, tender lymphadenopathy frequently is observed. The patient notes itching and pain, and lesions are spread by autoinoculation.

B. Complications include local extension of cellulitis, glomerulonephritis (if the infecting organism is a specific serotype), bacteremia, and distant metastatic spread. Although these events are uncommon, antibiotic therapy is recommended to reduce the risk.

C. Treatment consists of local care and antibiotics. Mechanical debridement should be instituted with antibacterial soaks (povidone-iodine or hexachlorophene).

While these measures produce a satisfactory cosmetic effect, there is little evidence that they alter the course. Antibiotics, however, have been shown to produce clinical and bacteriologic cures, although relapses are common. The treatment of choice is penicillin G. Higher response rates are noted with benzathine penicillin (single dose, IM, 1.2 million units). Oral penicillin can also be used (400,000 units qid for 10 days), although there are often problems with compliance. In penicillin-allergic individuals, oral cephalosporins can be used, unless the patient has a history of anaphylaxis; the alternatives, erythromycin and clindamycin, have also produced good results.

III. Erysipelas

A. Classically seen in infants and elderly people, erysipelas is a rapidly spreading acute **lymphangitis** of the skin. No primary site of entry can be found in most patients. The majority of cases occur in the flush area of the face, with a bilateral distribution forming a butterfly pattern. The extremities can also be affected, particularly in the presence of existing lymphatic obstruction due to trauma, postoperative effects (mastectomy lymphedema), or Milroy's disease. The infection begins as a small erythematous papule, usually painless, which enlarges circumferentially with an advancing red border and small tongues of erythema. Characteristically, the skin is elevated by edema that is caused by local lymphatic obstruction. There is clear demarcation between the advancing border and the healthy skin. The center becomes pale, and in severe cases, vesicles or bullae are produced and may advance to gangrene of the skin.

B. Diagnosis is based on clinical findings. Bacteriologic studies, including needle aspiration of the advancing edge, are almost always negative. It is helpful to draw a line with a ballpoint pen at the advancing border in order to observe the progression or improvement over the next several hours.

C. Treatment consistes of administration of penicillin G by the parenteral route. Large doses should be employed initially, since the disease may progress rapidly, with severe consequences. For adults, penicillin G, 3 million units IV q4h, is given. For patients with mild penicillin allergy (not anaphylaxis) a parenteral cephalosporin can be used. Alternatively, clindamycin, 600 mg IV q6h, has had success. It must be emphasized that penicillin is the best drug for erysipelas and should be used whenever possible.

Erysipelas usually responds rapidly to parenteral antibiotic therapy; after 2–3 days, oral medication with lower doses can be substituted. Treatment should be continued for at least 10 days. There is a marked tendency for erysipelas to relapse, often in the same site. Some individuals, particularly those with chronic lymphedema, suffer several relapses yearly; long-term daily administration of oral penicillin has reduced the incidence of attacks in such cases.

IV. Streptococcal cellulitis

A. *Strep. pyogenes* can be inoculated directly into a wound or small puncture site, producing cellulitis. This condition differs clinically from erysipelas in that cellulitis lacks the distinct, palpable border with elevation and edema. Instead, there is diffuse erythema, pain, tenderness and swelling of the entire area of skin. The feature that suggests involvement by group A *Streptococcus* is rapid spread of the process.

B. Treatment is the same as for erysipelas (see sec. **III.C**).

V. Streptococcal wound infections

A. Surgical incisions, even those associated with clean procedures, can be infected by *Strep. pyogenes*. The route of spread is direct inoculation into the wound from a carrier of the organism, usually someone in direct contact during or just after the operative procedure. Within the 1st 24 hours the wound becomes bright red, edematous, and painful. The erythematous border spreads rapidly, with a discrete advancing edge. There is often no drainage; at best, only a minimal amount. There are profound systemic manifestations, such as high fever, tachycardia, and hypotension. Bacteremia is commonly present and may be associated with severe hemolysis. This process has a high mortality unless the diagnosis is recognized early and antibiotic treatment is initiated.

B. The major mode of **treatment** is antibiotics, with penicillin G in high doses (3–5 million units IV q4h). Surgical intervention usually is not indicated, unless the margins of the wound are taut and swollen, in which case the suture line should be opened. The process spreads through the lymphatics and the bloodstream, without accumulation of pus or tissue debris.

VI. Streptococcal ulcers. *Strep. pyogenes* can cause discrete, round or oval ulcers, covered with a yellow crust and surrounded by erythema and induration. The lesion is mildly painful, with a paucity of systemic findings. Treatment is oral penicillin G, 400,000 units 4 times daily for 10 days.

VII. Streptococcal gangrene (Meleney's streptococcal gangrene, β-streptococcal gangrene)

A. Streptococcal infection can progress to cause severe destruction of the superficial layers of skin. This form of gangrene most frequently occurs on the extremities, associated with minor trauma, puncture wound or surgical incision, but can occur in postoperative abdominal incisions. The initial event is erysipelas, with the typical findings of pain, erythema, edema, and advancing border. Within 1–2 days the center of the lesion becomes dark red, then blue-black, with formation of bullae and gangrene of the skin and subcutaneous tissues. The surrounding tissue is fiery red, raised, and edematous. Deeper fascia and muscle may also be involved.

B. Surgical management involves debridement of the gangrenous skin and incision and drainage of the surrounding tissues and fascial planes. As it is important to release the pressure on the skin and subcutaneous tissues, the incisions should be extended beyond the areas of gangrene and far enough into the superficial fascia to establish good drainage. The limb should be elevated in order to promote drainage, and dressed with moist packs for superficial debridement. Although no discrete pockets of pus are to be found, there is significant oozing of tissue fluid, which must be made up by appropriate intravenous administration of fluids and colloids. High-dose penicillin G is given in doses of 3–5 million units IV q4h (see sec. **III.C,** therapy for erysipelas).

Anaerobic Streptococci

I. Definitions. Anaerobic gram-positive cocci can produce crepitant myositis, fasciitis, and several types of skin infections. These organisms are divided into two genera:

A. Peptostreptococcus, also known as **anaerobic streptococci.** These organisms form part of the normal flora of the oral cavity, gastrointestinal tract, and vagina.

B. Peptococcus, known as **anaerobic staphylococci,** since they appear as clumps or "a bunch of grapes" on Gram's stain. These organisms do not form gas and have no odor. They make up a major part of the anaerobic microflora of the skin. For this reason *Peptococcus* is involved frequently in infections of the integument and soft tissues, such as decubitus ulcers and diabetic foot ulcers.

II. Anaerobic streptococcal myositis

A. Clinical course. Myositis is a more indolent process than other streptococcal infections. Involvement of the muscle and fascial planes usually is associated with trauma or a surgical procedure. There may be severe local pain. The overlying skin appears as a gangrenous wound that emits a foul, watery, brown discharge. Bleb formation is common. Crepitus may be apparent in the surrounding tissue. The gas formation can be extensive, with tracking into the adjacent healthy tissues. Inspection of the muscle reveals redness and edema with some local destruction. There is no myonecrosis, however, and the muscle contracts under the scalpel. Although there is generalized toxicity and fever, the patient is not as ill as someone with gas gangrene.

B. Diagnosis. The initial approach to a crepitant skin infection is to obtain a sample of exudate for Gram's stain and open the wound for inspection of muscle and soft tissue. The major distinctions between the diseases caused by anaerobic streptococci and clostridia are as follows (Table 9-1):

1. Systemic effects are less prominent with the streptococcal form. This infec-

Table 9-1. Differential diagnosis of some anaerobic soft-tissue infections

Characteristic	Clostridial cellulitis	Clostridial myonecrosis (gas gangrene)	Anaerobic streptococcal myositis	Necrotizing fasciitis	Synergistic necrotizing cellulitis
Toxemia	±	+ + + +	+ +	+ +	+ +
Local pain	±	+ + + +	Occurs late	±	+ +
Local swelling	±	+ + +	+ + +	+ +	+ +
Gas	+ + to + + + +	+ +	+ +	±	±
Appearance of skin	Essentially normal	Tense, white or gangrenous with bullae	May be coppery	Brawny, pale red, or gangrenous	Swollen, red or gangrenous
Gross characteristics of exudate	Putrid, brown	Thin, serous; may be sweetish or putrid	Seropurulent, brown	Variable	Purulent, putrid
Gram's stain of exudate	Abundant PMNs Gram-positive rods	Few PMNs Gram-positive rods	Many PMNs Gram-positive cocci	Many PMNs Variable, sometimes mixed organisms	Variable PMNs Mixed organisms
Etiology	Clostridia	Clostridia	Anaerobic streptococci (± aerobic streptococci and staphylococci)	Aerobic and anaerobic streptococci and staphylococci; occasionally *Bacteroides*	Mixed: anaerobic streptococci, *Bacteroides*, and coliforms
Surgical therapy	Judicious incisions and debridement	Extensive removal of all infected muscle	Removal of necrotic muscle	Widespread filleting incisions if no response to antibiotics	Widespread filleting incisions

+ + + + Severe; + + + Moderate; + + Mild; ± May or may not be present.
PMN = polymorphonuclear leukocyte.

tion does not cause hypotension and renal failure, as does the clostridial disease.

2. Upon inspection, the involved muscle remains viable in the streptococcal disease, although there may be inflammatory reaction and edema. True myonecrosis is not found.
3. The anaerobic streptococcal form can produce considerable gas, which occurs early in the course; whereas clostridial infections tend to have less gas, and usually as a late development.
4. The discharge from the wound in streptococcal myositis is a thin, brown ooze which shows gram-positive cocci and multiple PMNs in the Gram's stain slide. By contrast, the discharge in gas gangrene shows gram-positive rods but few PMNs.

C. Treatment. Incision and drainage of the infected wound are critical. The necrotic tissue and debris are resected, but the inflamed muscle should not be removed, since it can heal and become functionally useful. The incision should be packed with moist dressings.

Antibiotic treatment is highly effective. These organisms are all sensitive to penicillin G, and this drug should be administered in high doses, 3 million units IV q4h, until the inflammatory reaction has abated. For patients allergic to penicillin G, alternative therapies are the cephalosporins, cefoxitin, and clindamycin.

III. Necrotizing fasciitis

A. Necrotizing fasciitis is a relatively rare infection involving subcutaneous tissues with extensive undermining and tracking along fascial planes. Although originally associated with hemolytic streptococci (group A *Strep. pyogenes*), it is apparent that the disease can be caused by other microorganisms, including anaerobic streptococci, *Staph. aureus, Bacteroides,* and a mixed anaerobic-aerobic flora.

B. Clinical features

1. Extension from a skin lesion is seen in 80% of cases. The lesion often is trivial, such as a minor abrasion, insect bite, injection site (in the case of heroin addicts), or boil. Rare cases have arisen in Bartholin's gland abscess or perianal abscess, from which the infection has spread to fascial planes of the perineum, thigh, groin, and abdomen. The remaining 20% of patients have no visible skin lesion.
2. The initial presentation is that of **cellulitis,** which advances rather slowly. Over the next 2–4 days, however, there is systemic toxicity with high temperatures. The patient is disoriented and lethargic. The local site shows the following features:

Clinical features	Percent of patients
Cellulitis	90
Edema	80
Skin discoloration or gangrene	70
Anesthesia of involved skin	Frequent (true incidence unknown)

3. The most distinguishing clinical feature is the **wooden-hard** feel of the subcutaneous tissues. In cellulitis or erysipelas the subcutaneous tissues can be palpated and are yielding. But in fasciitis the underlying tissues are firm, and the fascial planes and muscle groups cannot be discerned by palpation. It is often possible to observe a broad erythematous track in the skin, along the route of the fascial plane, as the infection advances cephalad in an extremity. If there is an open wound, probing the edges with a blunt instrument permits ready dissection of the superficial fascial planes well beyond the wound margins. There is remarkably little pain associated with this procedure.

C. Bacteriology

1. **Monomicrobial form.** Pathogens in this group are group A, β-hemolytic *Strep. pyogenes, Staph. aureus,* and anaerobic streptococci (*Peptococcus* and *Peptostreptococcus*). Staphylococci and hemolytic streptococci occur in about

equal frequency, and approximately one-third of patients will have both pathogens simultaneously. Most patients acquire their infection outside the hospital. The majority of these infections present in the extremities, approximately two-thirds in the lower extremity.

There is often an underlying cause, such as **diabetes, arteriosclerotic vascular disease,** or **venous insufficiency with edema.** In some instances a chronic vascular ulcer changes into a more acute process. The mortality in this group is high, approaching 50% in patients with severe vascular disease.

2. Polymicrobial form

a. An array of anaerobic and aerobic organisms can be cultured from the involved fascial plane: from 1 to 15 bacteria, with an average of 5 pathogens in each wound. The most common organisms, found in various combinations, are:

Anaerobes	**Aerobes**
Bacteroides	*E. coli*
Peptococcus	*Klebsiella*
Peptostreptococcus	*Citrobacter*
Clostridium	*Pseudomonas*

b. The polymicrobial infection is associated with four clinical settings:

(1) Surgical procedures, especially bowel resections and penetrating trauma, can be complicated by cellulitis, leading to a superficial fascial dissection.

(2) An infection proceeding from a decubitus ulcer, minor trauma, or a perianal abscess can involve the buttocks and perineum. Due to the proximity of the anus, contamination by fecal bacteria is universally present.

(3) In heroin addicts, the upper extremities are frequently involved at the site of injection. Because the needles and "works" are contaminated, unusual organisms such as *Citrobacter* and *Pseudomonas* can be isolated, in association with the anaerobes listed above.

(4) The lesion can spread from a Bartholin's abscess or a minor vulvovaginal infection. Some cases have been associated with pudendal block anesthesia during delivery. While mixed infections are usually noted in this setting, some cases are caused by a single pathogen, particularly anaerobic *Streptococcus*.

D. Diagnosis

1. It may not be possible to diagnose fasciitis upon first seeing the patient. Overlying cellulitis is a frequent accompaniment. That the process involves the deeper fascial planes is suggested by the following features:

a. Failure to respond to initial antibiotic therapy. Cellulitis usually improves, with lowering of fever and reduction in local signs, within 24–48 hours. Fasciitis is a more stubborn infection and shows little improvement in the initial few days.

b. Hard, wooden feel of the subcutaneous tissue, extending beyond the area of apparent skin involvement.

c. Systemic toxicity, often with altered mental status.

2. Another diagnostic consideration initially is **erysipelas.** However, erysipelas has raised, sharply defined, bright red borders, often associated with streaking lymphatics in a caudad direction. The overlying skin usually is tender. Most importantly, the red border advances rapidly, so that a mark made with a pen at the edge will demonstrate progression within 1–2 hours. Necrotizing fasciitis, on the other hand, moves more slowly, does not have a discrete border, and is not particularly tender—indeed, it may be anesthetic.

3. The most important diagnostic feature of necrotizing fasciitis is the appearance of the fascial planes. Upon direct inspection, the fascia is swollen and dull gray in appearance, with stringy areas of necrosis. A thin, brownish exudate emerges from the wound. Even upon deep dissection, there is no true pus. Extensive undermining of surrounding tissues is present, and the fascial planes can be dissected with a gloved finger or a blunt instrument.

4. A Gram's stain of the exudate demonstrates the pathogens and provides an early clue to therapy. Gram-positive cocci in chains suggest streptococcal disease (either group A or anaerobic); large, gram-positive cocci in clumps suggest *Staph. aureus* or *Peptococcus*. A mixed flora suggests polymicrobial infection.
5. **Cultures** are best obtained from the deep tissues. If the infection has emanated from a contaminated skin wound, such as a vascular ulcer, the bacteriology of the superficial wound is not necessarily indicative of the deep tissue infection. An array of coliforms, staphylococci, and various streptococci can be isolated from the ulcer, but the fascia may have a pure culture of a single organism, such as anaerobic streptococci or *Staph. aureus*. Direct needle aspiration of the advancing edge has been advocated as a means of obtaining material for culture, but this technique is nearly always unproductive. A definitive bacteriologic diagnosis can be established only by culture of the fascia at operation or by positive blood culture.

E. Treatment

1. **Surgical intervention** is the major therapeutic modality in cases of necrotizing fasciitis. It should be emphasized, however, that some patients can be treated with large doses of appropriate antibiotics and thereby avoid potentially mutilating surgery. The decision to undertake aggressive surgery should be based on the following:
   a. Failure to respond to antibiotics after a reasonable trial is the most common index. A response to antibiotics should be judged by reduction in fever and toxicity and lack of advancement.
   b. Profound toxicity, fever, hypotension, or advancement of the skin and soft tissue infection during antibiotic therapy dictates surgical intervention.
   c. When the local wound shows extensive necrosis with easy dissection along the fascia by a blunt instrument, more complete incision and drainage are required.
2. The patient should be well hydrated and adequately transfused before beginning the surgical procedure. Under general anesthesia, the skin is incised or the wound is widened down to the fascial plane for complete inspection. Finger dissection along the fascial plane determines the extent of the linear incision. Usually, multiple incisions or "filets" are required to delineate adequately the extent of involvement. Loose gauze dressings are packed into the wound and changed every 6 hours or as required. Wet-to-dry dressings are used in order to facilitate mechanical debridement. As the dressings are removed, the depth of the wound should be inspected by a gloved finger to determine any extension that requires further incision. It must be emphasized that the first procedure is almost never sufficient to determine the extent of involvement. As further tracts are discovered, the patient is returned to the operating room for additional incision and debridement. Although no discrete pus is encountered, these wounds can discharge copious amounts of tissue fluid. For this reason, aggressive fluid and colloid therapy is a necessary adjunct.
3. **Antimicrobial therapy,** when administered appropriately, can minimize the extent of, and even avert, surgical intervention, especially in those cases in which the distinction between cellulitis and fasciitis is difficult. The therapy must be **directed at the pathogens** and used in **high doses for a prolonged period of time,** usually 2–3 weeks. The appropriate regimens as as follows:
   a. **Streptococcal or staphylococcal disease.** These pathogens are suspected when the condition arises from a small lesion or when it occurs spontaneously in an extremity. In the first instance, it is usually impossible to distinguish whether staphylococci or streptococci are the cause. For this reason, initial therapy should be directed against both organisms.

When definitive culture reports become available, it is possible to delete one or the other drug. Recommended initial therapy is as follows:

Penicillin G	3–4 million units IV q4h
Semisynthetic penicillin (oxacillin, nafcillin)	2 gm q4h

b. Patients with **renal insufficiency** should receive lower doses of penicillin, depending on the degree of malfunction. In the event of penicillin allergy, a cephalosporin or clindamycin can be used.

c. The **response** to antibiotic therapy often is dilatory. In the initial few days there should be a gradual decline in fever and toxicity and a lack of advancement. The subcutaneous tissues should become softer and less inflamed. The condition slowly resolves over the next 1–2 weeks. Even at this stage, however, it may be necessary to incise and drain some areas, although the extent of linear incisions needed is usually minor in the later phases. After resolution, it is advised to continue oral antibiotic treatment for another 2–4 weeks, since there is a tendency for these infections to recur. If the organism has not been identified by this stage, an oral semisynthetic penicillin or cephalosporin should be administered.

d. Polymicrobial infections should be treated with a broad-spectrum regimen designed to suppress both aerobic and anaerobic bacteria. The suggested drugs, which would also encompass staphylococci and streptococci, are

Clindamycin, 600 mg IV q6h, **plus** an aminoglycoside (gentamicin, tobramycin, or amikacin)

Cefoxitin, 2 gm IV q6h; may be used as a single agent, unless *Pseudomonas* is suspected, in which case an aminoglycoside should be added

If the staphylococci or streptococci are found to be the only pathogens, the regimen should be changed to penicillin, as listed in **III.E.3.a.**

F. Risk factors. The overall mortality in necrotizing fasciitis is 20–30%. Adverse risk factors include

1. Diabetes
2. Advanced arteriosclerotic vascular disease
3. Lesions that involve an extremity and that then progress into the buttocks or back muscles or onto the chest wall.

Polymicrobial Skin Infections

I. Definitions

A. A group of skin infections with diverse pathophysiology are related to one another by clinical features, bacteriology, and therapeutic considerations. These include **diabetic foot ulcer, decubitus ulcer, pilonidal sinus,** and **hidradenitis suppurativa.** The clinical manifestations may be either acute or chronic.

B. The **acute** form is characterized by

1. A time of onset measured in days, rather than weeks as in the chronic form.
2. A lesion that displays a purulent discharge, with advancing erythema and cellulitis in the surrounding tissues. In the chronic form the erythema and tissue involvement are localized.
3. Systemic manifestations, especially if cellulitis is extensive.

C. A **chronic** lesion may be present as a prelude to an acute exacerbation of spreading cellulitis and fever.

II. Bacteriology. The acute form, involving tissue extension and cellulitis, is usually caused by *Staph. aureus* and group A *Strep. pyogenes,* present singly or in combination. The chronic form, certainly the most common type seen clinically, has a mixed anaerobic-aerobic flora. Multiple bacteria are isolated, and sampling from different sites reveals different organisms as well. The most common isolates in the chronic form are *Peptococcus* (anaerobic gram-positive cocci) and *Proteus*. The following table indicates the range of pathogens:

Anaerobes	**Aerobes**
Peptococcus	*Proteus*
Bacteroides	*E. coli*
Clostridium	*Klebsiella*
Fusobacterium	*Streptococci* (various types)
Peptostreptococcus	

III. Treatment

A. Treatment of the **acute** form should be directed at *Staph. aureus* and *Strep. pyogenes*. Semisynthetic penicillins (oxacillin, nafcillin, and cloxacillin) or cephalosporins are useful agents. Oral erythromycin can be used for the allergic patient. It should be emphasized that most acute episodes can be treated on an outpatient basis with warm soaks and oral antibiotics. Indications for hospitalization are systemic toxicity or extension from the local site with cellulitis and lymphangitis.

B. Antimicrobial therapy can do little for the **chronic** forms of these skin infections. The mainstay of treatment is surgical debridement and local care, including wet-to-dry dressings to encourage mechanical debridement. Even though a chronic decubitus or a diabetic foot ulcer is discharging pus, experience has taught that antibiotics cannot alter the course. The only indications for antibiotic therapy are

1. Systemic toxicity with fever and chills
2. Severe cellulitis and extension of the process beyond the wound margin. The surrounding skin is red, indurated, and painful.

In these settings, antibiotics should be administered for only short periods of time, usually 5–7 days, until the acute phase has passed. Prolonging treatment beyond this time only changes the local flora to drug-resistant bacteria and threatens the patient with drug toxicity. Since there are mixed aerobes and anaerobes in such chronic infections, the following regimens are recommended:

Clindamycin, 600 mg IV q6h **plus** an aminoglycoside (gentamicin, tobramycin, or amikacin)

Cefoxitin, 2 gm q6h, as a single agent, unless *Pseudomonas* is suspected, in which case an aminoglycoside is added

Synergistic Necrotizing Cellulitis

I. Definitions

A. This is a highly lethal polymicrobial infection that produces extensive necrosis of skin and soft tissues with progressive undermining along fascial planes. The process may be rather indolent at first, presenting after 7–10 days of mild symptoms. Patients are often afebrile or have only low-grade fever, lacking systemic toxicity in the early stages. The initial lesion in the skin is a small area of necrotic or reddish brown bleb with extreme local tenderness. However, the superficial appearance belies the widespread destruction of the deeper tissues. By direct inspection through skin incisions, there is extensive gangrene of the superficial tissues and fat, with gelatinous necrosis of fascia and muscle. The discharge is brown, rather thin and watery, with a foul odor; such exudate has been labeled "dishwater pus." Gram's stain reveals a mixed flora with abundant polymorphonuclear leukocytes. Gas can be palpated in the tissues in 25% of patients.

B. The most common **site of involvement** is the **perineum,** seen in one-half of patients. The major predisposing causes are **perirectal abscess** and **ischiorectal abscess;** these conditions track to the deeper structures of the pelvis, leading to a severe form of the disease. A more superficial form involves the buttocks without extension to deeper muscles.

C. Approximately 40% of patients have involvement of the thigh and leg. Some infections arise in the adductor compartment of the thigh, often extending from an infected amputation stump or diabetic gangrene. Lesions in the lower leg usually are associated with vascular disease or diabetic foot ulcers. The remaining 10% of cases occur in the upper extremities or in the neck, most frequently in patients with vascular disease or diabetes.

II. **Predisposing conditions.** Seventy-five percent of patients have diabetes mellitus, which may be relatively mild and only discovered at the time of admission. Some patients present with ketoacidosis. Cardiovascular and renal disease are seen in 50% of patients. Obesity is common, found in over 50% of patients.

III. **Bacteriology.** This is a mixed aerobic-anaerobic infection, consisting of organisms that have their origin in the intestinal tract. Of the aerobes, coliforms are most common, such as *E. coli, Klebsiella,* and *Proteus.* The anaerobes include *Bacteroides, Peptostreptococcus, Peptococcus, Clostridum,* and *Fusobacterium.* Approximately one-third of patients have positive blood cultures, usually a coliform, *Bacteroides* or *Peptostreptococcus.*

IV. **Differential diagnosis.** Several infections of the skin can be mistaken for synergistic necrotizing cellulitis.

A. **Gas gangrene.** This clostridial infection is more dramatic in presentation, often associated with renal failure, high fever, and severe toxicity. The most striking feature in gas gangrene is myonecrosis, in which the muscle initially is pale white, then mushy red color, and eventually black with gangrene. The overlying skin is extensively involved with blebs and hemorrhagic necrosis. Abundant gas is found in the subcutaneous tissues. Gram's stain of the exudate from gas gangrene shows **no** polymorphonuclear leukocytes and an abundance of large, gram-positive rods.

B. **Progressive synergistic bacterial gangrene (Meleney's gangrene).** This is an indolent process involving the skin and subcutaneous tissues, without extensive tracking into deeper structures. Gram's stain of the outer zones reveals gram-positive cocci.

C. **Necrotizing fasciitis.** Although systemic toxicity may be severe, the necrotizing component is confined to the fascial planes, with relative sparing of the superficial layers of skin and surrounding muscles. There is little exudate, and the pathogen on Gram's stain or culture is often a single organism, such as *Staph.,* group A *Streptococcus, Peptostreptococcus,* or *Bacteroides.*

V. **Treatment**

A. **Surgical management** of synergistic necrotizing cellulitis involves radical debridement of involved tissues, followed by wet-to-dry dressing and mechanical debridement. When the lower extremity is involved, as in diabetes, an amputation usually is required. In the perineum, infection that is confined to the buttocks can be managed with complete surgical excision; however, deeper infection in the pelvis, extending from perirectal disease, is difficult to approach by complete resection, and may require repeated sessions of debridement in the operating room to achieve adequate drainage.

B. **Antibiotic therapy** involves a spectrum broad enough to cover both aerobes and anaerobes. The following drugs are recommended:

Clindamycin, 600 mg IV or IM q6h **plus** an aminoglycoside (gentamicin, tobramycin, or amikacin)

Cefoxitin, 2 gm q6h with or without an aminoglycoside, depending on the presence or absence of *Pseudomonas*

Metronidazole, 500 PO or IV q8h **plus** an aminoglycoside

VI. **Complications.** There is a 50% mortality in this disease. The patients usually succumb to septic shock and circulatory collapse. Adverse risk factors include

A. Diabetes, especially ketoacidosis

B. Severe renal disease

C. Involvement of deep tissues of the pelvis and perineum

Nonclostridial Crepitant Cellulitis

I. Definitions. Gas-forming organisms can involve the skin, either primarily or as an extension from deeper structures. The origin of infection may be an abdominal wound, perianal disease, or operative incisions that have become secondarily infected. Tracking of gas-forming organisms from deeper sites of infection may also present as crepitant cellulitis without a break in the skin. This can be noted in the perineal area, associated with ischiorectal abscess, or in the flank, communicating with a perinephric abscess. Among the bacteria isolated are anaerobic organisms, such as *Bacteroides* or anaerobic streptococci (*Peptostreptococcus*), and/or coliform bacteria, especially *E. coli* and *Klebsiella*. Diabetics are more likely to acquire such infections, especially in the lower extremities. It should be emphasized that these emphysematous infections generally are not as serious as those associated with clostridia, since the nonclostridial pathogens do not liberate systemic toxins.

II. Treatment. The surgical approach should be aggressive, but tailored specifically to the underlying cause of infection. Extensive resection usually is not required, since the gas is not an index of underlying necrosis, but rather reflects tracking of the infection along the fascial or lymphatic planes. Antibiotic therapy is directed at a mixed aerobic-anaerobic flora, until culture reports are available.

III. Differential diagnosis. Noninfectious processes can be associated with gas in subcutaneous tissues:

A. On the chest wall, at the site of thoracentesis, chest tube insertion, or a thoracic procedure, there may be subcutaneous emphysema that tracks extensively along subcutaneous tissues.

B. A tracheotomy provides a portal for air to track along the tissues of the neck, even to the anterior chest wall. Transtracheal aspiration by a needle produces local emphysema in approximately 10% of cases.

C. On rare occasions, a thin column of gas is palpated or seen by x-ray along the course of an IV catheter in the arm. This is most likely caused by a central venous pressure line or a Swan-Ganz catheter. This is a benign condition, not associated with infection in the lines or the surrounding veins.

The relative benignity of noninfectious subcutaneous emphysema, in the situations just noted, is indicated by the paucity of changes in the skin (erythema, induration, pain) and the absence of systemic toxicity.

Fournier's Gangrene

I. Definitions

A. This is a variant of synergistic gangrene that involves the scrotum and penis and has an explosive onset. It occurs in relatively healthy men, usually 25–50 years of age, although rare cases have been reported in the neonate and in the elderly. One-half of patients have no preceding infection; the remaining individuals have one of the following conditions:

1. Ischiorectal abscess
2. Perianal fistula
3. Erysipelas of the perineum
4. Bowel disease (rectal carcinoma, diverticulitis)
5. Scrotal trauma
6. Prior urogenital surgery
7. Urogenital infections, especially involving the periurethral glands

B. In recent times, this disease has been observed in alcoholics who develop pressure sores of the scrotum and perineum by sitting in the same position in a drunken stupor. There is also an association with diabetes mellitus. Dissection of pancreatic juice through the retroperitoneum has on rare occasion presented as scrotal gangrene.

C. The route of infection is thought to be via Buck's fascia, spreading along the planes of the dartos fascia of the scrotum and penis. The infection may then extend to Colles' fascia of the perineum and even to Scarpa's fascia of the abdominal wall. At the outset, it tends to be superficial gangrene, limited to skin and subcutaneous tissue, extending to the base of the penis. The testes and spermatic cord usually are spared. There may be extension to the perineum and the anterior abdominal wall through the fascial planes.

II. Bacteriology

A. A single organism, most commonly *Staph. aureus* or anaerobic streptococci (*Peptostreptococcus* or *Peptococcus*), is often isolated. Improved techniques in recent years have revealed a mixed flora of aerobic and anaerobic organisms, similar to those noted in synergistic necrotizing cellulitis. *Pseudomonas* has been noted in some patients, as part of a mixed infection.

III. Treatment

A. Prompt **surgical debridement** should be instituted, with aggressive removal of all necrotic tissue, sparing the deeper structures when possible. The infection does not usually penetrate below the fascial planes of the scrotum, so the testes and spermatic cord can be preserved in early cases.

B. **Antibiotic therapy** is similar to that for necrotizing cellulitis (p. 194); if infection is due to a single organism, such as *Staphylococcus* or *Streptococcus,* one antibiotic, either a penicillin or cephalosporin, can be employed.

Progressive Bacterial Synergistic Gangrene (Meleney's Gangrene)

I. Definitions

A. This is a postoperative infection that typically occurs in the vicinity of retention sutures or in a drain site following an abdominal operation. Occasionally it occurs in other areas, such as an incision of the chest wall.

B. Meleney's synergistic gangrene is an indolent process characterized by poor wound healing with elevation and erythema of the surrounding skin. The diagnosis is recognized 1–2 weeks after operation, when the lesion has extended circumferentially with three zones of involvement:

1. A **central area** of necrosis
2. A **middle zone** of violaceous, tender, edematous tissue
3. An **outer zone** of bright erythema

C. Local pain and tenderness are nearly always present. However, fever and systemic toxicity usually are absent.

II. Bacteriology. This condition is caused by synergistic (cooperative) association between *Staph. aureus* and a microaerophilic or anaerobic *Streptococcus*. These organisms can be isolated from the outer zone of infection; sampling the central zone of necrosis, however, yields a mixed flora of coliforms that does not reflect the essential pathologic process.

III. Treatment

A. In the preantibiotic era, Meleney advocated extensive resection of all nonviable tissue, as well as extension of the incision beyond the area of induration and necrosis to include some healthy tissue. The availability of antibiotics has eliminated the requirement for such radical excision. It is now recommended that all necrotic tissue be removed, with inspection of subcutaneous structures for burrowing tracks. Wet-to-dry dressings should then be employed. Daily inspection should reveal any extension of the process that requires additional debridement. A heterograft or homograft may be necessary to cover the wound.

B. Antimicrobial therapy should be directed at the two major pathogens, *Staph. aureus* and the anaerobic *Streptococcus*. A semisynthetic penicillin (nafcillin or oxacillin) or a cephalosporin can be used.

Table 9-2. Sites of infection of bite wounds

	Site of infection (% of cases)				
Source	Hands	Arms	Legs and feet	Face	Trunk
Human	65	8	2	15	10
Cat	55	25	9	9	2
Dog	30	15	40	10	5

Bite Wounds

I. Definitions

A. Bite wounds of animal or human origin can lead to serious infections, tissue destruction, and even amputation and death. The mouth is an abundant source of pathogenic microorganisms. When these microbes are inoculated deep into tissues, as through a bite wound, they can spread via lymphatic and fascial planes, causing gross necrosis of supporting tissues, joints, and bones.

B. The most common bite wounds seen in the emergency room are as follows.

Source	Incidence (%)
Dog	65
Cat	15
Human	15
Miscellaneous*	5

C. The sites of infection are related to the type of animal inflicting the wound. Dog bites are most common on the lower extremities, whereas bites of cats and humans involve the hands (Table 9-2).

II. Complications

A. Dog bites carry the lowest risk of infectious complications, usually producing only mild cellulitis. Most dog bites are superficial lacerations that can be managed by debridement and primary closure. The major complications occur with human and cat bites.

Source	Incidence of infectious complications (%)
Human	30
Cat	25
Dog	3

B. Human bites have a high incidence of infectious complications and can produce severe sepsis. The most common cause of these bites is fisticuffs, in which the knuckles, especially those of the middle and index fingers, are cut in the process of striking the opponent's teeth. Human bites are also an occupational hazard for physicians, nurses, and dentists. There is a high risk in dealing with young children or with violent or mentally disturbed patients.

The usual infection with a human bite is on the knuckle of the hand. Although the entry may be tiny, the bite can penetrate the extensor tendon and even enter the joint. At first there is minimal pain, but 6–12 hours later the finger and dorsum of the hand swell and become painful, and the wound emits a thin, grayish, malodorous discharge. Pain on movement of the finger suggests involvement of the joint. The patient becomes febrile, although severe toxicity is unusual. Over the next few hours, the local process can progress up the arm, and may be associated with spreading lymphangitis and lymphadenopathy. The most

*Monkey, rat, raccoon, rabbit, mouse, bat, horse, mule, bear, and assorted wild animals.

serious human bites occur around the head and neck, although they are relatively uncommon.

III. Bacteriology. The mouth flora contains an enormous assortment of microorganisms, many of which are anaerobic and not susceptible to conventional culture techniques. The most common organisms in human or animal bites are α-hemolytic streptococci. In animal bites, especially those of dogs and cats, an unusual gram-negative pathogen is commonly present: *Pasteurella multocida.* Anaerobes are recovered in 50% of human and animal bites, and the most frequently found types are *Bacteroides* (*B. oralis* and *B. melaninogenicus*), *Fusobacterium, Peptostreptococcus,* and spirochetal organisms (usually not cultivable). *Staph. aureus* is found in one-third of primary bite wounds. Unusual gram-negative organisms are also encountered, including *Eikenella. Moraxella, Enterobacter,* and *Hemophilus.*

IV. Treatment

A. Dog bites should be rinsed with copious amounts of fluid. Deeper wounds are cleaned and irrigated with saline. Most dog bites do not require suturing, but those that are deep, with clean edges, should be primarily closed.

B. As a general rule, bites of humans, cats and monkeys **should not be sutured.** There are certain exceptions involving mutilating wounds of the face, especially around the nose, mouth, and eyelids, in which an experienced surgeon may attempt a primary closure following careful cleaning and debridement. This is done to avoid the gross deformity that would result from an open wound. However, it must be recognized that primary closures of these types of bites lead to a high incidence of infection in the suture line.

C. Antibiotic treatment is not required for most animal bites, since they are usually superficial.

1. Dog bites that are mild, not requiring sutures, should not be treated with antibiotics. On the other hand, when sutures are employed or when there is extensive tissue damage, antibiotics are indicated.
2. Human, cat, and monkey bites should be treated with antibiotics on most occasions. Only the most superficial scrapes do not require antibiotics. The initial treatment of choice for all bites, whether of human or animal origin, is penicillin or ampicillin. For outpatient therapy, conventional doses of either drug are employed, given by the oral route (ampicillin, 250 mg PO q6h). Patients who are hospitalized with severe bites should be given parenteral antibiotics (penicillin G, 2 million units IV q4h, or ampicillin, 2 gm IV q4h). A Gram's stain of the discharge should be used as a guide to additional antibiotics; for example, the presence of staphylococci would necessitate antistaphylococcal drugs (such as oxacillin, nafcillin, or cefazolin), while the presence of gram-negative rods would require an aminoglycoside. Subsequent culture reports should be checked for specific organisms and their antibiotic susceptibilities.
3. When a wound closure has been attempted and is later complicated by infection, the sutures should be removed and the wound inspected for necrotic tissue. Extensive debridement is not advised at the early stage, since the infection can often be managed by opening the wound and instituting antibiotic therapy. When a limb is involved, it should be immobilized and elevated in order to decrease tissue edema.

Rabies

Rabies is a rare disease in the United States, with only 1–5 reported cases yearly since 1960. Nevertheless, the management of people with possible exposure is of paramount importance, and thousands receive rabies prophylaxis each year. The following are revised recommendations by the Immunization Practices Advisory Committee (1980).*

*For specific queries the physician should consult the local or state health department, or the Centers for Disease Control.

I. **Species of biting animals**

A. **High risk.** Animals most likely to be infected with rabies virus are **carnivorous wild animals,** especially skunks, raccoons, foxes, coyotes, and bobcats. **Bats** have been responsible for most rabies cases in the United States since 1960. Patients **exposed** to these animals should receive prophylaxis, unless the biting animal is tested and shown not to be rabid (see sec. **II** definition of **exposure**). Treatment initiated prior to testing may be discontinued if tests are negative.

B. **Limited risk.** The incidence of rabies in domestic pets, especially **dogs and cats,** varies in different regions, so guidelines depend to some extent on the local experience.

C. **Very low risk.** Animals rarely infected are rabbits and rodents such as squirrels, hamsters, guinea pigs, gerbils, chipmunks, rats, and mice. Rabies prophylaxis is rarely indicated, although state or local health authorities may be consulted in unusual circumstances.

II. **Exposure.** The virus must be introduced into open cuts or wounds, or transmitted via mucous membranes. A **bite** means any penetration of the skin by teeth. **Nonbite exposure** refers to scratches, abrasions, open wounds, or mucous membranes exposed to either saliva or potentially infected material such as brain tissue. Casual contact such as petting a rabid animal does not constitute exposure.

III. **Nature of incident.** An unprovoked attack is more likely to indicate the animal is rabid.

IV. **Management of animal.** Domestic pets should be retained and observed for 10 days to detect signs of rabies. Wild animals with rabies do not reliably show clinical signs and should be killed for necropsy examination if responsible for exposures. The preferred diagnostic test in animals is a fluorescent-antibody examination to detect virus in the brain.

V. **Treatment of wound.** The most important preventive measure is immediate and vigorous cleansing of bite wounds or scratches with soap and water.

VI. **Prophylaxis** to prevent tetanus is discussed on p. 212.

VII. **Immunization.** Postexposure prophylaxis includes both passive and active immunization simultaneously. The only exception is a person previously immunized, with documented antibody levels, who should receive only vaccine. Prophylaxis should be initiated as soon as possible, although the decision to treat has been made as late as 6 months after exposure. Available preparations include

A. **Antisera** (one dose, preferably RIG)

1. **Rabies immune globulin (human) (RIG)** is the preferred antibody preparation for passive immunization. It is given once at the beginning of prophylaxis. The usual dose is 20 IU/kg, up to one-half infiltrated into the wound site and the rest given intramuscularly. Side effects are local pain and low-grade fever.
2. **Antirabies serum (equine) (ARS)** is given if RIG is not available. The usual dose is 40 IU/kg IM. Side effects with equine serum include serum sickness in up to 40% of patients and occasional cases of anaphylaxis. Patients should be skin-tested for sensitivity to equine serum prior to administration, although the skin test itself has been known to evoke anaphylaxis.

B. **Vaccine** (multiple doses, preferably HDCV)

1. **Human diploid cell rabies vaccine (HDCV)** is a recently introduced vaccine composed of inactivated virus grown in tissue-cultured cells. It has well-documented efficacy and is preferred over the older preparation, DEV. HDCV is available in 1-ml single-dose vials to be given intramuscularly in five doses—as soon as possible after exposure, then on days 3, 7, 14, and 28. Side effects are primarily local reactions such as pain, erythema, and swelling. These have been noted in 25% of recipients. Mild systemic effects are noted in 20% and include headache, nausea, abdominal pain, myalgias, and dizziness. There have been no serious reactions such as anaphylaxis or neuroparalytic reactions.
2. **Duck embryo vaccine (DEV)** is inactivated rabies virus grown in embryonated duck eggs. This should be used only when RIG is not available, as it carries an increased incidence of side effects. It is available in 1-ml single-

dose vials to be given subcutaneously in 23 doses—21 daily doses, or 14 doses in the 1st 7 days (two simultaneous injections given at separate sites) followed by 7 daily doses; then 2 booster doses at 10 and 20 days after the 21st dose. Subcutaneous injection sites should be rotated and include the abdomen, lower back, and lateral thighs. Side effects are common. Most patients have local pain, erythema, and induration at injection sites. Systemic symptoms of fever, malaise, or myalgias occur in one-third. The estimated incidence of neuroparalytic reactions is 1/25,000. Fewer than 1% develop anaphylaxis.

Gas Gangrene (Clostridial Myonecrosis)

I. General principles. Among the most serious surgical infections are those caused by the clostridia. Gas gangrene, produced by *Clostridium perfringens,* is a destructive process of muscle associated with local crepitance and systemic signs of toxemia. An antecedent event such as trauma, gunshot wound, frostbite, or intestinal surgical procedure exposes muscle and subcutaneous tissue to these ubiquitous organisms. Given the setting of tissue necrosis, low oxygen tension, and adequate concentrations of amino acids and calcium, the clostridial spores introduced from the external environment or the gastrointestinal tract germinate, with the production of the potent alpha toxin.

II. Bacteriology

A. Clostridia are gram-positive, spore-forming, obligate anaerobes widely present in soil and in animals. In humans, their normal residence is the gastrointestinal tract and the female genital tract, although they can be isolated occasionally from the surface of the skin and from the mouth. At present, there are over 60 recognized species of clostridia, in addition to many isolates that do not fit the accepted taxonomy.

B. The most important of the histotoxic species involved in gas gangrene is *C. perfringens.* The organism is relatively aerotolerant and exhibits "stormy fermentation" in milk. It is the fastest-growing clostridial species, with a generation of 8 minutes under ideal conditions. *C. perfringens* produces alpha toxin, which is a phospholipase C (lecithinase) that splits lecithin into phosphorylcholine and diglyceride. Its activity can be inhibited by specific antitoxin. The alpha toxin has been associated with gas gangrene; it is known to be hemolytic, to destroy platelets, and to cause widespread capillary damage.

C. Myonecrosis is caused by *C. perfringens* in 80% of cases. The remaining agents are *C. novyi, C. septicum,* and *C. bifermentans.* Other species that have been implicated are *C. histolyticum, C. sporogenes, C. fallax,* and *C. tertium,* but the proof of their etiologic role is rather tenuous. The wounds themselves are usually contaminated with a miscellany of aerobic and anaerobic bacteria.

III. Pathogenesis

A. The pathophysiologic setting of gas gangrene is necrosis of the muscle due to a compromised blood supply, either through direct injury or underlying vascular disease, in association with contamination by potential pathogens. The conditions for elaboration of toxin are a low oxidation-reduction potential, anoxia, tissue necrosis, and the presence of various peptides, amino acids, and calcium. These conditions are fulfilled in traumatic wounds associated with sepsis.

B. The history of gas gangrene has been intimately tied to warfare, since traumatic wounds, gross contamination, and delay in surgical management are characteristic of battlefield conditions. We have come to recognize that this disease also occurs in peacetime, although the epidemiology is somewhat different (Table 9-3). The current experience in metropolitan centers is that 60% of cases are related to trauma; one-half of these are caused by automobile accidents, while the remainder are crush injuries, industrial accidents, or gunshot wounds acquired in our urban combat zones. The other peacetime cases of gas gangrene occur postop-

Table 9-3. Peacetime gas gangrene

Cause	Percent
Trauma	60
Automobile accidents	
Crush injuries	
Industrial accidents	
Gunshot wounds	
Postoperative	35
Colon resection	
Ruptured appendix	
Perirectal infections	
Perforated bowel	
Biliary tract surgery	
Vascular insufficiency	5

eratively. Elective colon resections make up the largest category, followed in order of occurrence by ruptured appendix, perirectal infections, perforated bowel, and biliary tract surgery. A small group of cases of gas gangrene can be traced to vascular insufficiency, usually in diabetics who develop disease in the stump following amputation. Overall, the experience in peacetime is that two-thirds of gas gangrene cases occur in the extremities and one-third in the abdominal wall.

IV. Clinical features

A. The **incubation period** of gas gangrene is 8 hours to 20 days, with an average of 4 days, following the initiating event, which is either trauma or a surgical procedure. There is a sudden onset of pain in the wound, increasing in severity and extending somewhat beyond the original borders over the next several hours. The skin becomes edematous and tense. It changes in color from an initial pale appearance to a magenta hue, often accompanied by large, hemorrhagic bullae. A thin, watery discharge appears early in the course. It may have an unpleasant, foul-sweet odor, and microscopic examination reveals abundant gram-positive rods with a remarkable **paucity of inflammatory cells.** Initially the patient has a tachycardia that cannot be explained by the height of fever or circulatory changes. Subsequently shock and renal failure ensue.

B. The **appearance of the involved muscle** is characteristic in gas gangrene, being quite unlike any other soft-tissue infection. It must be viewed by direct surgical exposure, since many of the changes are not apparent when inspected through the edges of a traumatic wound. Initially the muscle is pale and edematous, looking like a piece of steak that has been seared over a charcoal fire. The muscle, however, does not contract under the scalpel; further dissection reveals beefy red, nonviable muscle tissue. As the disease progresses, the muscle becomes frankly gangrenous, black, and extremely friable, but by this time the patient is near death. It is important to establish the diagnosis of myonecrosis as early as possible in order to resect all devitalized, necrotic tissue.

C. The **mental status** of a patient with gas gangrene is an extraordinary feature of the disease process. Despite profound hypotension, renal failure, and advancing crepitance, patients may be remarkably alert, showing extreme sensitivity to their surroundings. They feel their impending doom, and a sense of terror can be read in their furtive gaze. This intense mental awareness is mercifully suspended just prior to death, when the patient lapses into toxic delirium and eventually into coma.

V. Diagnosis. The sine qua non for diagnosis of gas gangrene is **direct visualization of the muscle** to observe the characteristic appearance of the disease. The clinical features just described should arouse suspicion early in the course, so that the disease can be recognized and surgically managed with haste. Gas in the wound and surrounding tissue is a relatively late finding; by the time crepitance is appreciated, the patient may be beyond hope of survival. X-ray of the affected site reveals gas in the tissues and along the fascial planes, but, again, this tends to be a late finding. It is of great help to examine a Gram's-stained slide of the wound discharge for the presence of clostridia and the absence of inflammatory cells. Needle aspiration of the active margin of infection is helpful when wound discharge is not present. Approximately 15% of patients have positive blood cultures.

VI. Treatment

A. Surgical management is the most important part of therapy. As a general principle, all involved muscle should be resected in order to ensure survival. Clearly nonviable muscle, as demonstrated by lack of response to stimulus with the scalpel, should be removed. This may involve rather mutilating surgery, however, especially when a proximal limb or the abdominal wall is involved. Muscle that is marginally involved should be preserved as much as possible in order for medical therapy to exert its beneficial effect. Major attention should be paid to adequate excision; reconstruction can be planned at a later stage. Such decisions require fine surgical judgment based on the extent of myonecrosis. The commonest error of judgment in cases of this disease is delaying the incision that is required to inspect the involved muscle. Even a few hours delay can tip the balance against the patient.

B. Antibiotic treatment is directed at clostridia in the case of gas gangrene of the extremities, and at a mixed microflora in cases involving the abdominal wall. Penicillin G has excellent activity against nearly all strains of *C. perfringens;* only 5% of the other species that cause gas gangrene shows variable degrees of resistance. Clindamycin has been somewhat disappointing against clostridia, with 15–20% of strains resistant.

Gas Gangrene of the Extremities Penicillin G	3 million units IV q4h; reduce dose in the face of renal failure
Gas Gangrene of the Abdominal Wall Penicillin G	Same dose as above, **plus** broad-spectrum coverage: Cefoxitin and/or aminoglycoside Metronidazole and aminoglycoside Clindamycin and aminoglycoside

C. The use of gas gangrene **antitoxin** is **still controversial,** despite the rather convincing claims from war-time experiences. (It should be recognized that injured soldiers in World War I and II could not be given optimal surgical management due to battlefield conditions and the state of the art at the time.) Furthermore, there are limited supplies available now since the manufacturers have generally discontinued production. The antitoxin is believed to neutralize toxin circulating in the bloodstream. The disease in its classic form, however, is characteristized by compromised circulation and rapid fixation of toxin to tissue. It should be recalled that antitoxin is available only as a **horse serum** preparation; the large doses recommended for therapy carry a significant risk of immediate-type anaphylactic reactions, as well as the delayed-type reactions such as serum sickness. For these reasons, **we do not recommend** the use of antitoxin in treating gas gangrene, especially when optimal surgical management is available at an early stage.

Despite the disagreement concerning its use in conventional gas gangrene, antitoxin, in large doses, should be given to patients with clostridial toxemia who display marked hemolytic anemia with the attendent findings of hemoglobinemia, hemoglobinuria, disseminated intravascular coagulation, shock, and renal failure. Examination of a peripheral blood smear reveals crinkled and damaged red blood cells, indicating the destructive action of the alpha toxin. These findings are noted commonly in uterine gas gangrene and rarely in spreading clostridial cellulitis and rapidly advancing myonecrosis. It should be noted that these circumstances portend a high mortality. A few survivors of this condition have been reported, and antitoxin therapy does seem appropriate in this special situation. (**Dose:** 50,000 units of polyvalent gas gangrene antitoxin.)

D. Exchange blood transfusion can be performed on patients with severe hemolysis in order to remove the damaged red blood cells from the circulation. It goes without saying that the wound source of clostridial toxin must be managed surgically if transfusions or antitoxin therapy is to have any logical benefit. As with most other therapeutic modalities for this disease, there have been no controlled trials to assess the efficacy of exchange transfusion.

E. Hyperbaric oxygen. The therapeutic use in gas gangrene of hyperbaric oxygen (100%) under pressure of 3 atmospheres has its strong adherents and its skeptics. Under laboratory conditions, hyperbaric oxygen has generally, but not always, caused inhibition and even killing of clostridia. There is also inhibition of toxin production, even though the organism may survive. It is very difficult to judge the efficacy of this therapy from reading the literature, but this author (S.L.G.) can avow from personal experience that the effect of hyperbaric oxygen therapy in gas gangrene can be very dramatic. There are certain problems with such a therapeutic modality, however, not the least of which is the logistics of moving a desperately ill patient to appropriately equipped centers. In addition, hyperbaric oxygen has certain untoward effects. Oxygen toxicity produces complications in the central nervous system and lung that can be serious and even life-threatening. It would be reasonable to conclude that patients with gas gangrene should be treated with hyperbaric oxygen if a facility is readily available. To be sure, some centers without a hyperbaric chamber have reported acceptable mortality rates, indicating that expert surgical management and control of complications are the most important aspects of treatment of gas gangrene.

VII. Complications. The mortality of gas gangrene is 40–60%. It is highest in cases involving the abdominal wall and lowest in those affecting a single extremity. Among the signs that prognosticate a poor outcome are **leukopenia, low platelet count, intravascular hemolysis,** and severe **liver** or **renal** impairment.

Hypotension is an early sign of gas gangrene and can lead to **renal failure** and **irreversible shock.** Release of alpha toxin into the bloodstream can cause severe **hemolysis,** including hemoglobinemia, hemoglobinuria, and renal cortical necrosis. This diagnosis is established by measuring free hemoglobin in the urine and serum and by examining the peripheral blood smear for the characteristic red blood cells with crinkled, shaggy edges. Such hemolysis is more common in uterine gas gangrene, although it is occasionally seen in cases involving the limbs, in which there is extensive muscle involvement.

Other Clostridial Infections

I. Popular misconceptions. Much of the literature about clostridial infections has been written by microbiologists with little clinical experience or by archivists who uncritically review the literature. As a result, several misconceptions have been propagated for years, without a major attempt to update the classification of clinical disease on the basis of newer findings. These popular misconceptions include the belief that

A. The presence of clostridia in soft-tissue infections or in blood cultures necessarily signifies serious disease.

B. Anaerobic cellulitis due to clostridia is a relatively benign disease process without systemic signs of toxemia.

C. The single species *C. perfringens* accounts for the majority of infections in skin and soft tissues ascribed to clostridia.

The classification of clostridial infections in humans, as outlined in Table 9-4, attempts to update the expanding knowledge in this field.

II. Skin and soft-tissue infections

A. Simple contamination

Simple contamination, without clinical signs of sepsis, is by all accounts the most frequent setting for clostridia. Before the widespread use of antibiotics, clostridia could be cultured from 10–30% of wounds in civilians and from up to 80% of war wounds. In the Korean War experience, 27% of battle wounds were contaminated by clostridia without showing signs of suppuration. Even with treatment with

Table 9-4. Clinical presentations of clostridia in humans

Skin and soft tissues
Simple contamination
Suppurative infections
Intraabdominal
Cholangitis
Female pelvic tract
Pulmonary
Localized infections of skin and soft tissues
Anaerobic cellulitis
Stump infection in diabetics
Perirectal abscess
Diabetic foot ulcer
Decubitus ulcer
Suppurative myositis
Conjunctivitis and ophthalmitis
Diffuse, spreading cellulitis and fasciitis
Gas gangrene (myonecrosis)
Extremities
Abdominal wall
Uterus
Bacteremia
Associated with suppurative or localized infection
Underlying disease but apparently unrelated
Intestinal disorders
Food poisoning
Enteritis necroticans ("pig-bel")
Pseudomembranous colitis

Table 9-5. Species of *Clostridium* isolated from soft tissue

Species	Number of isolates
C. perfringens	20
C. ramosum	15
C. bifermentans	5
C. sphenoides	4
C. sporogenes	3
C. innocuum	3
C. difficile	3
C. butyricum	3
C. sordellii	3
C. limosum	2
C. subterminale	2
C. septicum	2
C. novyi	2
C. tertium	1
C. barati	1
C. cadaveris	1
C. beijerinckii	1
C. fallax	1
C. carnis	1
C. pseudotetanicum	1
C. ghoni	1
Unclassified	12
Total	87

Table 9-6. Source of isolates of *Clostridium* in soft-tissue infections

Source	Number of patients
Intraabdominal sepsis	28
Carcinoma	8
Empyema	8
Pelvic abscess	6
Subcutaneous abscess	5
Frostbite with gas gangrene	3
Infected stump	2
Brain abscess	1
Prostatic abscess	1
Perianal abscess	1
Conjunctivitis	1
Aortic graft	1
Total	65

antibiotics such as cephalothin and kanamycin, clostridia were isolated from 16% of penetrating abdominal wounds. There is no difference in the frequency with which clostridia are isolated from suppurating wounds as opposed to their frequency in well-healing open wounds in cases associated with trauma.

Recovery of clostridia from a wound does not determine its clinical status nor does it dictate a specific therapeutic decision. Clostridial infections (as opposed to contamination) are **clinical entities**, not bacteriologic diagnoses.

B. **Suppurative infections.** A wide range of clostridial species can be isolated from soft tissues (Table 9-5). *C. perfringens* is the most frequently encountered species, although it represents only one-fourth of the total isolates. *C. ramosum* is nearly as common, and a host of other species are seen with regularity. The organisms are usually present in polymicrobial situations. In our experience, 84% of soft-tissue infections harboring clostridia also had other bacteria, often as many as 5–10 different types. The clinical features of clostridial infections are extremely variable, and it has become apparent that, as our anaerobic technology improves, these organisms are being isolated with increasing frequency from a variety of infected sites (Table 9-6).

Clostridial species can be recovered from septic conditions that are characterized by a severe inflammatory process without the local or systemic signs of clostridial toxins. Indeed, it is impossible to separate the role of the clostridia from the multiple other organisms in the same location.

1. **Intraabdominal infections**, especially those associated with bowel perforation, are highly likely to harbor clostridia. In our study, 43 clostridial strains were isolated from 67 patients with intraabdominal infections. These strains included 16 known species and a number of nontypable ones. *C. ramosum* was the most common, followed by *C. perfringens* and *C. bifermentans*. None of the patients had gas gangrene, and it was impossible to differentiate on clinical grounds those with positive cultures for clostridia.
2. **Cancer.** There is an important association between suppurative intraabdominal infections involving clostridia and **carcinoma.** The usual scenario is carcinoma of the colon with a silent perforation that leads to intraabdominal abscess formation. Other cancers can be associated with clostridial infections of the abdomen, including carcinoma of the pancreas. It has been suggested that *C. septicum* is particularly common in patients with malignancies, either solid tumors, lymphomas, or leukemia. A strict association with this particular species has not been established, although the occurrence of several types of clostridia with malignancy has been widely documented.
3. **Gallbladder infections.** Using careful techniques, some investigators have recovered *C. perfringens* in 10–20% of diseased **gallbladders** during surgical procedures. A particularly severe form of cholangitis, termed **emphysema-**

tous cholecystitis because of gas formation in the biliary tract radicles, is known to be caused, in at least 50% of cases, by clostridial species (see Chap. 9). This disease has a higher mortality and is more often associated with diabetic patients than the usual form of biliary tract infection. There is, however, no evidence of muscle invasion nor of systemic signs of clostridial toxin. Patients appear to expire from septic shock with a clinical picture similar to that of severe biliary tract infection.

4. **Pelvic infections.** Clostridia can be associated with suppurative infections of the **female pelvic tract.** In three series of such infections in 200 patients, these organisms were isolated in 6% of cases. Clostridia were most frequently recovered in cases of tuboovarian and pelvic abscess. These organisms have also been isolated from suppurative discharges in women with septic abortion.
5. **Pulmonary infections**. Clostridia have been isolated from a variety of **pulmonary infections.** In our series of 162 patients with pulmonary infections related to aspiration, 10% were found to harbor these organisms in reliably collected specimens such as empyema fluid or transtracheal aspiration. This organism has been noted particularly often in patients with **empyema** due to traumatic injuries. It can also be found in empyema associated with underlying aspiration pneumonia. As in other suppurative infections, these patients usually show no sign of local or systemic toxin production. The disease, as it presents clinically, is indistinguishable from other cases of empyema not involving clostridia.

C. Localized infections of skin and soft tissues

1. Localized infections may involve clostridia, either in pure culture or in association with other bacteria. While such processes may be invasive and produce extensive local necrosis, the infection is rather indolent, spreading slowly to contiguous areas. The following conditions are included in this category: **clostridial anaerobic cellulitis, stump infections in amputees, perirectal abscess, diabetic foot ulcers,** and **decubitus ulcers.** When these infections involve muscle, they progress by an advancing border, producing a suppurative destruction that is quite different from myonecrosis.
   Crepitance may be present even in localized infections, but this finding does not indicate a severe prognosis. The harbinger of serious disease is extension of crepitance through subcutaneous and fascial planes and the appearance of systemic signs of clostridial toxemia.
2. A distinctive form of **suppurative myositis** has been seen in heroin addicts. The disease presents with local pain and tenderness, which eventually develop into a discrete area of fluctuance that requires surgical drainage. The major sites are the thigh and forearm, not necessarily related to areas of trauma or heroin injection. The pathology involves subcutaneous abscesses, purulent myositis, and fasciitis. The condition has been associated with pure cultures of clostridia or with mixed infections involving aerobes and anaerobes. Its clinical form resembles tropical myositis, although the tropical disease is caused by *Staph. aureus.*
3. Although the site is unusual, clostridia can be isolated from patients with **conjunctivitis** and **ophthalmitis.** The disease is mild in character, and the laboratory report of this organism is usually greeted with considerable skepticism due to the benign nature of the infection.

D. Diffuse spreading cellulitis and fasciitis

1. In contrast to the localized processes, a diffuse spreading cellulitis and fasciitis is also caused by clostridia. The disease may present with dramatic abruptness, spreading through the fascial planes with suppuration and widespread gas formation. There are systemic signs of overwhelming clostridial toxemia, often leading to rapid demise.
2. **Physical examination** reveals diffuse, subcutaneous crepitance with relatively little pain over the muscles. The gas spreads through contiguous fascial planes within a period of hours. The overlying skin, however, may

appear normal. The patient rapidly develops shock, renal failure, and intravascular hemolysis and usually expires within 48–72 hours of onset.

3. **Pathologic examination** fails to show severe muscle involvement such as the myonecrosis characteristic of gas gangrene. There may be a mild inflammatory reaction in the muscle groups adjacent to the affected fascial or subcutaneous planes.
4. This condition occurs in a variety of **clinical settings**. It can appear in association with a **silent carcinoma** of the large bowel, which heralds its presence by this devastating disease process. A discrete bowel perforation is not generally found, although it is suspected that the route of entry is by this mechanism. In some instances muscle invasion and myonecrosis are present, and this process is known as **nontraumatic gas gangrene.** Even in these cases the crepitant fasciitis spreads far beyond the confines of involved muscle.
5. Spreading cellulitis may arise from **contaminated injection sites**, particularly around the buttocks and in association with vasoconstrictor drugs such as epinephrine. It may also present with minor trauma to an extremity that provides a route of entry for the pathogen.
6. This fulminant process can occur without any antecedent event; the patient presents with crepitance in one limb, and the condition rapidly spreads over the next several hours to the trunk and thence to other extremities. Recent cases studied in our department have been associated with pure cultures of *C. perfringens*, *C. ramosum*, or *C. septicum* in soft tissues and in the bloodstream.
7. Spreading cellulitis and overwhelming toxemia should not be confused with gas gangrene. Myonecrosis is not present, and there is no diseased muscle to be surgically removed. Indeed, surgical intervention is usually unrewarding—the disease moves so rapidly that, by the time it is recognized, it is impossible to incise and drain all affected areas.

III. Bacteremia. In a large general hospital, clostridia was found in 0.3% of all blood cultures and represented 2.6% of the positive microbial isolates. The distribution of clostridia in blood cultures is somewhat different from the pattern in soft-tissue infections. *C. perfringens* accounts for approximately 60% of positive blood isolates, compared to an incidence of 25% in soft tissues.

Clostridial bacteremia shares a paradox with certain other infectious processes. Conventional wisdom would assume that a positive blood culture of this organism has profound clinical significance. Such is not always the case, however. Several reports have noted the often poor correlation between isolation of this organism in the bloodstream and clinical findings of sepsis. In a series of cases of septic abortion, positive clostridial blood cultures were found in 18–27%; the syndrome of uterine gas gangrene was relatively rare, and the majority of patients with positive cultures had a benign course. In our series of 29 patients with clostridial bacteremia, only 12 had a concurrent soft-tissue infection involving the organism. The remaining patients had "spontaneous" clostridial bacteremia, documented at the time of admission to the hospital for a variety of unrelated conditions (Table 9-7); most of these patients recovered from their primary illness, and the source of the clostridia was never detected. The lesson from these studies is clear: clostridial bacteremia must be interpreted in the entire clinical context, with careful attention to the status of the patient. This is especially important in cases in which clostridial bacteremia bears no apparent relation to the underlying illness.

IV. Treatment

A. Therapy of clostridial infections should be tailored to the specific clinical condition. **Simple contamination** by clostridia is managed with judicious surgical debridement and calculated avoidance of antibiotics. Many patients with clostridial bacteremia fall into a similar category; the clinical status of the patient at the time of discovery should guide the choice of treatment.

B. The **localized skin and soft-tissue infections** also can be managed by debridement and surgical dressings rather than systemic antibiotics, although these drugs are required when the process extends into adjacent tissues or when systemic signs of fever and sepsis are present.

Table 9-7. Underlying diseases in 29 patients with clostridial septicemia

Underlying disease	Number of patients
Aspiration pneumonia*	6
Decubitus ulcers (debridement)	4
Intraabdominal abscess	3
Septic abortion and pelvic abscess	3
Seizure disorder*	2
Pulmonary tuberculosis*	2
Spontaneous *E. coli* peritonitis*	1
Meningitis	1
Meningococcemia	1
Infantile gastroenteritis	1
Frostbite*	1
Carcinoma of colon	1
Leukemia	1
Neonatal septicemia	1
Empyema*	1

*Associated with chronic alcoholism.

C. Suppurative infections that involve clostridia are managed by the same surgical approach as if the organism were not present. Abscesses should be drained, necrotic tissue excised, tissue planes opened and drained, etc. In addition, it is necessary to use broad-spectrum antibiotics designed to suppress the aerobic and anaerobic bacteria that are invariable components of this infection. For aerobes, an aminoglycoside antibiotic such as gentamicin, tobramycin, or amikacin is indicated. The anaerobes in this setting can be treated with clindamycin, chloramphenicol, metronidazole, or cefoxitin. Occasionally clostridia resistant to one or more antimicrobial drugs may emerge as the dominant pathogen, but such examples have been relatively uncommon in these mixed infections.

D. Careful attention to the **antibiotic resistance** patterns of clostridia is demanded when the organism is causing rapidly spreading disease, myonecrosis, or systemic toxicity. Penicillin G has excellent activity against nearly all strains of *C. perfringens*, and only 5% of other species show variable degrees of resistance. Clindamycin has been somewhat disappointing against clostridia, since 15–20% of strains are currently resistant. The species that tend to be resistant to clindamycin are *C. ramosum, C. tertium,* and *C. sporogenes*; some resistant strains of *C. perfringens* have also been noted.

V. *Intestinal disorders*. Clostridia are known to cause three types of intestinal illness: **food poisoning, enteritis necroticans**, and **pseudomembranous colitis.** These diseases are entirely distinct: They are caused by different clostridial strains and their toxins, and each has its own epidemiology and pathogenesis.

A. Food poisoning associated with clostridia ranks 2nd or 3rd on the list of common forms in the United States. It may be even more frequent than recorded, since identification of the organism is difficult in small outbreaks. Epidemiologically, the disease is associated with a high attack rate, often 50–70%. The responsible vehicle is usually a poultry or meat product cooked one day, allowed to cool, then recooked, often in a stew or hash, and served the following day.

The most prominent clinical finding is moderate-to-severe midepigastric pain, crampy in nature and usually associated with watery diarrhea. Fever and vomiting are uncommon, although nausea is frequent. The incubation period is 8–24 hours, with the usual onset 8–12 hours after contact with contaminated food. Fortunately, the disease is rather mild, not lasting more than 24 hours. Surgical intervention is not indicated in this condition.

B. Enteritis necroticans is a severe, necrotizing disease of the small intestine and has a high mortality. The implicated organism is *C. perfringens*, type C, and the beta toxin appears to be the major pathogenic instrument. Many cases known as

"Darmbrand" were described in postwar Germany in the 1940s. Subsequently, large outbreaks of "pig-bel" were reported from New Guinea; the setting is an orgiastic pork feast in which the pig is slaughtered and cooked in a deep pit lined with hot stones. Large quantities of undercooked pork are consumed, and the disease ensues within 24 hours.

Clinical features include acute abdominal pain, bloody diarrhea, vomiting, shock, and, in approximately 40% of patients, peritonitis and death. The pathology is an acute ulcerative process of the bowel, usually restricted to the small intestine. The mucosa is lifted off the submucosa, forming large denuded areas. Pseudomembranes composed of the sloughed epithelium are commonly seen, and gas may dissect into the submucosa. There is very little experience with surgical management of this condition. Since vast areas of small bowel are involved in the severe cases, it is unlikely that survival would be improved by aggressive intervention.

C. Pseudomembranous colitis is a severe, necrotizing process involving the large intestine. It occurs as a complication of antibiotic therapy. Although the major antibiotic associated initially with the disease was clindamycin, most cases are now ascribed to ampicillin and cephalosporins. It is clear that nearly all antimicrobial drugs can cause this condition (Table 9-8).

1. **Bacteriology.** The responsible pathogen is *C. difficile*, a member of the normal flora which apparently overgrows to large populations in the presence of antibiotics. Many strains of this organism are resistant to antimicrobial agents, although the pattern of resistance is highly variable. However, all strains are sensitive to vancomycin. *C. difficile* elaborates a potent necrotizing toxin that is protein in nature, heat-labile, and acid-sensitive.
2. The **clinical features** can vary from mild diarrhea to necrotizing colitis that leads to perforation. The most common presentation by far is mild grinding diarrhea, lasting days to weeks. In some patients the progression from mild diarrhea to severe disease (pseudomembranous colitis) can be observed, but this course can be interrupted by stopping the offending antibiotic or by instituting appropriate therapy.
3. The **pathologic features** of pseudomembranous colitis are quite distinctive. Initial events are limited to the superficial mucosa, with necrosis and formation of a pseudomembrane composed of fibrin with a paucity of inflammatory cells. The underlying submucosa is denuded and hemorrhagic but lacks the inflammatory reaction that is seen with ulcerative colitis or bacillary dysentery. Severe cases of pseudomembranous colitis display sloughing of the pseudomembrane, transmural extension of the necrosis, and perforation through the serosa into the peritoneal cavity.
4. **Diagnosis** is initially based on the clinical setting of diarrhea, which is related temporally to antibiotic therapy. About half the cases occur during therapy, while the remainder represent patients whose symptoms begin after stopping the antibiotic, usually within the 1st week but occasionally up to 4 weeks later. **Sigmoidoscopy** reveals the characteristic appearance of an inflamed, friable mucosa. In more advanced cases there are a myriad of yellowish plaques or pseudopolyps, and a grayish membrane covers the mucosa in a patchy distribution. The late stages show a diffusely ulcerated mucosa. X-ray of the abdomen shows "fingerprinting" of the bowel wall with fine ulcerations. A laboratory test is available for rapid identification of toxin in the feces.
5. **Therapy** of antibiotic-associated diarrhea and pseudomembranous colitis is divided into several stages, depending on the severity of the disease.
   a. **Mild diarrhea** is treated by removing the offending antibiotic. If necessary, fluid and electrolytes should be administered to dehydrated patients. Pepto-bismol can be used to control the loose bowel movements. **Narcotic drugs and their analogues must be avoided.** These include paregoric, tincture of opium, Lomotil, and Imodium.
   b. **More severe** or **chronic** forms of **diarrhea** can be treated with vancomycin, 250 mg PO tid for 7 days. Metronidazole has been used effectively in

Table 9-8. Antimicrobial agents implicated in *C. difficile*-induced diarrhea and enterocolitis

Common	Occasional	Rare	Not reported
Amoxicillin	Erythromycin	Chloramphenicol	Bacitracin
Ampicillin	Penicillins	Metronidazole	Parenteral aminoglycosides
Cephalosporins	Carbenicillin indanyl sodium	Sulfasalazine	Vancomycin
Cefamandole	Dicloxacillin	Tetracycline	
Cefoperazane	Nafcillin	Rifampin	
Cefazolin	Oxacillin	Anticancer agents	
Cefoxitin	Penicillin G		
Cephalexin	Penicillin V		
Cephalothin	Ticarcillin		
Cephradine	Trimethoprim/sulfamethoxazole		
Parenteral cephalosporins combined with cephalexin			
Clindamycin			

some cases (500 mg PO tid), although it should be recognized that this drug has sometimes been a cause of pseudomembranous colitis. An alternative agent is bacitracin, 25,000 units PO tid; this drug is not licensed for use for this condition, but it has shown efficacy in a small group of patients.

c. Pseudomembranous colitis can progress to **toxic megacolon**, a condition that requires emergency surgical intervention. The procedure of choice is total colectomy; whenever possible, the rectal stump should be preserved with a Hartmann's pouch, since the disease would be expected to heal itself, and a reanastomosis might be possible at a later date.

d. **Corticosteroids** have had an unimpressive record in treatment of this condition. We have had some encouraging results, however, from treating toxic megacolon with large doses of prednisone (60 mg/day in four divided doses), thereby averting total colectomy. Short of this drastic situation, steroids are not recommended, since most patients would respond to vancomycin therapy.

e. **Cholestyramine** has been recommended for pseudomembranous colitis, but the results are variable.

f. Severely ill patients with pseudomembranous colitis may be unable to tolerate oral vancomycin; intravenous **metronidazole** should be employed in these cases, since the drug is delivered in sufficient concentrations to the bowel wall and lumen.

Tetanus

I. **General principles.** Tetanus is a tragic disease, not only because of its severity, but because it can be completely prevented by appropriate immunizations. At the present time in the United States tetanus occurs primarily in rural areas or where childhood immunizations are not performed routinely, and among heroin addicts who practice "skin popping" (thus introducing tetanus spores subcutaneously).

II. **Bacteriology.** *C. tetani* is a ubiquitous, gram-positive, anaerobic, spore-forming rod. In its spore state it is highly resistant to physical and chemical disinfectants.

III. **Pathogenesis.** Most cases of tetanus occur after puncture wounds, lacerations, and crush injuries. The organism finds a receptive environment in the presence of tissue necrosis, anoxia, and other bacterial contaminants. As it germinates, the organisms release **tetanospasm**, the toxin responsible for the clinical syndrome. The toxin interrupts neuromuscular transmission by inhibiting the release of acetylcholine. The clinical picture is similar to that of strychnine poisoning. The toxin is rapidly and irreversibly fixed by nervous tissue.

IV. **Clinical features.** The **incubation period** is variable, from a few days to several weeks. In general, a long latency is associated with more distal injuries and has a better prognosis. Three clinical forms of tetanus are recognized:

A. **Generalized tetanus**, responsible for about 80% of cases. Clinically, the disease descends, often beginning with trismus and progressing to neck stiffness, abdominal rigidity, and tetanic spasms of the extremities. Trismus can produce facial spasm known as **risus sardonicus**. As the spasm progresses, the back muscles are involved, with arching of the back known as **opisthotonos.** The two best signs of incipient generalized tetanus are trismus and rigid abdominal musculature.

B. **Cephalic tetanus** occurs with otitis media or traumatic injuries to the head. There is usually isolated cranial nerve involvement, especially the 7th nerve.

C. **Local tetanus**, involving the muscles in an area of injury. This is the mildest form.

Many diseases are confused with tetanus. Before making the diagnosis, the following conditions should be considered:

Generalized tetanus	Trismus	Opisthotonos
Phenothiazine reaction	Dental abscess	Strychnine poisoning
Bacterial meningitis	Mandibular fracture	Rabies
Hypocalcemic tetany	Tonsillitis	Perforated peptic ulcer
Retroperitoneal hemorrhage	Diphtheria	Vertebral osteomyelitis
Epilepsy	Mumps	
Decerebrate posturing	Trichinosis	
Narcotic withdrawal	Retropharyngeal abscess	
	Mandibular osteomyelitis	

V. **Diagnosis.** Tetanus is a **clinical diagnosis** based on the physical findings. The organism can be seen in Gram's stain of infected material, but it is often confused with other gram-positive rods, and it may be difficult to identify in the mixed flora of a grossly contaminated wound. Culturing the organism also is very difficult. Even experienced microbiologists have problems with isolating this strict, fastidious anaerobe from mixed cultures.

VI. **Complications.** The muscle spasms and seizures can lead to **fractures** of the spine and long bones. **Pulmonary embolism** has been a major problem with this disease. **Autonomic dysfunction** can occur, leading to hypertension and cardiac arrhythmias. A frequent complication and a major cause of death is **pulmonary infection** due to aspiration.

VII. **Prevention.** A "tetanus-prone" wound is characterized by tissue necrosis associated with gross contamination from the environment. Such wounds are at greatest risk of producing tetanus, but it must be emphasized that even minor puncture wounds or needle sticks have been the precursor to severe disease. While it is a matter of judgment who should receive preventive measures, it is best to err on the side of conservation, especially in unimmunized individuals. Table 9-9 indicates the current recommendations.

A most important feature of prevention is appropriate wound care, with debridement and cleansing in order to remove any pockets of necrotic tissue and anaerobic dead spaces. With regard to the use of toxoid and tetanus immune globulin (TIG) (see Table 9-9), the following points should be made:

A. **TIG** is human globulin; the older preparations of horse serum should not be employed unless TIG is unavailable. The **toxoid** should be the combined tetanus-diphtheria toxoid (Td, adult type), in the form of adsorbed toxoid (with aluminum adjuvant). Thus the patient can be immunized against diphtheria as well as tetanus.

B. The usual dose of TIG is 250 units, unless there is a severe injury, in which case 500 units can be employed. The TIG should be given in a different syringe and at a different site from the Td. In the event that this dose of Td constitutes a primary immunization, the patient should be instructed to return 28 days later to receive the second dose.

C. In general, a booster injection of adsorbed toxoid, following an adequate primary vaccination series, should provide protective antibody for 10 years, during which time booster doses are not required. This interval should be shortened to 5 years in the setting of a severe injury. Multiple injections of toxoid, prompted by frequent injuries, can lead paradoxically to lower levels of circulating antibody, so this practice is discouraged.

D. Antibiotic treatment and surgical debridement do not give adequate protection against tetanus. Thus, the immunization status of all patients with contaminated wounds must be ascertained, and appropriate treatment initiated, as indicated in Table 9-9.

VIII. **Treatment.** The treatment of tetanus is mainly a physiologic exercise in preventing complications. Any toxin that has been elaborated and already fixed to tissues is in an irreversible state, so the disease cannot be interrupted once it has started. Indeed, the spasms and increased muscular contractions can continue for several weeks after the organism has been eradicated.

The initial phases of treatment involve elimination of the organism by surgical

Table 9-9. Tetanus immunization

Immunization record	Wound	Recommendation
None / Incomplete / Unknown	Low risk	Toxoid—complete immunization
	High risk	Toxoid + TIG
No booster in the past 10 yr	Low risk	Toxoid
	High risk	Toxoid + TIG
Booster in the past 10 yr	Low risk	None
	High risk	Toxoid if no booster in the past 5 yr

High risk = severe, neglected for 24 hr; Toxoid = tetanus and diphtheria toxoid (adult type), 0.5 ml IM; TIG = tetanus immune globulin, 250 units IM.

debridement and antibiotics, and administration of antitoxin for circulating toxin that has not yet been fixed. The other modalities are directed at physiologic stabilization and nutrition.

A. Surgical debridement of any obvious wound should be undertaken in order to remove necrotic tissue and anaerobic dead spaces. In some patients with tetanus the wound may be very subtle, and in rare cases, never found. A careful search for puncture wounds, insect bites, otitis media, and scalp wounds should be undertaken when there is a cryptic focus.

B. Antibiotic therapy should be directed at the organism, and penicillin G is the treatment of choice (2–3 million units IV q4h). In the setting of a grossly contaminated wound, additional antibiotics should be used, according to the coexistent pathogens. The length of treatment is dictated by the extent of the traumatic injury, although in general short courses of therapy, over several days, should be sufficient.

C. Antitoxin should be administered in an attempt to bind any circulating toxin. TIG, 500 units, is given. (The treatment dose—500 units—is larger than the prophylactic dose—250 units.) During the course of the illness, a full immunizing schedule of toxoid should be provided in order to prevent a second attack.

D. Prevention of muscle contractions and spasm is achieved by short-acting barbiturates and muscle relaxants such as chlorpromazine. Diazepam may be used to control seizures. In severe cases curare-like drugs are required.

E. Environmental stimuli should be reduced to a minimum by placing the patient in a quiet, darkened room. Loud talking and slamming of doors must be prevented, since auditory stimuli can initiate a series of muscle contractions and seizures.

F. Tracheostomy should be considered for patients who have had a series of tetanic seizures. It is obviously necessary when curare-like drugs are employed.

G. Total parenteral alimentation is an important part of the management of patients with tetanus who may be unable to swallow due to trismus.

IX. Mortality is related to age, with the highest incidence in neonates and elderly patients. A rapid onset of generalized tetanus with continuous seizures has a poor prognosis. Overall, the mortality is 15–30%, although rates up to 60–80% have been reported in patients at the extreme ages of life.

Burns

I. General prinicples

A. Sepsis is the major cause of death in the severely burned patient, and usually develops after resuscitation from the initial shock phase. Even in relatively minor burns, infection can increase morbidity, compromise functional and cosmetic results, and produce life-threatening septic episodes.

B. The **burn wound** is the principal site of sepsis. Pneumonia caused by gram-negative organisms is also a common problem, especially in the patient with inhalation injury. Less frequently, septicemia with or without suppurative thrombophlebitis is a complication of indwelling intravascular catheters.

C. Early sepsis is difficult to recognize in the burned patient. A change in **mood** or **sensorium** may be the only signal of impending sepsis. Other characteristic findings include a rise or sudden fall in body temperature, chills, leukocytosis or leukopenia, glucosuria, tachycardia, or tachypnea. Late manifestations are nausea, vomiting, ileus, hypotension, oliguria, obtundation, and death.

In about 50% of cases of **burn wound sepsis**, blood cultures remain negative. This fact, coupled with the variability of presenting symptoms in the severely burned patient, increases the difficulty of early diagnosis.

D. Host resistance is diminished in a burned patient due to

1. Open wounds—an invitation to bacterial contamination and invasion of deeper tissues
2. Necrotic tissue with poor blood supply—a good environment for bacterial growth
3. Loss of fluids, proteins, and calories, leading to physiologic derangements, hypoproteinemia, and poor overall nutrition

The problems should be dealt with by excision of necrotic tissue and closure of deep burn wounds, appropriate fluid and electrolyte replacement, and total parenteral alimentation.

II. Pathology of the burn wound

A. Following a thermal insult, the vascular supply to the involved area is rapidly occluded. **In full-thickness burns**, vascular occlusion remains for 2–3 weeks before any appreciable circulation is restored. This causes coagulation necrosis of the involved tissue, resulting in the **burn eschar**. When the circulation becomes reestablished, it is localized in the granulation tissue at the interface of the burn eschar and the underlying, uninvolved tissue. Large accumulations of nonviable tissue that accompany a full-thickness burn provide an excellent culture medium for saprophytic and pathogenic microorganisms.

B. In **partial-thickness burns**, circulation in the involved area also ceases initially, but it returns within the 1st 2 days. If sepsis intervenes, however, there is progressive thrombosis of the reestablished circulation, and the wound may be threatened with full-thickness skin loss.

III. Bacteriology of burn sepsis

A. Bacterial invasion of the burn wound occurs both from the surface of the wound and from the deeper epidermal appendages.

B. Colonization on the surface of the burn wound is dominated in the initial 1–3 days by gram-positive organisms such as streptococci and staphylococci. By the 3rd postburn day, gram-negative bacilli such as coliforms, *Pseudomonas, Serratia, Proteus*, and *Providencia* make their appearance. In the absence of local antimicrobial therapy, gram-negative organisms invade the burn wound in large numbers by the fifth postburn day.

C. Burn wound sepsis is defined as invasion of the adjacent or subjacent unburned tissue along with proliferation of microorganisms in numbers exceeding 100,000/gm of tissue. Bacteriologic monitoring of the burn wound surface is usually not helpful in diagnosing burn wound sepsis; it is necessary to perform deeper qualitative and quantitative bacteriologic monitoring.

D. Septicemia is usually seen in the setting of burn wound sepsis; this complication carries a high mortality for several reasons:

1. The poor underlying condition of the patient, especially with compromised host defenses related in some unknown manner to the burn itself.
2. Inability to eradicate the focus of septicemia due to deep colonization of the pathogen in the burn wound.
3. Pathogens that are often resistant to commonly used antibiotics. The organisms isolated are the same as those responsible for burn wound sepsis. Historically, most septicemias were due to staphylococci, while in the last decade the gram-negative bacilli, such as *Pseudomonas aeruginosa* and *Providencia*

stuartii, have predominated. Recently, burn centers have reported an increase in *Candida* burn wound spesis. *Candida* sepsis usually follows alteration of the normal bacterial flora, which results from the topically and systemically administered antimicrobial drugs. Poor oral hygiene and the prolonged use of indwelling intravenous catheters favor the development of candidemia.

IV. Burn wound management

A. Initial mechanical treatment

1. Burned clothes should be removed as soon as possible. When possible, the burn wounds should be covered with freshly laundered linen, which is ideal because of its rather low bacterial count. The patient should be thus covered before being transported to the hospital, to decrease the possibility of contamination.
2. Once the patient has been hospitalized, the most immediate concern is for the ventilatory status and the restoration of circulation; these issues take priority over local treatment of the burn wound. Unnecessary delays, however, should be avoided. Early inspection and gentle washing with soap and water are done as soon as possible. Loose and obviously devitalized tissue should be debrided in a hydrotherapy tank full of water at 38°C. When found, blisters should be unroofed.

B. Follow-up mechanical treatment

1. Daily inspection, washing, and debridement of loose or separating tissue or eschar are essential.
2. First-degree and superficial second-degree burns require only topical agents and protection from cross-infection.
3. Deep second-degree (dermal) and all third-degree burns require rapid excision of devitalized tissue and immediate closure of the wound following excision. When this technique is employed, it is essential to provide intensive nutritional support as well as a controlled environment. The wound closure is accomplished by use of split-thickness skin grafts (autografts), if possible.
4. When larger, more extensive burns have been excised, closure with autografts is frequently impossible. Wound closure is then accomplished with the use of temporary skin substitutes. Some authorities have advocated the concurrent use of immunosuppression, as it may extend the period before rejection occurs, but this is not widely accepted.
5. Temporary skin substitutes include human allografts (homografts), such as cadavaric skin or amniotic membrane; various xenografts (heterografts); and synthetic materials, such as plastics or silicone. These skin substitutes decrease water and protein losses and provide an antiseptic barrier during the period before autografts can be applied. In the current state of the art, viable human allograft is the best skin substitute.

V. Topical antibacterial therapy

A. General concepts

1. The burn wound is vulnerable to infection because the microcirculation in the devitalized tissue is absent or decreased. The burn wound eschar presents a barrier to passage of antibiotic agents moving from either direction. Parenteral antibiotics do not reach the surface flora, and therefore their use should be reserved for infections that invade adjacent soft tissues or the bloodstream. On the other hand, topical antimicrobials reduce the flora of the burn wound, thereby promoting wound healing, facilitating graft "takes," and reducing the risk of burn wound sepsis and bacteremia.
2. Agents chosen should effectively control the bacteria usually found in burn wounds, have relatively low local and systemic toxicity, and facilitate the process of eschar separation.
3. The ideal topical antibacterial agent has not been developed. Nevertheless, effective agents are available, and they have been the single most important factor responsible for decreased mortality due to burn wound sepsis.

B. Topical agents (Table 9-10)

1. **Silver nitrate (0.5%).** This agent has a long history of use in topical burn

Table 9-10. Topical antibacterial agents in burn therapy

Agent	Control of burn wound microflora	Tissue penetration	Requires dressings	Bacterial resistance	Local pain or irritation	Acid-base or electrolyte problems
Silver nitrate	+	−	+	−	−	+
Silver sulfadiazine	+	+	−	±	±	−
Cerium nitrate–silver sulfadiazine	+	+	+	−	−	−
Sulfamylon	+	+	−	±	+	+
Gentamicin	+	+	−	+	−	−
Povidone-iodine	±	+	−	−	−	+

wound therapy. It offers a good spectrum of activity. Tissue penetration is poor, because the active silver ion is precipitated as silver chloride when it contacts body fluids. Thus, effective action requires that thick gauze dressings saturated with silver nitrate solution be kept in contact with the burn wound. The disadvantages of this agent include the dark, brownish staining of everything it touches, as well as the increased cost of the dressings. The main side effects involve fluid and electrolyte disturbances due to the hypotonicity of the dilute silver nitrate solution and the corresponding absorption of large amounts of free water. A rather rare occurrence is the development of methemoglobinemia, which results from the conversion of nitrate to nitrite by certain microorganisms in the burn wound, such as *Enterobacter cloacae*.

2. **Silver sulfadiazine.** This agent is a poorly soluble compound readily synthesized by reacting silver nitrate with sodium sulfadiazine. It is available in a water-soluble cream base in a concentration of 1%. The in vitro antimicrobial spectrum of this drug is excellent and includes *Staph. aureus*, Enterobacteriaceae, *E. coli*, and *Candida*. One disadvantage of long-term use is the development of bacterial resistance. Systemic absorption is rare, even in extensive burns. Cutaneous sensitivity reactions to silver sulfadiazine occur in fewer than 5% of patients and rarely are severe enough to warrant discontinuation. This agent is applied to the open burn, but it can be covered with a dressing.
3. **Cerium nitrate–silver sulfadiazine.** Recent evidence suggests that this agent has good clinical efficacy. It is available in a cream for topical use, usually being covered with dressings. The bacteriologic spectrum is similar to that of silver sulfadiazine. No systemic toxicity has been observed except for a rare case of transient methemoglobinemia. No resistance has been observed up to this time.
4. **Mafenide (Sulfamylon).** This drug is available as a 10% preparation in a water-miscible hydroscopic cream base. It has a good spectrum of activity, but superinfection with antibiotic-resistant *Providencia stuartii* is frequently reported. Absorption is rapid, requiring application every 12 hours. No dressings are required, and the drug has good penetration. Toxicity has limited its widespread usage. **Local burning and pain**, which commonly occur during the application of mafenide, are its main disadvantages. These symptoms can often be controlled with mild analgesics. Allergic reactions occur late, usually after the 2nd week of application. If the reaction is mild, it can be controlled with antihistamines without discontinuation of the agent. Acid-base imbalances are seen occasionally due to the agent's strong inhibitory effect on carbonic anhydrase. Compensatory hyperventilation can occur, with the resultant development of respiratory failure or pneumonia. Careful monitoring of acid-base balance and pulmonary function are essential when this drug is employed.
5. **Gentamicin sulfate**. This is a bactericidal aminoglycoside antibiotic that has been used topically in a 1% cream. Systemic absorption is great, and superinfection with resistant bacterial strains occurs rapidly. For this reason, it should **not** be used in the topical therapy of burns.
6. **Povidone-iodine.** This agent has a long record of clinical efficacy as an antiseptic for use on normal skin and mucous membranes. It is also available in a water-miscible cream base, in which the iodine content is 1%, for burn therapy. There is some evidence that protein binding of the iodine in an open wound may result in diminished in vivo antimicrobial effect. Lethal metabolic acidosis due to renal toxicity has been reported. More information is needed before povidone iodine can be recommended for topical burn therapy.

VI. Systemic antibacterial therapy. Systemic parenteral antibiotics cannot be substituted for local therapy in the initial treatment of the burn wound. The use of systemic antibiotics is indicated only for the treatment of burn wound sepsis or systemic infections that emanate from pulmonary infections, urinary sources, or intravenous catheter sites.

A. Prophylaxis. Systemic antibiotics such as penicillin are used in the immediate postburn period to avoid the occurrence of β-hemolytic streptococcal cellulitis. Most experts no longer recommend the routine use of prophylactaic penicillin in all burn cases. If marked spreading erythema does appear at the burn wound margins, cultures should be obtained and penicillin therapy begun. Some authorities recommend prophylactic antibiotics at the time of extensive excision and debridement, but this view is not universally accepted.

B. Therapeutic use. Systemic antimicrobials should be selected on the basis of Gram's stains, cultures, and sensitivity tests in cases of pulmonary and urinary tract sepsis. In **burn wound sepsis**, where the blood culture is frequently negative at the time therapy must be started, the least toxic wide-spectrum combination of drugs that cover the organisms known to be colonizing the patient or the burn unit should be chosen. Such treatment is aimed at both *Staphylococcus* and *Pseudomonas*. A semisynthetic penicillin (nafcillin or oxacillin) or a cephalosporin plus an aminoglycoside should be used in the beginning. If gentamicin-resistant strains are present, the use of amikacin would be indicated. Modification of the initial choice of antibiotics should be done when culture and sensitivity results are available. The usual duration of antibiotic therapy in burn wound sepsis is 10–14 days, but this varies with the clinical course and blood culture results. It is important to measure serum levels of the aminoglycoside to prevent toxicity and to assure therapeutic serum levels.

C. Fungal infections. Fungal infections in the burn patient have become increasingly more common since the advent of potent antibacterial therapies. The emergence of *Candida, Phycomyces*, and *Aspergillus* has usually been related to topical therapy failures and indwelling catheters, especially those used for hyperalimentation. *Phycomyces* and *Aspergillus* are ubiquitous contaminants, whereas *Candida* is a normal constituent of the human gastrointestinal tract. *Phycomyces* and *Aspergillus* can invade the burn wound, and diagnosis is confirmed by the biopsy finding of these organisms invading the adjacent dermal tissue. **Burn wound sepsis** or septicemias caused by these organisms are treated with amphotericin B (see pp. 281–282).

D. Herpes infections. Herpes simplex can invade a burn wound, with severe consequences. An episode of oral or genital herpes may occur in a burned patient, and the open wounds and wet dressings provide a good milieu for viral growth. Even bloodstream dissemination and systemic herpes can evolve, due to the debilitated state of the patient. There is no treatment currently established, although vidarabine and systemic acyclovir should be considered in life-threatening cases. The most important issue is prevention of spread (1) to other sites on the patient, (2) to personnel in attendance, and (3) to other patients in the unit.

VII. Adjunctive treatment techniques

A. Tetanus prophylaxis. A tetanus toxoid booster (0.5 ml) is given to all previously immunized patients with burns. To nonimmunized patients, human tetanus immune globulin (250 units) is given in addition to the toxoid (see pp. 212–213). Adequate surgical debridement of all devitalized tissue remains the best single prophylactic step in prevention of clostridial infection.

B. Subeschar antibiotic injection. A recently developed technique utilizes the direct deposit of appropriate antibiotic solutions into the tissue plane beneath a localized burn eschar. Clinical experience with this technique is limited, and its overall value remains unproved. Difficulty of administration and complications, including salt and fluid overload and local irritation, may limit its usefulness to cases of small burns, for which excision and closure still are the treatment of choice.

C. Antiserum therapy. The injection of polyvalent antigen derived from multiple strains of *P. aeruginosa* in an attempt to stimulate the patient's own antibody response has been successful in both experimental and clinical settings. Additional studies are necessary before general use can be advocated. If further studies prove the efficacy of this technique, vaccines may be developed for each of the organisms that commonly cause burn wound sepsis.

10 Head and Neck Infections

Sinusitis

I. General principles. Sinusitis refers to inflammation of the paranasal sinuses, a relatively common infection but also overdiagnosed. Many patients who complain of "sinus trouble" actually have uncomplicated conditions such as allergic rhinitis, viral rhinitis, or nonspecific vasomotor rhinitis due to dry air, smog, smoking, or local medication. An established diagnosis of sinusitis requires **localization of the inflammatory process to the sinuses** by history, palpation, rhinoscopy, examination of purulent excretions, or x-rays.

II. Pathophysiology

A. Classification. Sinusitis is classified as **acute, subacute,** or **chronic** on the basis of duration of symptoms. This temporal classification scheme is arbitrary and sometimes difficult to apply, but it is a useful tool in terms of clinical findings and therapeutic approach.

1. **Acute sinusitis** refers to cases of **less than 3 weeks' duration.** There is hyperemia of the mucosal surfaces, sloughing of epithelial cells, and a polymorphonuclear leukocyte exudate. The periosteum and underlying bone are not involved. Fever to 38–38.5°C is common and helps to distinguish acute sinusitis from uncomplicated rhinitis. Localized pain results from positive pressure due to collection of edema fluid or negative pressure due to air absorption following osteal occlusion. With successful resolution of the infectious process, the edema fluid is reabsorbed, the epithelium regenerates, and the normal mucosal surface is reconstituted.
2. **Chronic sinusitis** refers to cases of **more than 3 months' duration.** Clinically, there is chronic nasal discharge and nasal obstruction; fever and localized pain are seldom seen. Histologic studies show a mononuclear leukocyte infiltrate, necrosis, and mucosal proliferation. Additionally, there may be metaplasia, polyp formation, scarring, periostitis, and osteitis. Surgery is the most important aspect of successful management of chronic sinusitis.
3. **Subacute sinusitis** refers to cases of **3 weeks' to 3 months' duration.** It represents an intermediate stage between acute and chronic forms in terms of clinical findings and pathologic changes. The subacute form may respond to medical treatment or go on to the irreversible changes of chronic sinusitis.

B. Protective mechanisms. The sinuses are normally protected by a mucociliary blanket that constantly wafts foreign particles and microorganisms toward the ostia. This defense mechanism is analogous to the mucociliary system found in the lower respiratory tract. Additional protection is provided by a leukocytic response to microbial invasion and by lysozyme, immunoglobulins, and other antimicrobial properties of sinus secretions.

C. Predisposing causes. Infection of the sinuses occurs when the defense barriers break down, usually due to injury of the sinus epithelium or interference with osteal drainage. Infection results from spread of microorganisms from the nose to the directly continuous sinuses.

1. Viral infections of the upper respiratory tract and nasal allergy are the most common predisposing causes of sinusitis.

2. Obstructing lesions can also lead to sinusitis. They include nasal polyps, hypertrophied nasal turbinates, deviated nasal septa, neoplasms, foreign bodies (especially in children), choanal atresia, hypertrophied adenoids, cleft palate, and nasal packs used to control epistaxis.
3. Acute pressure changes in the sinuses, such as feet-first water diving, rapid ascent with scuba diving, and rapid descent in an airplane can cause sinusitis.
4. Chemical and environmental insults can be related to sinusitis, e.g., local medications, changes in humidity, and inhaled irritants.
5. Direct extension from dental infections or oroantral fistulae can cause infection in maxillary sinuses.
6. Trauma, especially a facial fracture, can be an inciting cause.
7. Certain systemic conditions are associated with an increased incidence of sinusitis. They include bronchiectasis, Kartagener's syndrome (triad of sinusitis, bronchiectasis, and situs inversus), cystic fibrosis, hypogammaglobulinemia, Hurler's syndrome, and blood dyscrasias.

III. Clinical features

A. Symptoms. Those suggesting sinusitis are nasal obstruction and anterior or posterior purulent nasal discharge. Headache, constitutional symptoms, and fever are generally found only with acute sinusitis. The headache is characteristically worse in the morning due to overnight accumulation of exudate, and it improves during the day as the upright posture facilitates drainage.

B. Physical examination. Palpation usually reveals tenderness over the sinus, which is acutely inflamed. The sphenoid sinus cannot be palpated or visualized; a clue to involvement of this structure is headache over the top of the head. Anterior and posterior rhinoscopy are performed to detect erythema, edema, and purulent discharge. Anterior rhinoscopy to visualize the middle meatus is facilitated by shrinking mucous membranes with topical application of 1–3% ephedrine or 0.25–0.5% phenylephrine hydrochloride (Neo-Synephrine).

IV. Diagnosis

A. Transillumination is valuable in detecting involvement of the frontal and maxillary sinuses. Variations in symmetry are common in normal persons, however, so the changes must be interpreted with caution.

B. Sinus **x-ray** should include four views: posteroanterior or Caldwell view, Waters' view, lateral view, and basal or submentovertical view. Of these the most useful is the Waters' view, with the head tilted backward and the x-ray directed 20 degrees upward. Abnormalities to be found include sinus obliteration, air-fluid levels, and thickening of mucous membranes to > 8 mm. Up to 20–30% of normal persons have roentgenographic evidence of membrane thickening, polyps, or cysts. Therefore these changes must be carefully correlated with clinical findings. The principal uses of x-ray are to (1) identify the sinuses involved; (2) follow serial changes during treatment; (3) identify underlying lesions, such as cysts and tumors; and (4) detect complications, such as osteomyelitis.

C. Aspiration of sinus discharge or sinus lavage for cell count, cell analysis, Gram's stain, and culture. Normal sinus secretions have fewer than 100 white cells/ml and either no bacteria or counts of less than 10^2/ml.

1. In acute suppurative sinusitis the discharge shows > 5,000 white cells/ml, predominantly polymorphonuclear leukocytes (PMNs); such cell counts are correlated with the presence of bacteria in concentrations exceeding 10^5/ml.
2. A dominance of mononuclear cells suggests subacute or chronic sinusitis.

D. Methods of localizing the sinus(es) involved. Most cases involve more than one sinus. Localization to a single sinus suggests an underlying anatomic abnormality, such as a foreign body, cyst, tumor, or choanal atresia. Clinical clues to localization of infected sinuses are noted in Table 10-1.

V. Bacteriology. The most common bacterial pathogens in **acute sinusitis** are *Streptococcus pneumoniae* and *Hemophilus influenzae* (Table 10-2). Less frequently present are *Streptococcus pyogenes, Staphylococcus aureus,* and anaerobic bacteria. Cultures of carefully collected sinusitis exudate are sterile in 20–40% of cases; a

Table 10-1. Clinical clues to localization of sinusitis

Sinus	Head pain	Tenderness	Nasal discharge
Maxillary	Cheek and upper teeth (bite pain)	Over maxilla	Low in middle meatus
Frontal	Supraorbital	Frontal or upward pressure under eyebrow	High in middle meatus
Ethmoid	Retroorbital, pain with eye movement	Medial canthal region	Superior meatus
Sphenoid	Occipital; often variable or vague	—	Superior meatus

negative culture suggests a nonbacterial disease (i.e., viral infection), the effect of previous antibiotics, or inadequate culture techniques.

The major organisms that are found in **chronic sinusitis** are anaerobic bacteria. Again, 20–30% of these cultures are sterile, even when rigorous culture techniques are used.

The practice of obtaining cultures in the routine evaluation of sinusitis is controversial because

A. Bacteriologic patterns are generally predictable, thereby allowing empiric antibiotic selection in most cases.

B. The usual culture techniques are generally inadequate to provide specimens uncontaminated by the resident nasal flora. For example, nasal discharge or irrigations evacuated through the nose invariably yield nasal contaminants. Specimens appropriate for meaningful cultures are

1. Exudate obtained directly from a sinus during a surgical procedure

2. Aspirates collected via a polyethylene catheter passed through a larger-bore needle that has been inserted into the sinus

VI. Treatment

A. Medical

1. Antimicrobial drugs are selected on the basis of Gram's stain and culture of carefully collected specimens. Trimethoprim/sulfamethoxazole, 80/400 mg PO bid, or ampicillin, 500 mg PO qid, is likely to be effective in acute sinusitis. Continue treatment for 5–7 days after symptoms have cleared and sinus washes (if done) fail to yield pus. Local instillation of antibiotics into a sinus cavity has not been adequately evaluated to establish efficacy. Chronic sinusitis generally does not respond to antimicrobial therapy.

2. Irrigation with warm sterile saline is indicated for cases of maxillary or frontal sinusitis that fail to respond to oral antibiotics. This procedure should not be employed until systemic antimicrobials have been administered for several days, as it might extend the infection.

3. Nonspecific measures include analgesics and nasal decongestants (oral agents such as triprolidine hydrochloride [Actifed], qid, or topical drugs such as 0.25–0.5% Neo-Synephrine, qid). The use of topical decongestants is controversial due to possible "rebound phenomena" and **rhinitis medicamentosa;** use of these agents should be restricted to 1 week.

4. Treatment of **underlying problems,** especially allergies, is a necessary adjunct.

B. Surgical intervention. A surgical procedure is seldom indicated in acute sinusitis but is frequently required for a chronic infection with irreversible destructive changes. Goals of surgery are to **establish drainage** or to **obliterate the sinus.** Indications are

1. Underlying anatomic defects, e.g., deviated nasal septa or nasal polyps

Table 10-2. Bacteriology of and therapeutic guidelines for infections of the upper airways

Condition	Most likely pathogen	Empiric antimicrobial selection
Pharyngitis	*Streptococcus pyogenes* *Neisseria gonorrheae* Infectious mononucleosis Viral	Penicillin Erythromycin
Laryngitis	Viral	
Epiglottitis	*Hemophilus influenzae*	Ampicillin Chloramphenicol
Sinusitis		
Acute	*Strep. pneumoniae* *H. influenzae*	Ampicillin or amoxacillin Sulfamethoxazole/trimethoprim
Chronic	Anaerobic bacteria	
Otitis media		
Acute	*H. influenzae* *Strep. pneumoniae* *Strep. pyogenes*	Ampicillin or amoxacillin Erythromycin & sulfonamide Sulfamethoxazole/trimethoprim
Chronic	Coliforms *Pseudomonas aeruginosa* Anaerobes, including *Bacteroides fragilis*	
Cervical adenitis		
Acute	*Staph. aureus* *Strep. pyogenes* Anaerobes	Penicillinase-resistant penicillin Cephalosporin
Sialadenitis	*Staph. aureus*	Penicillinase-resistant penicillin Cephalosporin
Perimandibular space infections	Anaerobes Streptococci	Penicillin G or V Clindamycin
Dental infections	Anaerobes	Penicillin G or V Clindamycin (serious infections)
Postoperative infections		
Oral surgery	Anaerobes Streptococci	Penicillin G or V Clindamycin
Nasal surgery	*Staph. aureus* Streptococci Anaerobes	Penicillinase-resistant penicillin Cephalosporin Clindamycin
Neck dissection	Gram-negative bacilli *Staph. aureus*	Aminoglycoside, **plus** Cephalosporin **or** penicillin-resistant penicillin **or** clindamycin

2. Persistent symptoms or repeated attacks after an adequate trial of conservative measures
3. Local complications, such as osteomyelitis, pyocele, or mucocele
4. Extension of the infection beyond the confines of the sinus, causing orbital cellulitis, fistulae, or intracranial complications.

VII. Complications. The major complications of sinusitis involve extension of the infection into orbital soft tissues, adjacent bones, or the central nervous system. The bacteriology of these infections is similar to that described for acute and chronic sinusitis, the predominant pathogens being streptococci, *H. influenzae, Strep. pneumoniae,* and anaerobes. Although *Staph. aureus* is relatively uncommon, it is important to recognize it as a pathogen due to its unique antibiotic susceptibility patterns, especially its frequent resistance to penicillin and ampicillin.

A. Orbital involvement. The orbits are surrounded by the paranasal sinuses except in the lateral direction. Infection may extend through the sinuses, causing edema or displacement of the orbital contents. Orbital involvement in sinusitis (other than reactive edema) threatens vision and may impinge on the central nervous system. Patients with such involvement require hospitalization for treatment with intravenous antibiotics and decongestants. Surgical drainage of sinuses should be undertaken for cases in which signs of sepsis fail to resolve (or even progress) beyond 24–48 hours of antimicrobial treatment.

1. **Orbital edema** with painless swelling of the eyelids is generally due to reactive inflammation and obstructed venous drainage, which can occur in the course of maxillary, ethmoid, or frontal sinusitis. This is the only form of orbital involvement that does not require hospitalization, since most cases resolve rapidly with oral antibiotics combined with decongestants.
2. **Orbital cellulitis** presents as tender, erythematous edema of the eyelids and chemosis; proptosis may be present, depending on the extent of posterior orbital involvement. Vision is usually intact but may be decreased due to pressure on the optic nerve. Most cases are secondary to posterior ethmoid or sphenoid sinusitis.
3. **Orbital abscess** causes proptosis, visual impairment, chemosis, and ophthalmoplegia. The abscess forms in the orbital fat; the extent of ocular findings is related to the degree of retroorbital involvement. There may be permanent loss of vision and even intracranial spread. When fluctuance is not detected, it is difficult to distinguish orbital cellulitis from abscess. In these cases orbital exploration and emergency drainage of the sinuses should be performed if there is no response to parenteral antimicrobial treatment within 8 hours.
4. **Subperiosteal abscess** is a purulent collection between the periosteum and the bony wall of the orbit. This condition is a complication of frontal, maxillary or ethmoid sinusitis. The orbital contents typically are displaced laterally and inferiorly. Depending on the size of the abscess, there may be proptosis, ophthalmoplegia, and loss of visual acuity.
5. **Superior orbital fissure syndrome** complicates inflammation or mass lesions of the sphenoid sinuses. These sinuses are close to the superior orbital fissure, through which pass the third, fourth, sixth, and first division of the fifth cranial nerves. Initially there is a sixth cranial nerve palsy, followed by pain in the forehead and eye (fifth cranial nerve), exophthalmos, and finally complete ophthalmoplegia. X-rays should include laminagraphy of the sphenoid sinuses. Treatment is immediate exploration and drainage, along with parenteral antibiotics.

B. Osteomyelitis. This complication may occur in any of the bony structures adjacent to the sinuses, but it is most common with frontal sinusitis. The course may be acute or chronic. With **acute frontal bone osteomyelitis,** there is fever; headache; and extension, either posteriorly, leading to a pericranial abscess, or anteriorly, causing a doughy swelling of the forehead ("Pott's puffy tumor"). Death may occur rapidly, due to sepsis and intracranial involvement. **Chronic frontal osteomyelitis** is a more insidious process, with low-grade fever and a tender frontal swelling. Osteomyelitis of the **superior maxilla** is a complication of maxillary sinusitis; it presents with the usual symptoms of sinusitis, combined with marked tenderness and edema of the cheek. **Sphenoid osteomyelitis** is rare and usually is not detected until intracranial complications occur.

The treatment of osteomyelitis complicating sinusitis consists of surgical drainage and parenteral antimicrobial agents. These drugs should first be given intravenously, then orally after fever and other signs of sepsis resolve.

C. Intracranial infection

1. **Cavernous sinus thrombosis.** Since the ophthalmic and facial veins communicate with the cavernous sinuses, any infection of the orbit or sphenoid sinus potentially leads to septic thrombophlebitis of the cavernous sinus. The findings include proptosis; ophthalmoplegia; engorgement of the retinal veins; paralysis of the third, fourth, fifth (first and second divisions), and sixth cranial nerves; loss of vision; high spiking fevers; and meningitis. This condition can be unilateral, but it commonly spreads to bilateral involvement. Mortality is high; survivors often have loss of vision or blindness and frequently suffer neurologic deficits. The evaluation should include blood cultures and examination of cerebrospinal fluid. *Staph. aureus* is a common pathogen in this condition. Preferred antibiotics are nafcillin combined with either ampicillin or chloramphenicol, until cultures are available.
2. **Meningitis.** This is most frequently a complication of acute frontal sinusitis; less common (in order of frequency) are infections of the sphenoid, ethmoid, and maxillary sinuses. Patients present with headache, stiff neck, and altered mental status. Cerebrospinal fluid examination shows low sugar, high protein, and pleocytosis with a predominance of PMNs; bacteria can usually be seen in the Gram's-stained slide. Pleocytosis with sterile cultures suggests a parameningeal infection (e.g., epidural or subdural abscess), brain abscess, or partially treated meningitis.
3. **Abscess.** Epidural, subdural, or brain abscess can occur by extension of the infection through the bony confines of the sinus (**contiguity**) or by spreading through vascular channels or nerve tracts (**continuity**). The onset of symptoms is acute or insidious, but most patients have symptoms referable to the central nervous system, such as headache, changed mental status, and focal neurologic deficits. Fever is not invariably present. Cerebrospinal fluid examination may be entirely normal or may show a spectrum of abnormalities. Bacteria are not usually present in the CSF.

Epiglottitis

I. General principles. Acute epiglottitis is a potentially disastrous infection that is considered a medical emergency because of possible airway obstruction. Most cases occur in children aged 1–4 years, and the usual pathogen is *H. influenzae,* type B. Occasional pathogens, especially in adult cases, are *Staph. aureus, Strep. pneumoniae,* and *Strep. pyogenes.* A viral infection also can cause epiglottitis.

II. Clinical features. The disease begins with fever, sore throat, and coryza, and has the appearance of a common cold. After 1–4 days there is dysphagia and dyspnea, which may progress to total airway obstruction within hours. The patient is unable to lie supine, as that position causes closure of the airway by gravitation of the edematous epiglottis. The accompanying dysphagia results in drooling and gurgling respirations. The composite picture in the advanced stage is an acutely ill, restless, febrile patient, sitting upright, with air hunger, gurgling respirations, inspiratory stridor, and drooling saliva.

III. Diagnosis. The diagnosis is established by visualization of the epiglottis, which shows intense hyperemia and edema. Children often have sufficient swelling so that the epiglottis can be seen on oral examination; in adults visualization usually requires indirect laryngoscopy. Lateral neck x-rays are also useful in demonstrating epiglottal edema with a narrowed glottic aperature. If x-rays are taken, the patient should be accompanied to the radiology department by a person prepared to do emergency tracheostomy or intubation.

IV. Differential diagnosis. The principal diagnosis to exclude in children is croup, since its prognosis and treatment are entirely different from those of epiglottitis. Croup is a viral infection characterized by typical croupy cough, normal or erythematous epiglottis, and a relatively benign course.

Angioneurotic edema or a foreign body impinging on the epiglottis may produce similar respiratory symptoms, but these conditions are not accompanied by evidence of systemic infection.

V. Microbiology. Cultures of the throat or epiglottis are of limited value, since the most common pathogen, *H. influenzae,* is a component of the normal throat flora. The relevance of such cultures is improved if the available laboratory can type *H. influenzae,* since type B is the usual pathogen, while most colonizing strains are nontypable. Bacteremia occurs in approximately 50% of cases, and all patients should have blood cultures. Rare cases are caused by *Strep. pyogenes.* Viral infections account for a considerable number of cases.

VI. Treatment

A. When the diagnosis of epiglottitis is established, serious consideration should be given to immediate **tracheostomy or intubation.** The prognosis is favorable when these procedures are performed electively, and experience indicates that progression to total airway obstruction can occur in a matter of several hours. Many authorities currently favor intubation over tracheostomy, since the hazards of tracheostomy are greater, and swelling usually subsides quite promptly with antimicrobial treatment and humidity. Before performing tracheostomy or intubation, a trial of medical management is carried out. Obviously, bradycardia or respiratory arrest requires an emergency tracheostomy or intubation.

Intubation should be performed transorally under direct vision, using a nonreactive plastic tube with a high-volume, high-compression cuff. The patient may be extubated when epiglottic swelling has subsided according to direct visualization or x-ray; this usually requires 2–5 days. The alternative to routine tracheostomy or intubation is antimicrobial therapy and humidity. Young children should be placed in a plastic tent with high humidity. Every effort is made to quiet the child and to reduce noise or outside stimuli that may cause alarm and increase respiratory effort. For older children and adults, a "cold" humidifier should be used within a tent, if available. Sedatives should be avoided. Rigorous monitoring of vital signs is mandatory, since the patient's condition may deteriorate.

B. Antimicrobial treatment for children consists of parenteral ampicillin, 300 mg/kg/day. Chloramphenicol, 100 mg/kg/day, is an alternative agent in penicillin-allergic patients. Adults with epiglottitis should receive parenteral ampicillin, perhaps with nafcillin or oxacillin, if *Staph. aureus* is suspected. Antibiotics are continued until the patient is afebrile and asymptomatic for 2–3 days.

C. Corticosteroids are sometimes advocated, but their efficacy is not established. Indeed, several studies have shown that these drugs have no effect on the course of this disease.

VII. Complications and associated conditions. Airway obstruction is the most common serious complication. Approximately 25% of patients develop pneumonitis, and a similar number develop cervical adenitis. Tonsillitis, otitis media, and meningitis are infrequent complications.

Infections of the Spaces of the Face, Perioral Cavity, and Neck

I. Anatomy. Infections of the face, perioral cavity, and neck are often confined to potential spaces within fascial planes. There are **two fascial planes,** which encircle the face and neck, and **two fascial sheaths.**

A. The **superficial fascia** surrounds the head and neck from the scalp to the thorax. Contents include facial muscles of expression and the platysma muscle. This fascial plane is separated from the deep cervical fascia by a potential space (Grodinsky's space #1), which contains superficial lymph glands, nerves, and vessels, including the external jugular vein.

B. The **deep cervical fascia** is divided into three layers:

1. The **superficial (or external) layer** extends anteriorly from the temporal fascia to the clavicle. Posteriorly, it attaches to the vertebral spines inferiorly and to the occiput and mastoid processes superiorly. Structures enveloped by this fascia include the sternocleidomastoid muscles, trapezius muscle, parotid gland, submaxillary gland, supersternal space (Burns' space) in the midline, and subvaginal space in the lower posterior triangle. Between the parotid and the submaxillary glands, it forms the stylomandibular ligament—a thick sheath connecting to the styloid process. In the face, the superficial layer of the deep fascia envelops the ramus of the mandible and the masseteric muscle and extends upward over the temporal muscle.
2. The **middle layer** of the deep cervical fascia is prevertebral and contains both muscular and visceral divisions. The anterior or muscular division contains the strap muscles and extends from the hyoid bone and thyroid cartilage to the sternum, clavicle, and scapula. The deeper visceral division envelops the esophagus, trachea (pretracheal fascia), larynx, and thyroid gland (prethyroid fascia).
3. The **deep layer** of the deep cervical fascia surrounds the spinal column and its associated musculature. Anteriorly, it forms a prevertebral layer from the base of the skull to the coccyx. The carotid artery and jugular vein lie anterior, and the phrenic nerve is just beneath it. The alar fascia is a portion of this layer and this fascia extends from the transverse processes to the visceral fascia, separating the retropharyngeal and pharyngomaxillary spaces.

C. The **carotid and axillary sheaths** are derived from the cervical fascia but function as anatomic units.

1. The **carotid sheath** contains the carotid artery, internal jugular vein, and vagus nerve. It extends from the base of the skull, through the posterior pharyngomaxillary space, along the prevertebral fascia, and into the chest, where it divides along with its component parts.
2. The **axillary sheath** is a lateral extension of the prevertebral fascia that surrounds the brachial plexus, subclavian artery, and subclavian vein.

II. Clinical features. Space infections usually arise from dental infections (palpitis) or following dental procedures, or from tonsillitis. Occasionally, an infection of the skin, such as furuncle or impetigo, can penetrate to an underlying space.

In most instances the signs of infection are both systemic and local. Systemic signs include variable degrees of fever, leukocytosis, and constitutional symptoms. Localizing findings are pain, tenderness, erythema, and swelling at the infected site. Abscess formation generally follows acute or subacute inflammation by at least 5–7 days. Associated symptoms, depending on the site involved, include trismus, dysphagia, and referred pain.

III. Bacteriology

A. Specimens. Direct needle aspirates of the involved site are most reliable if collected percutaneously, since intraoral aspirates may be contaminated by the oral flora. Anaerobic cultures should be performed on all specimens that are devoid of oropharyngeal contamination. The physician should be prepared for lack of laboratory confirmation of anaerobic infections, however, since many clinical laboratories are unable to cultivate these fastidious organisms. Blood cultures should be obtained from all septic patients.

B. Pathogens. The responsible bacteria are those that normally colonize the oral cavity and are involved in the initial dental infection (Table 10-2). In most instances the infecting flora is complex, with the dominant organisms being *Fusobacterium, Bacteroides melaninogenicus,* and multiple species of streptococci (both aerobic and anaerobic). *Staph. aureus* and *Staph. pyogenes* are less frequent, and they are usually associated with a skin infection on the face. Aerobic gram-negative bacilli are rare.

IV. Treatment

A. Parenteral antibiotics for initial therapy are

1. Penicillinase-resistant penicillin, such as oxacillin or nafcillin, 1–2 gm IV q4–6h.
2. Clindamycin, 600 mg IV q6–8h.
3. Cephalosporin, such as cefazolin, 500 mg–1 gm IV or IM q6–8h.
4. Aqueous penicillin G, 500,000–1 million units IV q4–6h. This is the preferred treatment, if *Staph. aureus* can be excluded by Gram's stain or culture.

Antibiotic therapy is continued at least 10–14 days; more prolonged treatment is indicated when there are complications, such as delayed resolution, osteomyelitis, metastatic abscesses, or jugular vein thrombophlebitis.

B. Surgical drainage is the cornerstone of treatment when abscess formation has occurred. Clinical clues to the presence of abscess are

1. A fluctuant mass
2. Failure to respond to intensive antimicrobial therapy
3. Recurrence of symptoms after antibiotics have been discontinued

In these cases, incision is performed under local anesthesia, shortly after initiation or reinstitution of antimicrobial treatment. An exception is masticator space abscesses, which generally drain spontaneously; if this does not occur within 1 week, incision is necessary to prevent osteomyelitis. Space infections can often be drained intraorally, thus avoiding disfiguration.

C. Dental therapy (extraction or root canal treatment) should be undertaken when feasible. The presence of acute pyogenic infection is not considered a contraindication to such dental procedures.

V. Complications

A. Osteomyelitis, usually at sites of dental infections. Roentgenographic evidence of osteomyelitis requires about 3 weeks. X-rays should be taken initially to detect underlying dental lesions and to serve as a baseline for future studies.

B. Septicemia, usually with anaerobic bacteria or *Strep. pyogenes;* less commonly, with *Staph. aureus*.

C. Hemorrhage, usually from the carotid artery (posterior compartment of the pharyngomaxillary space), temporal artery (superficial temporal space), or internal maxillary artery (deep temporal space).

D. Airway obstruction (submandibular space—see next discussion, Ludwig's Angina).

E. Extension to adjacent spaces, such as mediastinitis or secondary spread to the retropharyngeal space.

F. Venous septic thrombophlebitis, especially of the internal jugular vein; seen with pharyngomaxillary space infection or peritonsillar abscess.

Ludwig's Angina

I. General principles. Ludwig's angina is a rapidly spreading indurated cellulitis involving the floor of the mouth and upper cervical area. The disease was originally described in 1836, when it was usually fatal due to suffocation, hence the term ***angina.*** In recent years this term has been somewhat loosely applied to many infections involving the neck. For prognostic and therapeutic purposes it is best to restrict the diagnosis of Ludwig's angina to cases conforming to the classic description:

A. The infection is always bilateral.

B. Both the submaxillary and sublingual spaces are involved. These spaces extend from the floor of the mouth to the muscular and fascial attachments at the hyoid bone. They are separated by the mylohyoid muscle, with the sublingual compartment above and the submaxillary compartment below.

C. Extension is by contiguous spread along fascial planes rather than through lymphatic channels.

D. The infection starts in the floor of the mouth. Infections that begin in the throat, pharynx, tonsils, or cervical lymph nodes may secondarily involve the submandibular space and resemble Ludwig's angina in later stages.

II. **Clinical features.** The usual complaints are local pain, dysphagia, and dyspnea. Fever, leukocytosis, and systemic toxicity are generally present and may be severe. On physical examination there is tender, indurated edema of the submandibular region and swelling of the floor of the mouth, with elevation of the tongue. Frequently the intrinsic muscles of the tongue are secondarily involved, resulting in lingual swelling. Regional lymph nodes are spared, and abscess formation is seldom noted.

III. **Underlying conditions.** Dental infections, particularly recent molar extraction and apical abscesses, account for 60–80% of cases. The 2nd and 3rd molars are most frequently implicated, apparently because the apices of these teeth extend below the mylohyoid ridge, and the lingual cortical plate is relatively thin. These factors facilitate perforation and spread of the infection to the submaxillary space. Injuries such as compound fracture of the mandible and laceration in the floor of the mouth account for a small portion of cases. In some instances dental evaluation is entirely normal and no predisposing factor is detected.

IV. **Bacteriology.** The most extensive bacteriologic studies were performed in the prechemotherapeutic era, when this disease was far more common. These indicated that the infecting flora was complex and that multiple anaerobic bacteria were responsible. Several types of aerobic bacteria have also been cultivated on occasion, but their role in the pathogenesis of this disease is not established.

V. **Treatment**

A. A high parenteral dosage of antibiotics should be given immediately. Recommended agents are (1) penicillin G, 1–2 million units IV q4h, or (2) clindamycin, 600 mg IV q6h.

B. Supportive and symptomatic measures include local application of hot soaks, analgesics, and hydration.

C. External incision and drainage is sometimes performed routinely. Most patients, however, respond to antibiotics, and operative intervention should be reserved for those who fail to respond to conservative measures. The operative approach consists of a single transverse incision across the neck or three separate incisions—one below each angle of the mandible, with the third in the midline below the symphysis. Vertical openings are made to ensure drainage of the sublingual space. Purulent collections are seldom found, and the principal purpose of incision is to relieve tension.

D. Preservation of an adequate airway is a most important factor in therapy, since respiratory obstruction can occur precipitously. If there is evidence of airway obstruction, a tracheostomy should be performed or the patient should be intubated. Intubation should be undertaken only when facilities are available for immediate tracheostomy.

VI. **Complications.** The major complication is respiratory tract obstruction due to displacement of the tongue and pharynx. Additional potential complications include dehydration, aspiration pneumonia, pharyngomaxillary space infection, mediastinitis, mandibular osteomyelitis, and septicemia.

Pyogenic Infections of the Salivary Glands

I. **Acute suppurative sialadenitis** usually involves the parotid gland in elderly patients. Contributing factors are dehydration, cholinergic drugs, and debility. The gland and duct itself are usually normal prior to onset of symptoms. Younger patients are more likely to have submandibular gland involvement secondary to obstruction by stone or stricture.

A. **Clinical presentation** is acute unilateral tender swelling of a salivary gland with systemic signs of sepsis. Rarely, the infection is bilateral. Purulent material can be expressed from Stenson's or Wharton's duct to establish the diagnosis.

B. *Staph. aureus* is the usual pathogen.

C. Treatment

1. Local heat, hydration, and discontinuation of cholinergic drugs.
2. **Antimicrobial treatment** is selected on the basis of Gram's stain and culture of pus expressed from the duct. Since most cases involve *Staph. aureus,* appropriate initial treatment is a penicillinase-resistant penicillin (nafcillin or oxacillin) or a cephalosporin. These should be given intravenously and continued until evidence of inflammation resolves—usually 7–10 days.

Nafcillin or oxacillin	1–2 gm IV q6h
Cefazolin	1.5–2.0 gm IV q6h

3. **External surgical drainage** is indicated when the patient has failed to improve after 4–5 days of antimicrobial treatment. Long-standing infection with fluctuance is another indication for drainage.
4. Some authorities recommend early radiation of the salivary gland in debilitated patients in order to minimize the inflammatory reaction. A total dose of 600 R is given in four to six divided daily doses.
5. Stones located near the duct orifice should be removed intraorally after antimicrobials have been started. Stones in the proximal duct or gland should be removed externally after inflammation subsides.

II. Chronic sialadenitis is characterized by chronic inflammation with persistent or recurrent salivary gland swelling. There may be pain and tenderness, but systemic symptoms are lacking. Pus may be expressed from the involved gland duct, and cultures usually reveal *Staph. aureus.*

It is necessary to distinguish **nonobstructive** and **obstructive** forms by careful examination, plain x-rays, sialography, and duct probing. Nonobstructive forms are treated conservatively with local heat and with systemic antibiotics for acute exacerbations. The following obstructive forms are treated by removal of the underlying lesion.

A. Salivary calculi involve the submandibular gland. Their cause is unknown, and there is no apparent relationship to calcium or uric acid metabolism. Symptoms are variable, consisting of acute sialadenitis, recurrent chronic sialadenitis, or asymptomatic tumor mass. Many patients complain of swelling and pain associated with meals. About 75% of stones are radiopaque and are detected with plain x-rays. Sialography for radiolucent stones shows dilatation of the proximal duct system and delayed emptying or complete obstruction.

B. Duct stricture may be primary (congenital) or secondary (infection, trauma, or neoplasm). Symptoms are similar to those of calculi. The stricture is demonstrated by sialography or duct probing.

C. Sialectasis results from long-standing recurrent sialadenitis or may be congenital. Sialograms show dilated ducts with saccules, similar to the changes noted with bronchiectasis. Excision of the gland is indicated for severe forms.

III. Miscellaneous causes of salivary gland enlargement

A. Granulomatous diseases—sarcoidosis and tuberculosis

B. Actinomycosis

C. Alcoholism or diabetes

D. Sjögren's syndrome (may be complicated by pyogenic sialadenitis)

E. Drug reaction, especially to iodines

Pyogenic Cervical Adenitis

I. Clinical features. Most cases occur in children 1–4 years old. Complaints are often localized, with a tender or fluctuant mass and little or no systemic toxicity. One-third to one-half of patients are febrile, and most have leukocytosis. Associated conditions and nodal localization patterns are as follows:

Table 10-3. Differential diagnosis of cervical adenitis

Tuberculosis adenitis
Atypical tuberculosis adenitis
Cat scratch fever
Infectious mononucleosis syndromes
Epstein-Barr virus
Toxoplasmosis
Cytomegalovirus infection
Tularemia
Rubeola, rubella, varicella
Postvaccination
Fungal
Aspergillus
Cryptococcus
Histoplasmosis
Coccidioidomycosis
Syphilis
Dilantin hypersensitivity
Collagen vascular disease
Lymphoproliferative disorder
Carcinoma of head or neck

Underlying condition	**Lymph node**
Tonsillitis and pharyngitis	Upper deep cervical
Dental infection	Upper deep cervical, submandibular
Skin or scalp infection	Superficial posterior cervical
Nonapparent	Submandibular

II. Bacteriology

A. There are four common bacteriologic patterns:

1. *Strep. pyogenes*
2. *Staph. aureus*
3. Anaerobic bacteria, especially *Peptostreptococcus* and *Fusobacterium*
4. Combinations of these

B. Nose and throat cultures are unreliable. Node aspirates may be obtained as follows:

1. Prep and drape skin.
2. Anesthesize with 2% lidocaine or ethylchloride spray.
3. Aspirate with a #18–20 gauge needle and 10-ml syringe.
4. If no aspirate is obtained, inject 1–2 ml sterile saline (without preservative).
5. Specimens are submitted for stains (Gram's and AFB) and culture (aerobic, anaerobic, and mycobacteria).

III. Differential diagnosis. Several infectious and noninfectious conditions should be considered in the diagnosis of cervical adenitis, especially when the clinical features or bacteriology are not typical of the infections already mentioned (Table 10-3).

IV. Treatment

A. Medical. Most patients respond to antimicrobial treatment. Adenopathy associated with streptococcal pharyngitis should be treated with a 10-day course of penicillin or erythromycin. If the etiology is less apparent, or if penicillin fails, an agent for *Staph. aureus* should be used. Parenteral agents of choice are penicillinase-resistant penicillins (nafcillin or oxacillin), a cephalosporin, or clindamycin. Oral agents likely to be effective are dicloxacillin, cephalexin, erythromycin, and clindamycin. Treatment should be continued until evidence of inflammation resolves, usually in 10–14 days.

B. Surgical. Drainage is seldom required. Indications are node fluctuance or failure to respond after 4–5 days of appropriate antimicrobial therapy.

Cervicofascial Actinomycosis

I. General principles. Cervicofascial actinomycosis is an inflammatory mass usually involving the cheek, mandible, or submandibular region. There is considerable variation in clinical presentation: At one extreme is the most typical form, a chronic, fibrosing, indurated ("woody hard"), often painless mass at the angle of the mandible. The mass enlarges over several months and eventually forms draining sinuses. The differential diagnosis includes tuberculosis and tumor. The other end of the spectrum is an acute, painful swelling that rapidly progresses to abscess formation and resembles other suppurative bacterial infections. Lymph node involvement and osteomyelitis are seldom seen with actinomycosis.

II. Microbiology. The most common pathogen is *Actinomyces israelii,* which is an anaerobic, filamentous, branching gram-positive bacillus. *A. naeslundii, A. viscosus, A. odontolyticus,* and *Arachnia propionica* produce actinomycosis less frequently. These bacteria are normal constituents of the oral flora. They gain entry into the soft tissues following local trauma, as with periapical dental abscess, dental extraction, fractured jaw, or foreign body. Extraction of a third molar is a particularly common antecedent event, although the onset of symptoms may be delayed for several months after the procedure.

III. Diagnosis

A. Other conditions can produce a mass in the neck (Table 10-4), so it is important to base the diagnosis on recovery of one of the agents of actinomycosis from the lesion. Care must be taken to obtain a specimen uncontaminated by the normal oral flora. The most reliable culture sources are draining fistulae to the skin, percutaneous aspirates, and biopsy material. Many of the agents of actinomycosis grow microaerophilically, although optimal growth is achieved in anaerobic conditions. Failure of the laboratory to recover these organisms may be due to inadequate anaerobic culture techniques, failure to hold plates for an extended period, misidentification as "diphtheroids," or preceding antimicrobial therapy. Additional bacteria are virtually always present, the most common being *Actinobacillus actinomycetemcomitans, B. melaninogenicus,* and anaerobic or microaerophilic streptococci.

B. Gram's stain of specimens shows filamentous, branching gram-positive bacilli.

C. "Sulfur granules" are often seen. These structures are macroscopic yellow particles noted on dressings or with filtration of the exudate through gauze. On microscopic examination the sulfur granule is a tangled mass of filaments encircled by radiating "clubs." Sulfur granules may also be present in nocardiosis and are not invariably present in actinomycosis.

IV. Treatment

A. Medical. Penicillin G is the preferred antibiotic. Severe infections should be treated with 5–10 million units/day given intravenously for at least 2–3 weeks; this is followed by 2–4 gm/day (penicillin G or penicillin V) for 3–6 months. Tetracyclines and clindamycin are alternative agents with established efficacy.

B. Surgical. Indurated lesions generally respond to medical treatment, although sinus tracts may eventually require excision. Abscesses should be drained. Underlying dental lesions should be treated, when present.

Tuberculous Cervical Lymphadenitis (Scrofula)

I. General principles. Cervical lymph nodes are the most frequent sites of extrapulmonary tuberculosis. Excisional biopsy is required to establish the diagnosis, and it is also the preferred method of treatment for certain types of infection.

Table 10-4. Differential diagnosis of neck mass

Cause	Diagnostic test
Malignancy Leukemia—lymphoma Carcinoma	Biopsy for histologic study
Pyogenic infection Actinomycosis	Needle aspiration or incision for culture and Gram's stain
Infectious mononucleosis	Mono spot test; atypical lymphocytes in peripheral blood smear
Benign mass Aneurysm Bronchial cyst Carotid body tumor Salivary gland enlargement	Physical exam; history (duration of lesion); x-rays; scans, arteriograms
"Reactive hyperplasia"	Biopsy (etiology often unknown; usually considered to be a viral infection, but some cases represent early tuberculosis)
Granulomatous disease	
Tuberculosis*	Excisional biopsy, culture, AFB stain, skin test, chest x-ray
Sarcoid	Chest x-ray, other sites of involvement, diagnosis of exclusion
Fungal infection	Principally histoplasmosis, coccidioidomycosis, blastomycosis; culture, stains, serology
Brucellosis	Culture, complement fixation >1:16; contact with goats, cattle, swine, sheep
Tularemia*	Agglutination titer for *Francisella tularensis* >1:640; animal contact
Cat-scratch disease*	History of cat contact, biopsy
Syphilis*	Serologic test for syphilis
Hodgkin's disease	Biopsy, anergy

*Pathology may show central necrosis.

II. Clinical features. The typical setting is a slowly progressive, painless mass in the neck with few or no constitutional symptoms. A single node or multiple nodes may be involved. Initially the nodes are firm, discrete, and slightly tender. Subsequently they become rubbery and fixed to surrounding tissue (periadenitis). Late in the course there are likely to be draining sinus tracts overlying a "cold abscess" (i.e., a creamy, white discharge that has a paucity of cellular elements).

III. Diagnosis

A. Differential diagnosis. The major causes of firm, enlarged lymph nodes restricted to the cervical region are metastatic carcinoma from an upper respiratory source, hematologic malignancy, and tuberculosis (Table 10-4). Needle aspiration or excisional biopsy is the preferred diagnostic maneuver.

B. Diagnostic criteria

1. **Cultures and smears.** Biopsy specimens provide a positive culture of the organism in 30–60% of all cases. Smears are frequently positive for acid-fast bacilli, even when cultures are negative. Fluid obtained by needle aspiration gives a significantly lower yield. (The reason for poor success in recovering the organism, even from biopsies, in cervical tuberculosis is enigmatic. It probably relates to the small number of viable organisms in the tissues.)
2. **Histologic studies** showing granulomas are suggestive, but many other conditions also produce this type of tissue reaction (Table 10-4). **Caseating granulomas,** however, are more specific.
3. **Therapeutic response** to antituberculous agents is highly suggestive of

Table 10-5. Tuberculous cervical lymphadenitis: typical vs. atypical mycobacteria

	Mycobacterium tuberculosis	Atypical mycobacteria
Age group	5–40 yr	1–4 yr
Predominant sites	Posterior triangle, submandibular	Submaxillary and submandibular
PPD skin test	Nearly always positive	Often negative or weakly reactive
Chest x-ray	Abnormal in 50–70%	Usually normal
Early suppuration	Rare	More common
History of contact with tuberculosis	Common	Rare
Response to antituberculous medication	Common	Rare
Preceding infection in upper respiratory tract	Rare	Common

tuberculous adenitis, but regression of adenitis often requires 2–3 months, and spontaneous cure of other conditions may have occurred concurrently.

4. Skin tests and chest x-rays provide ancillary supportive data. Nearly all patients with cervical adenitis due to *Mycobacterium tuberculosis* have positive intermediate-strength PPD skin tests, and 50–70% have x-ray changes compatible with pulmonary tuberculosis. About 5–10% of patients have sites other than the lung involved with tuberculosis, such as bones, joints, kidneys, or peripheral (noncervical) lymph nodes.

C. Atypical mycobacterial cervical adenitis. There is no way to distinguish typical from atypical mycobacterial disease by histologic criteria. Skin tests for atypical mycobacteria are not available commercially. Culture is the optimal diagnostic test but may require 3–6 weeks. Clinical features that suggest atypical mycobacterial cervical adenitis are summarized in Table 10-5.

IV. Microbiology

A. *M. tuberculosis* causes the vast majority of cases. Usually there is evidence of tuberculosis in other areas of the body, especially the lungs. This suggests that cervical involvement represents either direct extension from a pulmonary focus or hematogenously disseminated disease.

B. Atypical mycobacteria are less common but account for a significant portion of cases in children 1–4 years of age. The most common pathogens, in order of prevalence, are *M. scrofulaceum* (group 2), *M. avium* (group 3), *M. intracellulare* (group 3), and *M. kansasii* (group 1). In contrast to those cases caused by *M. tuberculosis,* there is seldom evidence of distant disease with atypical mycobacteria. Many cases are preceded by an upper respiratory tract infection or are associated with salivary gland involvement. These findings indicate that atypical mycobacterial infection of the cervical nodes is a localized process that has spread from an oral portal of entry.

C. *M. bovis* accounted for 10–30% of scrofula cases in the era when tuberculosis in dairy herds was poorly controlled and many people ingested unpasteurized milk. In recent years this organism has become extremely rare.

V. Treatment

A. *M. tuberculosis.* The relative roles of chemotherapy and surgical intervention are disputed. Some authorities feel that surgical intervention should be restricted to biopsy for diagnostic purposes and drainage of cold abscesses. They argue that drug therapy can quite successfully cure the lymph node disease and draining sinuses with minimal cosmetic disturbance. The other opinion favors excisional biopsy, since it is easily accomplished and avoids the sinus tracts that may complicate a limited incision for biopsy. According to this argument, lymph nodes regress slowly with medical treatment; sinus tracts, once formed, are especially delayed in responding.

Regardless of the extent of the surgical procedure, INH, ethambutol and rifampin should be given for 12–18 months (see pp. 276–281 for doses). This recommendation is based on the supposition that tuberculosis also resides in other areas of the body, even though it may not be readily apparent.

B. Atypical mycobacteria. Here the extent of surgical procedure is more clearly defined. Excision of all involved tissue is required, since the response to medical treatment in lymph node disease has been uniformly poor. The disease is generally restricted to the cervical area, and the necessity for postoperative chemotherapy is not established.

11 Neurosurgical Infections

It is important to recognize and treat promptly infections occurring after neurosurgical procedures or head trauma, as they can lead to a devastating outcome. Besides the risk of central nervous system infection, such patients develop sepsis at other sites, including pneumonia, urinary tract infection, and catheter-associated bacteremia. Infections of the central nervous system are of the greatest concern, however.

I. Nonpenetrating head trauma

A. Pathophysiology. Nonpenetrating trauma to the central nervous system can produce a dural tear leading to a cerebrospinal fluid (CSF) leak. This event is important in the development of bacterial meningitis. Basal skull fractures, temporal bone fractures, and cribiform plate fractures are predisposing causes. CSF otorrhea and rhinorrhea signal the likelihood of dural tear and act as harbingers of meningitis. If a fracture occurs in the middle fossa, the likelihood of otogenous meningitis is increased. Cribiform plate fractures lead to rhinorrhea, and meningitis can occur via the nasopharyngeal route. The incidence of meningitis after such injuries is 5–10% in the 1st week after the dural tear.

B. Clinical features. The clinical findings of posttraumatic bacterial meningitis are abrupt onset of fever, stiff neck, changes in personality, either somnolence or increased activity, and positive meningeal signs. It is important to look carefully for persistent drainage from the ear canal or the nares. The CSF leak is continuous, although in some cases it can stop spontaneously, at least for a short period of time. A simple means of differentiating CSF from nasal discharge is a glucose dip-stick: CSF has a high glucose content, which gives a positive result on the dip-stick, while normal nasal discharge is negative.

C. Bacteriology. The origin of the infecting microorganisms is the sinuses or middle ear, depending on the location of the fracture. Pneumococci account for the vast majority of cases (80–90%) of posttraumatic bacterial meningitis. The other cases are caused by *Hemophilus influenzae, Neisseria meningitidis,* and some gram-negative organisms such as *Escherichia coli.* These organisms can be identified presumptively by Gram's stain of the CSF.

D. Treatment should be guided by the CSF appearance.

Penicillin (for pneumococci or *Neisseria*)	2 million units IV q2h
Chloramphenicol (for *Hemophilus*)	750 mg IV q6h
Moxalactam or cefotaxime (for unidentified gram-negative organisms)	2 gm IV q6h

Initially there is no surgical intervention, since many of these CSF leaks stop spontaneously. If there is a persistent leak, diagnostic studies should be undertaken to determine its source, and surgical repair is indicated sometime in the future.

E. Prophylactic antibiotics. Because meningitis often follows a basal skull fracture and dural leaks, it is common practice to administer prophylactic penicillin at the time of admission. Some studies show that this practice reduces meningitis in patients with posttraumatic CSF rhinorrhea. Several failures have been reported, however, and should meningitis break through the prophylactic regimen, the organism is likely to be a resistant strain. In addition, when diagnosed and treated properly, the outcome of posttraumatic meningitis is favorable. Hence, an acceptable alternative is to avoid prophylactic antibiotics, instead relying on careful observation and aggressive diagnosis and therapy.

II. Infections after penetrating head trauma

A. A **variable flora** is introduced at the time of penetrating head trauma. There is an assortment of aerobic and anaerobic organisms, reflecting those found on the scalp, face, or in contaminated materials associated with the penetrating instrument. To complicate matters, there is often necrosis of brain tissue with hematoma formation, a situation that provides an excellent substrate for polymicrobial growth.

B. Antibiotic treatment should be initiated promptly for contaminated penetrating head trauma. It is difficult to predict the bacteriology, but broad-spectrum drugs should be used. Some of the recommended combinations are as follows:

Nafcillin or oxacillin	2 gm IV q6h
plus Chloramphenicol;	750–1,000 mg IV q6h
or	
Moxalactam or cefotaxime	2 gm IV q6h

C. Surgical intervention is critical in these situations to remove devitalized tissue and to drain pus.

III. Surgical wound infections

A. Clinical features. Approximately 5% of craniotomy procedures are associated with postoperative wound infections. The initial presentation can be rather subtle, with slight redness at the border of the sutures, increased edema, and low-grade fever. These events usually make themselves apparent 3–5 days after the procedure. In some cases a subgaleal collection of pus develops, and the entire operative site is warm and edematous. High fever and sepsis suggest deeper penetration of the infection or bacteremic spread.

Most surgical infections are restricted to the wound itself, but some can produce postoperative meningitis. Meningeal involvement is a more serious complication, carrying a mortality of approximately 50%.

B. Wound infections are caused either by *Staphylococcus aureus* or gram-negative bacilli, with about equal frequency, depending on the particular neurosurgical unit. In some centers, *Staph. aureus* is still the predominant cause of localized wound infections and subgaleal collections.

C. Postoperative meningitis has a somewhat different spectrum of organisms. Eighty percent of such cases are caused by gram-negative bacilli, in particular *Enterobacter, Klebsiella, Serratia, Pseudomonas,* and *E. coli.* In 20% of cases there is a diverse group, including *Staph. aureus, Streptococcus,* and anaerobes.

D. Choice of drugs is problematic, as those agents that are active against the responsible pathogens penetrate the meninges rather poorly. If the offending microorganisms are sensitive to chloramphenicol, 750 mg IV q6h, this is the drug of choice. Unfortunately, many of the hospital-acquired organisms are resistant. The third-generation cephalosporins penetrate the CNS rather better than any of the other β-lactam antibiotics. Thus far, experience with these drugs has been very favorable, in the setting of a sensitive organism. Our recommendation for gram-negative meningitis is:

Moxalactam or cefotaxime	2 gm IV q6h

For *Pseudomonas aeruginosa* or other sensitive organisms, carbenicillin or ticarcillin can be administered. The aminoglycoside antibiotics (gentamicin, tobramycin, and amikacin) have been used in the past, but their penetration is very poor, even when the drugs are administered intrathecally.

Because the bacteriology is often complex, it may take a few days to sort out the sensitivities. In the interim, the patient may be given such drugs as moxalactam or cefotaxime alone, chloramphenicol plus ticarcillin, moxalactam or cefotaxime, or ticarcillin plus an aminoglycoside, IV and intrathecally.

IV. Shunt-associated infections

A. The use of ventriculoatrial and ventriculoperitoneal shunts has created an **etiologic niche** for infection, with a risk of about 10–20% becoming infected at some time.

B. The **clinical presentation** can be acute or subacute. Virtually all patients are febrile, but the fever may be intermittent, lasting over a period of months. Symptoms specifically referable to the central nervous system are usually absent. Patients complain of malaise, anorexia, fatigue, and sometimes headache.

C. Diagnosis. If a ventriculoatrial shunt is in place, most patients have positive blood cultures for the infecting organism. A lumbar puncture is often abnormal, but the pathogen is usually not present. The single most helpful diagnostic test is aspiration of fluid from the shunt itself; not only can the organism be seen on Gram's stain and grown in culture, but there is also a pleocytosis. Occasionally, inflammatory cells are absent when the organism is present.

D. Bacteriology. *Staph. epidermidis* is the most common pathogen, being encountered in over 90% of cases. Other organisms of low virulence are occasionally seen, such as *Propionibacterium* and diphtheroids. *Staph. aureus* and gram-negative bacilli are rare pathogens.

E. The choice of **therapy** depends on the susceptibility of the organism and the ability of the drug to penetrate the meninges. For staphylococci, oxacillin or nafcillin, 2–3 gm IV q6h, is employed.

Cephalosporin antibiotics and clindamycin should be avoided because of poor penetration into the CNS. (An exception is a third-generation cephalosporin, i.e., moxalactam or cefotaxime, which can be used in special cases, such as a gram-negative pathogen.)

Administration of the antibiotic directly into the shunt has been utilized to achieve higher levels at the infected site.

Rifampin, 600 mg PO once daily, has been recommended by some authorities, along with another antistaphylococcal agent (nafcillin or oxacillin), in an effort to provide increased killing of organisms associated with a foreign body. This drug should not be used alone because of the high frequency of resistant organisms.

Some authors have reported cures in 10–20% of shunt infections treated with antibiotics alone. However, most observers believe that complete removal of the shunt and replacement with a new one is the most certain way of eradicating infection. While it might be worth waiting for some time to see if antibiotics can effect a cure, we would recommend an operative approach, unless there are technical reasons that preclude the surgery.

F. A curious **complication** of infected ventriculoatrial shunt is diffuse glomerulonephritis. This has been found to be associated with hypocomplementemia, circulating immune complexes, and bacterial antigens within the renal glomeruli. It responds to treatment of the underlying infection.

V. Noninfectious causes of fever. Like other postoperative patients, neurosurgical patients may develop noninfectious fever due to atelectasis, sterile phlebitis, or drugs. These patients also are subject to special situations that give rise to fever.

A. Posterior fossa surgery is associated with meningismus, cerebral spinal fluid pleocytosis, and high fever, often accompanied by a depressed CSF glucose concentration. This **aseptic meningitis** appears to respond to judicious use of systemic steroids. Differentiation from bacterial meningitis can be difficult initially, but Gram's stain and culture of the CSF should be positive in bacterial meningitis. Another special circumstance is aseptic meningitis after pneumoencephalography; this condition subsides with no specific therapy.

B. Subdural or intracranial hematomas can produce a fever of noninfectious origin. Hypoglycorrhachia has been noted after subdural hematomas. This situation can represent a perplexing problem to the clinician, who is faced with CSF findings that include polymorphonuclear leukocytes and low glucose. An appropriate history (e.g., head trauma or anticoagulation) and adjunctive studies such as radionuclide brain scan and CT scan assist in discriminating pyogenic infection from these other conditions. In equivocal situations, empiric therapy for meningitis should be given and subsequently discontinued if cultures remain negative.

C. Arachnoiditis is rare but can follow intrathecal administration of contrast agents or anesthetic drugs. The diagnosis usually is not difficult because of the temporal association with the procedure. This aseptic inflammatory process is accompanied by high fever, headache, pronounced CSF pleocytosis, and low CSF glucose, mimicking a bacterial infection. When a patient manifests signs of an inflammatory process affecting the meninges after lumbar puncture, with or without prior use of contrast material or drugs, CSF examination is mandatory. If no bacteria are seen on Gram's stain, empiric antibiotic therapy may be withheld unless the patient is desperately ill. Steroids have been employed with apparent success in this form of arachnoiditis, although the natural history of the process is predictable, and spontaneous recovery is the rule.

12 Antimicrobial Agents

Penicillins

Multiple penicillins are available, and selection of a particular agent is largely determined by variations in spectrum of activity, pharmacokinetics, and oral absorption (Table 12-1).

I. Penicillin G

A. Spectrum. Highly effective against most gram-positive and some gram-negative microorganisms. Drug of choice for *Streptococcus pneumoniae, Strep. pyogenes, Strep. viridans, Bacillus anthracis* (anthrax), *Corynebacterium diphtheriae* (diphtheria), gonococci, meningococci, *Treponema pallidum,* and most anaerobes other than *Bacteroides fragilis.* Enterococci and *Hemophilus influenzae* are relatively resistant, unless penicillin is combined with an aminoglycoside. Penicillinase-producing *Staphylococcus aureus* are highly resistant. Some gram-negative enteric bacteria are susceptible to penicillin G in relatively high concentrations. These include most *Proteus mirabilis* and many *Escherichia coli, Salmonella,* and *Shigella, Klebsiella, Enterobacter, Pseudomonas,* and *Serratia* are highly resistant.

B. Mechanism of action. Inhibits cell wall synthesis, resulting in osmotic lysis of bacteria. Penicillins are bactericidal and are active only against rapidly growing organisms.

C. Pharmacokinetics

1. **Absorption.** Degraded by gastric acid. Under optimal conditions, only about one-third is orally absorbed by patients with normal gastric acid. Serum and urine levels in achlorhydric patients approximate those achieved with the same dose IM.
2. **Distribution.** Well distributed in serosal fluids, interstitial fluid, synovial fluid, bone, bile, and placenta. Cerebrospinal fluid (CSF) levels are low except in the presence of inflammation, in which case they are still low, but adequate for highly sensitive bacteria. Very high concentrations are achieved in urine.
3. **Levels.** Highly variable, depending on preparation and route of administration (see Table 12-1).
4. **Excretion.** Rapidly excreted, primarily by renal tubular resorption. Sixty to ninety percent is recovered in the urine, and ten to twenty-five percent is metabolized by the liver. In anuric patients most of the drug is excreted by the biliary tract. Probenecid, 0.5 gm q6h, competes with the tubular mechanism for excretion, producing one and one-half to twofold increase in serum levels of all penicillins.

D. Preparations

1. **Oral.** Potassium penicillin G or sodium penicillin G. Usual dose is 250–500 mg (400,000–800,000 units) 3–4 times daily one-half hour before meals or 2 hours after meals. This gives variable peak serum levels, usually 0.5–3 units/ml. With normal renal function, urine concentrations are 200 μg/ml, which is satisfactory for many uncomplicated urinary tract infections involving *E. coli, Pr. mirabilis,* or enterococci.

Table 12-1. The penicillins

Agent	Oral absorption	Penicillinase resistance	Broad spectrum	*Pseudomonas aeruginosa*
Penicillin G	±	−	−	−
Penicillin V	+	−	−	−
Methicillin	−	+	−	−
Nafcillin	±	+	−	−
Oxacillin	±	+	−	−
Cloxacillin	+	+	−	−
Dicloxacillin	+	+	−	−
Ampicillin	+	−	+	−
Amoxicillin	+	−	+	−
Bacampicillin	+	−	+	−
Carbenicillin	−	−	+	+
Indanyl carbenicillin	±	−	+	+
Ticarcillin	−	−	+	+
Mezlocillin	−	−	+	+
Piperacillin	−	−	+	+
Azlocillin	−	−	+	+

2. **Parenteral.** Available as the potassium (1.7 mEq K/million units) or sodium salt (2.0 mEq Na/million units). Dosage ranges from 1.2 to 40 million units/day in 4–8 divided doses depending on the nature of the infection and the pathogen involved. Peak serum level with bolus injection of 1.2 million units is 100 units/ml. With normal renal function this rapidly decreases to 10 units at 2 hours and to barely detectable levels at 4 hours. Half-life is approximately 30 minutes in normal persons, 10 hours in anuric patients, and up to 30 hours with combined hepatic and renal insufficiency.
   a. **Aqueous** (crystalline) penicillin G. **Advantage.** High peak levels. **Disadvantages.** Rapid excretion and painful with IM injection.
   b. **Repository penicillin G.** For deep IM injection only. Purpose is to provide slow absorption that gives prolonged levels, thus permitting less frequent administration. Peak levels, however, are relatively low. These forms should not be injected subcutaneously, intravenously, or into body cavities.
      (1) **Procaine penicillin G.** A single IM dose of 600,000 units gives peak plasma levels of 1.5 units/ml and levels of $<$ 0.4 units/ml for 24 hours. Usual daily dose is 1.2–2.4 million units in 1–3 divided doses. For uncomplicated gonorrhea, 4.8 million units (2 injection sites) combined with 1 gm oral probenecid is recommended.
      (2) **Procaine penicillin G in oil and aluminum monosterate suspension.** A single 300,000-unit dose gives a low peak plasma level (0.25 units/ml) but sustained levels of 0.03 units/ml for 4–5 days.
      (3) **Benzathine penicillin G** (Bicillin-LA). An IM dose of 1.2 million units results in a peak level of only 0.2 units/ml but sustained levels of 0.03 units/ml for 28 days. Chief use is for rheumatic fever prophylaxis. It is painful on injection, and allergic reactions may be severe and prolonged. **Advantage.** Prolonged serum levels. **Disadvantage.** Low peak serum levels.

E. **Dose modification in hepatic failure.** None.

F. **Dose modification in renal failure.** Usually none, although dose interval may be extended, and massive doses ($>$ 20 million units/day) should be avoided. In severe renal insufficiency (GFR $<$ 20 ml/min), doses of 10–12 million units/day may cause toxicity.

G. Side effects

1. **Hypersensitivity.** Incidence is approximately 5–10% and is higher in adults than in children, in persons with a history of atopy, and with parenteral rather than oral administration. Persons allergic to one form of penicillin must be regarded as allergic to all penicillins. A careful history is the best method of detecting hypersensitivity, although many patients with well-documented reactions are no longer sensitive. The optimal skin test requires both penicilloyl-polylysine (PPL) and minor determinants (MDM). PPL (pre-pen) is available; MDM is not available but can be approximated by placing a drop of penicillin G diluted to 1,000 units/ml on a superficial scratch on the forearm. A positive wheal and flare reaction occurs in 15–20 minutes. A negative reaction should be followed by an intradermal injection of 0.01 ml of the diluted penicillin. Epinephrine and a tourniquet should be available during skin testing. Negative results from both major and minor determinants give 98.5% assurance that an immediate (anaphylactic) reaction will not occur.
   a. **Immediate reaction.** Type 1 or IgE-mediated anaphylactic reactions, including laryngeal edema, generalized pruritis, urticarial skin rash, flushing, hypotension, and/or shock. These types of reaction usually occur within 20 minutes of administration and are far more common with parenteral than with oral therapy. The incidence of fatal reactions is 1–2/100,000 patients.
   b. **Delayed reactions.** Rash: morbilliform, erythematous (common); erythema nodosum, erythema multiforme, eczematous or vesiculobullous (uncommon). Serum sickness; drug fever; eosinophilia. Serum sickness, drug fever, and possibly cutaneous reactions are type 3 reactions that appear to represent immune-complex disease.
   c. Hemolytic anemia (positive Coomb's test, dose-related); marrow suppression with thrombocytopenia or leukopenia; or interstitial nephritis with proteinuria, hematuria, and acute renal failure. These are rare type 2 reactions reflecting complement-dependent cytolysis. There may also be altered platelet function and bleeding, which are most common with anti-*Pseudomonas* penicillins—carbenicillin, ticarcillin, piperacillin, mezlocillin, and azlocillin.
2. **CNS toxicity.** Patients at particular risk are those with neurologic disease, impaired renal function, or receiving massive doses, usually > 40 million units/day in patients with normal renal function or > 10 million units/day in azotemic patients. Findings are decreased consciousness, twitching, myoclonic jerks, hyperreflexia, or seizures. Owing to slow clearance of the drug from the CSF, symptoms may continue for extended periods after discontinuation of the drug. This is a relatively benign reaction that clears after the drugs are stopped.
3. **Hyperkalemia.** Seen in azotemic patients receiving K salts of penicillins in large doses. Rapid IV infusions, particularly via central venous catheters, may cause arrhythmias and even cardiac arrest.
4. **Hypokalemia.** With high doses of penicillins, especially the anti-*Pseudomonas* penicillins.

II. Phenoxymethyl penicillin (penicillin V) and phenoxyethyl penicillin. Principal advantages are acid stability and better oral absorption than penicillin G, giving peak serum levels after a 500-mg dose of 2–6 μg/ml. Activity against pneumococci, *Strep. pyogenes* and anaerobic bacteria is comparable to that of penicillin G; it is less effective against enterococci, gonococci, *H. influenzae, Pr. mirabilis,* and *E. coli.* Usual dose is 250–500 mg (400,000–800,000 units) 3–4 times daily.

III. Penicillinase-resistant penicillins

A. Spectrum. Agents of choice for treatment of infections caused by penicillinase-producing *Staph. aureus*. Use should be restricted to infections in which *Staph. aureus* is an established or a suspected pathogen, for three reasons:

1. These agents are often less effective than other penicillins for bacteria other than penicillinase-producing *Staph. aureus*. Against *Strep. pneumoniae,* for

example, methicillin is substantially less active than penicillin G. All are relatively inactive against enterococci, gram-negative bacteria, and anaerobes.

2. Overuse may result in the emergence of resistance. Methicillin-resistant *Staph. aureus* is especially prevalent in large university-affiliated hospitals, suggesting that epidemiologic spread is promoted by patient and physician transfers. These organisms are resistant to all penicillinase-resistant penicillins, and they should be regarded as resistant to cephalosporins regardless of in vitro sensitivity test results. All strains are sensitive to vancomycin. (A report of methicillin-resistant *Staph. aureus* should be carefully confirmed, since the methicillin disc for susceptibility testing is relatively unstable.)
3. Side effects appear to be greater than with penicillin G, especially renal and hematopoietic complications.

B. Pharmacokinetics. Distribution, activity, and renal excretion are determined to some extent by serum protein binding. Protein-bound drug is bacteriologically inactive, is retained in the vascular space, and is not excreted by glomerular filtration. (Tubular resorption, the principal route of excretion for penicillins, is not affected). Methicillin is about 40% bound, compared with 80–96% for nafcillin, oxacillin, cloxacillin, and dicloxacillin. Despite the variations in protein binding, there is little evidence that these drugs differ in clinical effectiveness when recommended doses are used.

C. Preparations

1. **Methicillin** (Staphcillin), 3 mEq Na/gm. Inactivated by gastric acid and available only for parenteral use. About one-fiftieth as active as penicillin G against pneumococci, streptococci, and nonpenicillinase-producing staphylococci. Interstitial nephritis with proteinuria, hematuria, azotemia, eosinophilia, fever, and/or rash may occur. This reaction is related to both dose and duration of therapy and is more common with methicillin than with other penicillins. Recommended dose is 6–24 gm/day in 4–6 divided doses. Maximum dose in renal failure is 12 gm/day.
2. **Nafcillin** (Unipen, Nafcil), 2.3 mEq Na/gm. More active than methicillin against gram-positive cocci other than *Staph. aureus* and rarely causes nephritis. Owing to less rapid renal clearance and high blood levels, the recommended dose is one-half that of methicillin—3–12 gm/day in 4–6 divided doses. Up to 90% is excreted in the bile, some for enterohepatic circulation; 30% appears in the urine. Half-life is 1 hour and is minimally affected in renal failure. Nafcillin precipitates in solutions with pH < 5.6; therefore, solutions for prolonged intravenous administration should be slightly alkaline. It is available in 250-mg capsules for oral administration, but absorption is unpredictable.
3. **Oxacillin** (Prostaphlin), 2.3 mEq Na/gm. Shares advantages with nafcillin. More active than methicillin against gram-positive cocci other than *Staph. aureus* and rarely implicated in nephritis. Large doses may cause drug-induced hepatitis. Serum half-life is one-half hour and is minimally prolonged in renal failure. Recommended parenteral dose is 3–12 gm/day in 4–8 divided doses. Available in 250-mg or 500-mg capsules, but oral absorption is unpredictable.
4. **Cloxacillin** (Tegopen). Spectrum and pharmacokinetics are similar to those for nafcillin. It is available only in oral form, and absorption is good. Usual dose is 0.5–1 gm 4 times daily, preferably one-half hour before meals or 2–3 hours after meals.
5. **Dicloxacillin.** Principal advantage is excellent oral absorption, giving serum levels approximately twice those of cloxacillin. Possible disadvantage is high protein binding—96%. Usual oral dose is 0.25–1 gm 4 times daily, preferably one-half hour before meals or 2–3 hours after meals.

IV. Ampicillin

A. Spectrum. Activity against most gram-positive bacteria, *Neisseria* (gonococci and meningococci), and anaerobic bacteria is comparable to that of penicillin G. It is inactivated by penicillinase, so that most *Staph. aureus* are resistant. Ampicillin is 4–8 times more active on a weight basis than penicillin G against enterococci and certain gram-negative bacilli, including *H. influenzae, Salmonella, Shigella, Pr. mirabilis,* and susceptible *E. coli*. Ampicillin resistance among *H. influenzae* is 20–30% of strains in most locations.

B. Pharmacokinetics. Acid-stable and 35–50% absorbed with oral administration. Peak levels following 500 mg PO are about 3 μg/ml, and following 500 mg IV are 20 μg/ml. Excretion is mainly renal, but high concentrations (approximately 10 times serum levels) are also attained in bile. Renal clearance is less rapid than that of penicillin G, so that serum levels are more prolonged after a single dose. Half-life of 1–1.5 hours increases to 10–15 hours in anuria.

C. Preparations

1. **Oral.** 2–4 gm/day in 4 divided doses, preferably one-half hour before meals or 2–3 hours after meals; for children: 50–200 mg/kg/day.
2. **IM or IV.** 0.5–2 gm q4–6h. In severe renal disease (creatinine > 5) the maximum dose is 3–6 gm/day. The usual pediatric dose is 50–200 mg/kg/day; for serious infections, up to 400 mg/kg/day can be administered every 2–4 hours.

D. Principal advantages. Good oral absorption, more prolonged blood levels than aqueous penicillin G or oral penicillin V, and greater activity against enterococci and certain gram-negative bacilli than penicillin G. **Principal disadvantages.** High incidence of skin rash. Approximately 10% of patients develop a morbilliform rash that may be unrelated to penicillin hypersensitivity and may resolve despite continued use of this drug. This rash is seen in nearly all patients with infectious mononucleosis. Diarrhea is more common than with penicillin G or V. The incidence of antibiotic-associated diarrhea is 5–10% with ampicillin, and this drug is a relatively common cause of pseudomembranous colitis.

E. Indications. Principal use is for infections involving *H. influenzae* (especially pediatric infections and exacerbations of chronic bronchitis); enterococcal infections; acute cholecystitis; chronic typhoid carriers; nonhospital-acquired urinary tract infections; and gram-negative infections in which susceptibility tests indicate efficacy. Ampicillin should not be used as a single agent for serious gram-negative infections unless susceptibility tests are known.

V. Amoxicillin. Similar to ampicillin with the advantage of better oral absorption. Blood levels are approximately **twice** those achieved with the same dose of ampicillin, and gastric absorption is not decreased by food ingestion. The incidence of diarrhea and nausea also appear to be less with amoxicillin. Amoxicillin should not be used for shigellosis, but it is effective in typhoidal syndromes. It is available only in oral form. Recommended dose is one-half that of ampicillin: 250–500 mg 3–4 times daily, usually 250 mg tid.

VI. Broad-spectrum penicillins

A. Carbenicillin disodium (Geopen, Pyopen). 5.3 mEq Na/gm.

1. **Spectrum.** Principal advantage is greater activity than other penicillins against *Pseudomonas aeruginosa,* indole-positive *Proteus,* and *Providencia. E. coli, Pr. mirabilis,* and *H. influenzae* are usually sensitive to both ampicillin and carbenicillin. Less active than penicillin G against gram-positive cocci and *Neisseria*. Most *Klebsiella* are resistant. Acquired resistance may develop during therapy, especially when carbenicillin is used as a single agent. Its activity against anaerobes is comparable to that of penicillin G; about 95% of *B. fragilis* are sensitive to levels achieved in the serum with the usual doses.
2. **Pharmacokinetics.** IV infusion of 5 gm gives serum concentrations > 150 μg/ml. These levels are required for many *Ps. aeruginosa* strains, but other gram-negative bacilli are usually susceptible to lower concentrations (i.e., 10–50 μg/ml). The drug is excreted primarily by tubular resorption—80% of unchanged drug appears in the urine. Serum half-life is 1 hour with normal renal function, 10–15 hours in anuric patients, and > 20 hours with combined anuria and hepatic insufficiency. Doses exceeding 40 gm/day in normal or improperly adjusted dosages result in neurotoxic levels in renal failure patients.

3. **Preparations and dosages**
   a. **Oral.** Carbenicillin disodium is not absorbed and not available for oral therapy. *Carbenicillin indanyl sodium* (Geocillin) is the oral form—approximately 50% is absorbed. Use is restricted to urinary tract infections, since blood levels are low with this agent. Usual dose is 0.5–1 gm q6h. Renal insufficiency (creatinine > 2 or creatinine clearance < 20 ml/min) produces inadequate urine levels and contraindicates this agent.
   b. **IM.** 1–2 gm q6h. This gives serum levels of only 20–50 μg/ml and should be reserved for urinary tract infections and systemic infections in patients with renal insufficiency.
   c. **IV.** Usual dosage is 20–40 gm/day in 4–6 divided doses; 30–40 gm/day should be used in infections in which *Ps. aeruginosa* is a known or suspected pathogen; 4–8 gm/day may be used in uncomplicated urinary tract infections.
   d. **Pediatric.** 50–200 mg/kg/day IV.
   e. **Dose modification in renal disease.**

Creatinine (mg/100 ml)	Creatinine clearance (ml/min)	Dose/day (gm)
1.5–3	> 50	20–30
3–6	10–50	4–16
> 6	< 10	4–6

   f. **Dose modification in hepatic disease.** Usually none. With combined severe hepatic and renal failure (creatinine > 6 or creatinine clearance < 10 ml/min) maximum daily dose is 2 gm.
4. **Indications.** Serious infections involving relatively resistant bacteria, particularly *Ps. aeruginosa* and indole-positive *Proteus*. This drug is usually used in combination with an aminoglycoside because (1) the agents are often synergistic; (2) carbenicillin is not active against some gram-negative bacteria (especially *Klebsiella*), and therefore carbenicillin alone does not provide adequate coverage in suspected gram-negative sepsis; (3) resistance may develop during therapy if carbenicillin is used as a single agent. Other penicillins are preferred for infections involving gram-positive cocci. Large sodium content (4.7 mEq Na/gm) may contraindicate this agent for patients requiring sodium restriction (Table 12-2).

B. **Ticarcillin disodium** (Ticar)
1. The antibacterial **spectrum** and **pharmacokinetic properties** are identical to those of carbenicillin, except that ticarcillin is somewhat more active against some gram-negative bacilli, including *Ps. aeruginosa*. Therefore, the usual dose is one-half that of carbenicillin. The sodium load (5.2 mEq/gm) is consequently reduced by approximately one-half, which may be important in some cases. The usual maximum dose in adults with serious infections in which *Ps. aeruginosa* is a suspected or established pathogen is 18 gm/day.
2. **Dose modification in renal insufficiency**

Creatinine (mg/100 ml)	Creatinine clearance (ml/min)	Maximum dose
< 1.5	> 40	3 gm q4h
1.5–5	20–40	3–4 gm q8–12h
> 5	< 20	3–4 gm q12h
> 5 with hepatic failure		2 gm q24h

C. **Mezlocillin monosodium** (Mezlin). A broad-spectrum penicillin with properties similar to those of carbenicillin and ticarcillin, except for the following:
1. **Spectrum.** Increased activity against Enterobacteriaceae (especially *Klebsiella*) and enterococci. Activity against *Ps. aeruginosa* and *B. fragilis* is comparable to that of ticarcillin. Synergistic activity with aminoglycosides

Table 12-2. Sodium content of penicillins

Agent	Na content	Usual dose	Total Na/day mEq	Total Na/day gm
Penicillin G	2 mEq/mu	12 mu	24	0.5
Ampicillin	2.9 mEq/gm	8 gm	24	0.5
Carbenicillin	4.7 mEq/gm	36 gm	170	3.8
Ticarcillin	5.2 mEq/gm	18 gm	94	2.2
Mezlocillin	1.8 mEq/gm	18 gm	33	0.8
Piperacillin	1.8 mEq/gm	18 gm	33	0.8
Azlocillin	2.2 mEq/gm	18 gm	50	0.9

against aerobic gram-negative bacilli is also similar to that of ticarcillin. (Penicillinase-producing strains of *Staph. aureus* are resistant, as with carbenicillin and ticarcillin.).

2. **Pharmacokinetic** properties and volume of distribution are similar except that 20–25% is eliminated by biliary excretion. Thus, the drug is less likely to accumulate in renal failure, in which it has an elimination half-life of 2.5 hours compared to 10–15 hours for carbenicillin.
3. **Dose** recommendation for serious infections in adults and children older than 7 days is 100–300 mg/kg/day at 4–6-hour intervals in the presence of normal renal function; 75 mg/kg/day is advocated for children less than 7 days old. With a creatinine level of 1.5–5 mg/100 ml in adults the usual dose is given at 8-hour intervals, and for creatinine of > 5 the usual dose is given at 12-hour intervals.
4. **Sodium load** is reduced for mezlocillin.
5. **Piperacillin.** A broad-spectrum penicillin with advantages compared to carbenicillin and ticarcillin that are similar to those of mezlocillin. Either piperacillin or mezlocillin, but not necessarily both, may possess increased activity against a given strain of *Ps. aeruginosa*. Piperacillin appears somewhat more active against some strains of *Enterobacteraceae*. As with carbenicillin, resistance is likely to emerge during therapy of serious *Pseudomonas* infections, so piperacillin (or ticarcillin or mezlocillin) should not be used as a single agent in this setting. Pharmacokinetic properties and dose recommendations are similar to those noted for mezlocillin.
6. **Azlocillin.** Similar to piperacillin and mezlocillin except for somewhat higher serum levels (~150–250 μg/ml 1 hour after IV infusion of 5 gm) and better activity against *Ps. aeruginosa*. The elimination half-life of 1 hour in the presence of normal renal function increases to 6 hours in complete renal failure. The recommended dose for serious infections is 200–350 mg/kg/day in 4–6 divided doses (usually 18 gm/day for adults with normal renal function); dose adjustment with a stable serum creatinine of 1.5–5.0 (creatinine clearance of 10–30 ml/min) is 2 gm q8h, and for a creatinine clearance of < 10 ml/min is 2–3 gm q12h. Patients undergoing hemodialysis should receive 3 gm after each dialysis and then this dose q12h. As already noted, none of the anti-*Pseudomonas* penicillins should be used alone to treat serious infections or infections prone to relapse.

Cephalosporins

Cephalothin became available in 1964, and numerous derivatives have been introduced since (Table 12-3). The cephalosporins produced before November 1979 have similar spectra of activity; the major differences between them relate to oral absorption and pharmacokinetics. Cefoxitin, cefamandole and cefuroxime are considered **second-generation** cephalosporins, since they have an expanded spectrum. **Third-generation** compounds have an even wider spectrum that includes most aerobic and anaerobic bacteria.

I. Spectrum. Cephalosporins are effective against most gram-positive bacteria including staphylococci, pneumococci, and streptococci other than enterococci. *H. influenzae* is usually sensitive to cefamandole, cefaclor, cefuroxime, and 3rd generation cephalosporins but not to other cephalosporins. *E. coli, Klebsiella* (community-acquired strains), *Pr. mirabilis,* and *Salmonella* are susceptible to most cephalosporins. Some *Klebsiella, E. coli,* and other gram-negative bacilli other than pseudomonads are resistant to first-generation cephalosporins but are sensitive to cefoxitin and/or cefamandole. Third-generation cephalosporins, the most active agents in this class against gram-negative bacilli, are somewhat less active against gram-positive bacteria. Cephalosporins are active against most penicillin-sensitive anaerobes; 90–95% of *B. fragilis* are sensitive to cefoxitin and moxalactam but are variably resistant to most other cephalosporins. Those resistant to all cephalosporins include enterococci, methicillin-resistant *Staph. aureus, Legionella, Mycoplasma,* and *Chlamydia.*

II. Indications. Cephalosporins are greatly overused. Penicillins are considered the agents of choice for most infections involving gram-positive bacteria. Aminoglycosides (gentamicin, tobramycin, or amikacin) are favored when these organisms are suspected in serious infections requiring therapy before culture results are available. Principal uses for cephalosporins are (1) for infections involving gram-positive cocci other than enterococci in patients allergic to penicillin, (2) for gram-negative infections when culture results indicate efficacy, (3) in combination with an aminoglycoside for selected cases of serious sepsis, (4) for prophylaxis in a variety of surgical procedures (see Chap. 13), and (5) for gram-negative bacillary meningitis (moxalactam, cefotaxime, or cefoperazone).

III. Mechanism of action. Inhibits synthesis of bacterial cell walls; bactericidal.

IV. Pharmacokinetics

A. Oral absorption, serum levels, and half-life of various cephalosporins are summarized in Table 12-1.

B. Distribution. Distributed throughout tissues and body fluids except for the central nervous system. CSF levels of active drug are low except for most 3rd generation drugs; other cephalosporins should not be used in meningitis. In the absence of biliary tract obstruction, bile levels are generally high; this especially applies to cefamandole and cefoperazone.

C. Excretion. The major route of elimination of cephalosporins is renal excretion. Approximately 30–50% of cephalothin, cefotaxime, and cephapirin are deacetylated by the liver to a metabolite not found for the other cephalosporins listed. Probenecid, 500 mg q6h, competes for tubular secretion, thereby increasing blood level and half life for most cephalosporins other than 3rd generation drugs. Half-life increases in renal failure, necessitating dosage modifications that vary according to pharmacokinetic properties. With cephalothin, cefotaxime, and cephapirin, most of the circulating drug is in the less active deacetylated form in the presence of renal failure.

V. Toxicity

A. Hypersensitivity reactions occur in 2–5% of patients. There may be hypersensitivity to the beta-lactam moiety, indicating allergy to all cephalosporins; alternatively there may be hypersensitivity to a side-chain component, in which case a patient may react to one agent but not others in the class. Cephalosporins also have structural similarities with penicillins. The incidence of cephalosporin reactions in patients with a history of penicillin sensitivity increases three- to fivefold and reached as high as 17% in one study. It is uncertain whether this reflects true cross-sensitivity or simply an increased rate of reactions in allergy-prone individuals. Cephalosporins are generally considered safe for subjects with a previous history of delayed hypersensitivity reaction to penicillin, i.e., moribilliform rash, fever, eosinophilia. However, these individuals should be carefully observed. Cephalosporins are to be avoided when the penicillin reaction appears to be IgE-

Table 12-3. Pharmacokinetic properties of cephalosporins

	Peak serum level (μg/ml) obtained with 1 gm/mg IV or 0.5 gm PO	Serum half-life (hr)		Protein binding (%)	Recommended dosage interval (normal renal function)	Daily dose (gm) based on serum creatinine*		
		Normal renal function	Anephric			<1.5	1.5–5	>5
First generation								
Short-acting								
Cephalothin (Keflin)	30–40	0.6	10	65	4–6 hr	4–12	3–8	2–3
Cephapirin (Cefadyl)	30–40	0.7	2	50	4–6 hr	4–12	3–8	2–3
Cephradine (Velosef, Anspor)	20–30	0.8	10	15	4–6 hr	4–12	3–8	2–3
Long-acting								
Cephaloridine (Loridine)	70	1.2	20	20		3–4	Contraindicated	
Cefazolin (Kefzol, Ancef)	90–110	1.8	55	85	8–12 hr	2–6	1–2	5
Oral								
Cephalexin (Keflex)	10–20	0.9	20	12	6–8 hr	1–2	1	0.25–0.5
Cephradine (Velosef, Anspor)	10–20	0.8	10	15	6–8 hr	1–2	1	0.25–0.5
Cefaclor (Ceclor)	10–20	0.8			6–8 hr	1–2	1	0.25–0.5
Second generation								
Cefamandole (Mandol)	70–30	0.8	8	75	4–8 hr	4–12	3–8	2–3
Cefoxitin (Mefoxin)	70–30	0.8	12	75	6–8 hr	4–8	3–6	1–1.5
Third generation								
Moxalactam (Moxam)	100	2.0	19	50	8–12 hr	2–12	1–6	0.5–2
Cefotaxime (Claforan)	100	1.0	4	50	6–8 hr	2–12	2–12	1–6
Cefoperazone (Cefobid)	150	2.0	4	90	8–12 hr	2–6	2–6	2–4

*Assumes stable renal function in adults. Creatinine < 1.5 indicates creatinine clearance > 40 ml/min; 1.5–5: 10–30 ml/min; creatinine > 5: < 10 ml/min.

mediated, i.e., immediate or anaphylactic. The principal types of cephalosporin hypersensitivity reactions are similar to those with penicillins—skin rash, fever eosinophilia, serum sickness, and anaphylaxis.

B. Hematologic reactions. Positive results of the direct Coomb's test are common especially with large doses; hemolytic anemia is rare. The incidence of positive Coomb's test results appears to be less with cefazolin. Neutropenia (often transient) and thrombocytopenia are rare.

C. Irritative reactions. Phlebitis at IV injection sites is common and appears to occur with nearly equal frequency with all parenteral cephalosporins Cephalothin is extremely painful with IM injection; cefazolin is generally regarded as the best-tolerated cephalosporin for intramuscular administration.

D. Nephrotoxicity is infrequent except with cephaloridine. Cephalosporins potentiate the nephrotoxicity of aminoglycosides, especially the combination of cephalothin and gentamicin.

E. GI reactions. Diarrhea and pseudomembranous colitis may occur with any cephalosporin.

F. Elevated serum glutamic-oxaloacetic transaminase (SGOT), serum glutamic-pyruvic transaminase (SGPT), and alkaline phosphatase, as well as prolonged prothombin time, have been reported.

G. Superinfection with resistant bacteria.

VI. Preparations

A. Cephalothin (Keflin)

1. **IM.** 0.5–1 gm q4–6h (often extremely painful).
2. **IV.** 4–12 gm/day in 4–8 divided doses, usually 1–2 gm q4–6h.
3. **Pediatric dose.** 40–80 mg/kg/day.
4. **Dose modification in renal failure.** Usual dose in moderate renal failure (creatinine 1.5–5) is 1–2 gm q6–9h; and in severe renal failure (creatinine > 5) is 0.5–1 gm q8–12h.
5. **Dose modification in hepatic failure.** None.

B. Cephapirin (Cefadyl). No important difference from cephalothin.

C. Cephradine (Velosef, Anspor): Parenteral form shows no important difference from cephalothin. Oral form shows no important difference from cephalexin (see **H**).

D. Cephaloridine (Loridine)

1. **Spectrum.** Similar to that of cephalothin but somewhat more active against anaerobic bacteria.
2. **Principal advantages.** Relatively pain-free with IM injection; higher blood levels than cephalothin; prolonged half-life. **Principal disadvantages.** Dose-related nephrotoxicity indicated by proteinuria, hyaline casts, decreased urinary output, and/or rising creatinine. This risk, and the availability of cefazolin with similar advantages, limits the usefulness of cephaloridine.
3. **Dosage.** 1–4 gm/day in 3–4 divided doses. **Pediatric dosage.** 100 mg/kg/day up to a maximum of 4 gm/day. Contraindicated in renal failure.

E. Cefazolin (Ancef, Kefzol)

1. **Spectrum.** Similar to that of cephalothin but somewhat more active against some strains of *E. coli*.
2. **Principal advantages**
   a. Blood levels are 3–4 times higher than those achieved with the same dose of cephalothin, and 2 times those achieved with cephaloridine. Half-life is prolonged, permitting less frequent administration.
   b. Less painful than cephalothin with IM injection.
   c. Negligible risk of the nephrotoxicity associated with cephaloridine.
   d. Not metabolized to a less active compound.
   e. Higher biliary tract excretion than with most other cephalosporins.
3. **Dose.** 1–6 gm/day in 2–3 divided doses by IM or IV administration, usually 2–4 gm/day. In renal failure, adult dose with creatinine 1.5–3 is 0.5–1 gm q8–12h; with creatinine 3–5, 0.5–1 gm q24h; with creatinine > 5, 0.25–0.5 gm q24h. Pediatric dose with normal renal function is 25–100 mg/kg/day.

F. Cefamandole (Mandol)

1. **Expanded spectrum** compared to other cephalosporins. Bacteria susceptible to cephalothin are also sensitive to cefamandole; some coliforms that are resistant to cephalothin are susceptible to cefamandole, especially *Enterobacter,* indole-positive *Proteus, E. coli,* and *Klebsiella.* Most strains of *H. influenzae* are sensitive, including some ampicillin-resistant strains. *Ps. aeruginosa, Serratia, B. fragilis,* methicillin-resistant *Staph. aureus,* and enterococci are resistant.
2. **Pharmacokinetic properties** are similar to those of cephalothin, except that the half-life is slightly longer and bile levels are much higher.
3. **Advantages.** Active against *H. influenzae* and some facultative gram-negative bacilli that are resistant to other relatively nontoxic drugs (e.g., cephalothin and ampicillin). Cefamandole is useful in treating pneumonia caused by sensitive gram-negative bacteria, particularly those infections acquired in the hospital. **Disadvantages.** Increased cost compared to ampicillin and cephalothin.
4. **Dosage.** Usual parenteral dose is 0.5–1 gm q4–8h with a maximum daily dose of 12 gm daily for serious infections.

G. Cefoxitin (Mefoxin)

1. **Expanded spectrum** compared with other cephalosporins. Some organisms resistant to cephalothin are sensitive to cefoxitin, including indole-positive *Proteus, E. coli, Klebsiella, Providencia,* some *Serratia,* and most *B. fragilis.* A major advantage is that 90–95% of strains of *B. fragilis* are susceptible to levels that can be achieved with maximum recommended doses. Cefoxitin is less active than other cephalosporins against some gram-positive organisms, especially *Staph. aureus* and streptococci.
2. **Pharmacokinetic properties** are similar to those of cephalothin with a somewhat longer half-life.
3. **Advantages.** Principal advantage is activity against *B. fragilis* or facultative gram-negative bacilli resistant to other antimicrobials, including other cephalosporins and penicillins. **Disadvantage.** Higher cost than most beta-lactam antibiotics other than 3rd generation cephalosporins.
4. **Dosage.** Usual parenteral dose is 1–2 gm q4–6h.

H. Cephalexin (Keflex). **Oral** cephalosporin, acid-stable and 80–100% absorbed.

1. **Principal uses**
   - **a.** Oral therapy of infections previously treated with parenteral cephalosporins.
   - **b.** Oral treatment of infections involving *Staph. aureus.*
   - **c.** Treatment of urinary tract infections involving organisms resistant to alternative (and cheaper) oral agents, especially those involving *Klebsiella.*
2. **Principal disadvantage.** Expense, and availability of alternative (more specific) agents for many common pathogens.
3. **Dosage.** 1–2 gm/day in 4 divided doses, usually 250–500 mg q6h. The usual dose is given at 8–12-hour intervals when creatinine is 1.5–5, and q48–60h when creatinine is > 5.
4. Most frequent **adverse effects** are nausea, vomiting, and diarrhea.

I. Moxalactam (Moxam). Third-generation cephalosporin with potential advantages of expanded spectrum against aerobic gram-negative bacilli, prolonged half-life, and good penetration into the central nervous system.

1. **Spectrum.** Active against most Enterobacteriaceae, including *E. coli, Klebsiella, Enterobacter, Moraxella, Serratia, Proteus, Salmonella,* and *Shigella.* This includes most strains of these organisms that are resistant to first- and second-generation cephalosporins. Even strains that are susceptible to cephalothin are likely to be substantially more sensitive to moxalactam, although there is no documented benefit from this improved activity for most infections. Gonococci and *H. influenzae* (including penicillinase-producing strains) are highly susceptible. Most anaerobes are sensitive, although *B. fragilis* is somewhat more susceptible to cefoxitin or clindamycin, and clos-

tridia are relatively resistant. Gram-positive bacteria are more sensitive to cephalothin, although moxalactam is generally adequate for methicillin-sensitive *Staph. aureus*. Resistant organisms include 30–50% of *Ps. aeruginosa, Acinetobacter,* enterococci, *Legionella,* most *Staph. epidermidis,* all methicillin-resistant *Staph. aureus,* 3–5% of Enterobacteriaceae, *Chlamydia,* and *Listeria monocytogenes.*

2. **Pharmacokinetic properties.** Peak serum levels are approximately 100 μg/ml when 1 gm is given intravenously, and 250 μg/ml when 3 gm is given. The drug diffuses well into tissue and body fluids, including the central nervous system, where peak spinal fluid levels are 10–20% of peak serum levels. Moxalactam is primarily (90%) eliminated by the urinary tract. The serum half-life is approximately 2 hours with normal renal function and increases to nearly 20 hours in anuria. Bile levels are 2–3 times serum levels in the absence of biliary obstruction.
3. **Side effects.** Similar to those of other cephalosporins, including phlebitis in 4%, hypersensitivity reactions in 3%, diarrhea in 2%, and *Clostridium difficile*–induced colitis. An unusual side effect is an Antabuse-like reaction with alcohol ingestion. Moxalactam can interfere with hemostasis through three different mechanisms: hypoprothrombinemia, platelet dysfunction, and rarely, immune-mediated thrombocytopenia. A total of 2.5% of patients enrolled in clinical trials treated for 4 or more days experienced a bleeding event, most of which were serious. Bleeding associated with hypoprothrombinemia can be prevented by administering vitamin K, at a dose of 10 mg/wk. The platelet-related bleeding episode is dose related and is seen mostly in patients receiving more than 4 gm/day for longer than 3 days. An additional complication is the somewhat high rate of superinfections with resistant organisms (especially enterococci) and the emergence of resistance during treatment (especially with *Ps. aeruginosa, Enterobacter,* and *Serratia*).
4. **Indications**
   a. Moxalactam is effective for gram-negative bacillary meningitis involving sensitive strains (other than *H. influenzae,* which can be treated with ampicillin and/or chloramphenicol).
   b. Infections with gram-negative bacteria resistant to other antibiotics. Moxalactam may be preferred over aminoglycosides (except for *Pseudomonas* infections, which have a high failure rate with moxalactam).
   c. Mixed aerobic-anaerobic infections of the abdomen and female genital tract. Other agents, such as cefoxitin and the combination of clindamicin or metronidazole plus an aminoglycoside, can also be used.
   d. Moxalactam is not the preferred agent for any infection involving purely anaerobic bacteria, gram-positive bacteria, or cephalothin-sensitive gram-negative bacilli (except for CNS infection).
   e. The drug is relatively expensive, and widespread use is likely to engender resistance. It should be used with caution as a single agent against *Ps. aeruginosa, Serratia,* and *Enterobacter,* even with sensitive strains, due to the potential for emergence of resistance during treatment.
   f. Some authorities believe that there is limited utility of moxalactam due to bleeding complications.
5. **Dosages.** Available for parenteral use only.
   a. **Adults.** Recommended IV dose is 1–2 gm given q8–12h (usually 4 gm/day) and up to 4 gm q8h for serious infections involving less sensitive strains.
   b. **Dose modification in renal failure**

Creatinine (mg/100 ml)	Creatinine clearance (ml/min)	Regimen
1.5	> 40	0.5–4 gm q8–12h
1.5–3	20–40	0.5–3 gm q8h
3–5	10–20	0.25 gm q12h–2 gm q8h
> 5	< 10	0.5–1 gm q8–24h

c. **Pediatric**

0–1 wk	50 mg/kg q12h
1–4 wk	50 mg/kg q8h
Infants	50 mg/kg q6h
Children	50 mg/kg q6–8h

J. **Cefotaxime** (Claforan). A 3rd-generation cephalosporin sharing properties noted for moxalactam except for modest variations in in vitro activity, considerable difference in pharmacokinetic properties, and infrequency of bleeding complications.

1. **Spectrum.** Similar to that of moxalactam except (1) most *Acinetobacter* are susceptible, (2) activity against many gram-positive bacteria is better (especially against *Staph. aureus, Staph. epidermidis,* and streptococci), (3) it is less active against *B. fragilis,* (4) strains of Enterobacteriaceae or *Ps. aeruginosa* may be susceptible to cefotaxime and resistant to moxalactam (the reverse also applies), and (5) synergy with aminoglycosides against gram-negative bacilli may be seen with moxalactam or cefotaxime but not necessarily with both.
2. **Pharmacokinetic properties.** Following 1 gm IV the peak serum level is 70–90 μg/ml and there is minimal detectable drug at 4 hours. As with cephalothin, about 30% is metabolized in the liver to a clinically active desacetyl form. There are also two other inactive urinary metabolites. Urinary recovery accounts for approximately 60% of the administered dose.
3. **Side effects.** Similar to those of other cephalosporins; unlike the effects of moxalactam, these do not include prolongation of the prothrombin time or antabuse-type reactions.
4. **Indications.** Similar to moxalactam (except that efficacy in mixed abdominal and female pelvic infections is not well established). Cefotaxime is useful in gram-negative bacillary meningitis.
5. **Dosages.** Recommended adult dose is 0.5 mg–3 gm IV q4–6h, usually 4–5 gm/day. One-half the usual dose should be given in the presence of renal insufficiency with creatinine > 3.

K. **Cefoperazone** (Cefobid): Similar to moxalactam and cefotaxime except for

1. **Spectrum.** Improved activity vs. *Ps. aeruginosa;* less active than cefotaxime vs. methicillin-sensitive *Staph. aureus;* less active than moxalactam vs. *B. fragilis;* less active than either vs. many *Enterobacteraceae.*
2. **Serum levels** with comparable doses are somewhat higher (Table 12-3).
3. **Serum half-life** is 2–2.5 hr. Thus, the proper dosage is 2–6 gm/day q8–12h.
4. The drug is largely eliminated by the enterohepatic route (70%), so minimal change is needed for the recommended dosage regimen in the presence of renal failure (Table 12-3). This excretory route produces high levels in bile and in the intestine; one consequence may be an increased incidence of diarrhea with cefoperazone, which has been reported by some investigators.
5. **Complications.** Side chain similar to that of moxalactam implicated in bleeding diathesis.

Aminoglycosides

Aminoglycosides are amino sugars linked to another moiety by a glycoside bond. Compounds in this class include, in order of their introduction to the market, streptomycin, neomycin, kanamycin, gentamicin, tobramycin, and amikacin (Table 12-4). These agents act by binding bacterial ribosomes to prevent protein synthesis. Other shared properties are

1. Insolubility in lipids, with poor penetration into the eye, prostate, and central nervous system.
2. Poor absorption with oral administration.
3. Reduced activity in an acid or anaerobic milieu.
4. Negligible activity against anaerobic bacteria.

Table 12-4. Dosage regimens and pharmacokinetics of aminoglycosides

Agent	Half-life (hr)		Desired serum level (μg/ml)		Usual dose (mg/kg)		Renal toxicity	Ototoxicity	
	Normal renal function	Anephric	Peak	Trough	Initial	Maintenance daily dose (normal renal function)		Vestibular	Hearing
Gentamicin	2–3	30–60	5–8	1–2	2	5	+ +	+ +	+
Tobramycin	2–3	50–70	5–8	1–2	2	5	+	+ +	+
Kanamycin	2–3	40–80	20–30	5–10	7.5	15	+ +	+	+ +
Amikacin	2–3	40–80	20–30	5–10	7.5	15	+ +	+ +	+ +
Streptomycin	2–3	100–110	20–40	<5	15	15	±	+ +	+

5. Elimination by glomerular filtration.
6. Low therapeutic-toxic ratio, indicating that levels required for antibacterial activity are relatively close to those considered toxic. All agents in this class are ototoxic and nephrotoxic, although these effects are independent of each other. Renal toxicity results from active transport of the drug into proximal tubular cells, with proximal tubular cell damage. Ototoxicity results from damage to neurosensory hair cells in the cochlea, leading to hearing loss, and damage to semicircular canals, leading to vestibular dysfunction. The propensity to cause these complications varies with different agents in the class (Table 12-4).

The major use of aminoglycosides is for therapy of infections caused by aerobic gram-negative bacilli. Gentamicin, tobramycin and amikacin are active against 90% of these organisms, although there are variations within hospitals from this pattern. Kanamycin is weakly active, and streptomycin is considerably less active. Bacterial resistance is usually because of the production of inactivating enzymes, which cause adenylation, phosphorylation, or acetylation of the drugs. As these enzymes act at different sites on the molecule, they produce varied susceptibility patterns. The least susceptible to enzyme inactivation is amikacin, which is the most predictably active drug in the class against gram-negative bacilli. A less common mechanism of resistance is a barrier to penetration into the bacterial cell; organisms with this barrier are generally resistant to all aminoglycosides. Resistance owing to inactivating enzymes is usually encoded by plasmids. This indicates that overuse of these drugs may result in resistance to multiple agents in the class.

I. Gentamicin (Garamycin)

A. Spectrum. Active against most *E. coli, Klebsiella, Enterobacter, Proteus* (both indole-positive and indole-negative), *Ps. aeruginosa,* and *Serratia.* Most *Staph. aureus* and *Staph. epidermidis* are sensitive. Pneumococci, streptococci, and virtually all anaerobes are resistant. Enterococci are sensitive when gentamicin is combined with a penicillin. Activity is markedly decreased when pH is below 6 and increased in alkaline conditions.

B. Indications. The principal advantage of gentamicin is its activity against gram-negative bacilli that are often resistant to other commonly used antimicrobials, especially *Ps. aeruginosa, Serratia,* indole-positive *Proteus, Enterobacter,* and certain hospital-acquired strains of *E. coli* and *Klebsiella.* It is a good agent for empiric therapy of serious gram-negative infections, particularly those that are hospital-acquired. When culture results are available, less toxic agents should be used according to susceptibility tests. Overprescribing gentamicin means encouraging emergence of resistant bacteria and should be avoided. The narrow toxic-therapeutic ratio of gentamicin demands careful observation and appropriate dosage adjustment according to renal function. Although most *Staph. aureus* are susceptible, alternative agents (penicillinase-resistant penicillins, cephalosporins, or clindamycin) are preferred for infections involving this organism.

C. Mechanism of action. Binds bacterial ribosomes and causes misreading of the genetic code; bactericidal. Cell entry is by an aerobically generated transport system, so that antimicrobial activity is reduced in anaerobic conditions.

D. Pharmacokinetics

1. **Absorption.** Not absorbed with oral administration.
2. **Distribution.** Peak blood levels of 5–8 μg/ml follow maintenance doses of 1.7 mg/kg at 30–90 minutes. The drug does not penetrate fat well and is mostly restricted to the extracellular volume, which constitutes about 30% of lean body weight. Protein binding is nil. Levels in bile are relatively low. CNS and ocular penetration are poor, necessitating intrathecal or intraocular injection to ensure adequate levels.
3. **Excretion.** Excreted principally by renal glomerular filtration. Half-life of 2–3 hours increases to 30–60 hours in anephric patients.

E. Preparations and dosages

1. **Parenteral**

   a. **IM.** 1.0–1.7 mg/kg q8h. The lower dose may be used in urinary tract infections. Higher doses (2.0 mg/kg initially, followed by 1.7 mg/kg q8h) are recommended in serious infections, especially when relatively resistant organisms such as *Ps. aeruginosa* are established or suspected pathogens. The drug is poorly lipid-soluble and does not penetrate fat, so doses for obese patients should be based on lean body water + 0.4 (total body water − lean body water).

b. IV. 1.0–1.7 mg/kg q8h infused over 30 minutes. Again, the initial dose should be 2 mg/kg for seriously ill patients, the usual maintenance dose is 1.5–1.7 mg/kg, and doses for obese patients should be based on lean body mass or ideal body weight.

c. Dose modification in renal failure. The usual dose (1.0–2.0 mg/kg) is given initially, and subsequent doses or dosing intervals are modified according to renal function. The half-life of gentamicin is approximately 4 times the serum creatinine in hours. The following formulae can be used:

(1) Maintenance doses may be the usual dose given every 2½ half-lives (1–1.7 mg/kg at an interval of 8–10 times the serum creatinine).

(2) One-half the usual dose may be given twice as often (0.8 mg/kg at an interval of 4–5 times the serum creatinine). Some authorities prefer this latter method for serious infections, since it decreases the duration of time of subtherapeutic levels between doses. An example of these dose-interval adjustments for a 70-kg patient with a creatinine of 2.4 gm/100 ml is a loading dose of 115–140 mg followed by maintenance doses of

(a) 115 mg q24h (1.8 mg/kg at intervals of 10 times serum creatinine)

or

(b) 60 mg q12h (0.8 mg/kg at intervals of 5 times serum creatinine).

These dose-interval formulas are based on stable renal function. Patients with rapidly rising creatinine levels or oliguria should receive the usual dose every 2–4 days, one-half the usual dose every 24–48 hours, or, preferably, dose regimens based on serum levels. Patients undergoing hemodialysis should receive one-half to one-fourth the usual loading dose after each procedure.

(3) Serum levels. The optimal method of monitoring therapy in renal failure is to measure gentamicin serum levels. "Peak levels" are obtained immediately after intravenous infusions or 45–60 minutes after intramuscular injections. These should show concentrations of 5–10 μg/ml to ensure therapeutic levels and levels of < 12 μg/ml to reduce toxicity. A more accurate index of potential toxicity is the predose ("trough") level taken just before administration of the next dose. Trough levels exceeding 2 μg/ml following full doses suggest drug accumulation, and the dose should be reduced or the dosing interval extended. Aminoglycoside levels are routinely recommended for patients with renal failure, those receiving prolonged courses (over 10–14 days), and those with suspected ototoxicity or nephrotoxicity.

d. Dose modification in hepatic failure. None.

2. Topical. Available in 0.1% cream and ointment. Topical gentamicin encourages the emergence of resistant organisms, particularly gentamicin-resistant *Pseudomonas*. Widespread use may result in loss of effectiveness of a valuable agent for systemic infections. Topical gentamicin should be avoided or should be restricted to cases of extensive burns, and burn patients so treated should be isolated to avoid transmission of resistant strains to other patients.

3. Intrathecal and intraventricular. Usual daily adult dose is 4–6 mg as a solution of 2–5 mg/ml in preservative-free physiologic saline.

F. Side effects

1. Toxicity

a. Ototoxicity. May cause hearing loss and, more commonly, vestibular damage. Clinically overt ototoxicity is seen in approximately 2% of patients receiving usual doses for < 2 weeks; patients with vestibular dysfunction may compensate, but the damage is not reversible. Usual findings are nystagmus, nausea, vomiting, and vertigo. Hearing loss is usually in the high frequency range. Predisposing factors to ototoxicity are high trough levels (over 2 μg/ml), impaired renal function, age > 60 years, total dose > 1 gm, anemia, previous hearing or vestibular impairment, exposure to other ototoxic drugs, repeated exposure to aminoglycosides, and concurrent administration of ethacrynic acid, furosemide, mannitol, or other diuretics.

b. Nephrotoxicity. Aminoglycosides accumulate in the renal cortex in levels that exceed serum concentrations and persist for several days after a single dose. Damage is to proximal tubular cells, with sparing of glomeruli. The incidence of mild nephrotoxicity with gentamicin is 8%, and of severe, 2%; renal damage is nearly always reversible if the drug is discontinued with early signs of renal dysfunction. Usual signs are proteinuria, tubular cells in urine, and rising creatinine with or without oliguria. The risk of renal damage is augmented by the same predisposing factors as ototoxity, with the additional one of concurrent use of cephalosporins such as cephalothin.

c. Neuromuscular blockage. Rare; reversible with calcium salts given intravenously.

2. Hypersensitivity. Fever, rash, pruritus, eosinophilia, or urticaria (1–3%). Anaphylaxis is rare.

II. Tobramycin (Nebcin)

A. Spectrum. The antibacterial spectrum is similar to that of gentamicin with a few exceptions. Compared with gentamicin, tobramycin is generally less effective against *E. coli* and *Serratia* and is more effective against *Ps. aeruginosa*. Most gram-negative bacilli resistant to one of these aminoglycosides are resistant to the other as well. These comparative susceptibility patterns may vary between different institutions.

B. Indications. Identical to those for gentamicin.

C. Pharmacokinetics. Serum levels, distribution, and excretion are essentially identical to those of gentamicin.

D. Dosage. Dose recommendations and modification of dosage in renal failure are the same as for gentamicin.

E. Toxicity. Similar to that of gentamicin, although the incidence of nephrotoxocity appears to be less.

F. Disadvantage. Tobramycin is considerably more expensive than gentamicin.

III. Kanamycin (Kantrex)

A. Spectrum. Good activity against many gram-negative bacteria, including *E. coli, Enterobacter, Klebsiella, Pr. mirabilis,* and *Providencia*. Resistance may develop during therapy but, unlike the case with streptomycin, this usually occurs only with extended courses. *Ps. aeruginosa* and occasional other gram-negative bacilli (especially hospital-acquired strains) are resistant. *Staph. aureus* is usually sensitive. Many other gram-positive organisms (streptococci and pneumococci) and essentially all anaerobic bacteria are resistant. Enterococci are often sensitive when kanamycin is combined with penicillin, but other penicillin-aminoglycoside combinations are often preferred. *Staph. aureus* is usually sensitive; this varies at different institutions, and other antimicrobials are preferred.

B. Indications. Effective parenterally in most infections involving susceptible gram-negative bacilli. Alternative less toxic agents should be used when susceptibility tests indicate efficacy. Oral kanamycin may be useful for preoperative bowel preparation, hepatic coma, or enteritis involving susceptible bacteria.

C. Mechanism of action. Identical to that of gentamicin.

D. Pharmacokinetics

1. Absorption. Poorly absorbed orally. Absorption from IM injection sites is excellent. Plasma level after usual IM dose is 20–30 μg/ml at 1 hour, decreasing to 5–10 μg/ml at 8 hours.

2. Distribution. Volume distribution and tissue penetration are similar to those of gentamicin.

3. Excretion. Excreted by glomerular filtration. Half-life of 2–3 hours increases to 2–4 days in anephric patients.

E. Preparations and dosages

1. **Oral.** Since oral absorption is poor, may be used for preoperative bowel preparation, intestinal infections, or hepatic coma. Usual dose is 1.0–1.5 gm q4–6h (50–100 mg/kg/day). Blood levels are generally low or unmeasurable except with renal failure or with extensive bowel ulceration. In such cases the patients may develop ototoxicity or nephrotoxicity with large oral doses or extended courses.
2. **IM.** 5.0 mg/kg q8h or 7.5 mg/kg q12h; maximum 1.5 gm/day. Total dose should not exceed 15 gm.
3. **IV.** 5.0 mg/kg q8h or 7.5 mg/kg q12h by IV infusion over 1–2 hours. Use only for serious infections.
4. **Dose modification in renal failure.** Usual loading dose (7.5 mg/kg) administered IM or IV every third half-life, which equals an interval of 8–9 times the serum creatinine in hours; an alternative is 3.5 mg/kg at an interval of 4 times the serum creatinine. Therefore, a 70 kilogram patient who has a creatinine of 2.0 and who has stable renal function should receive 500 mg every 18 hours.
5. **Dose modification in hepatic failure.** None.
6. **Intraperitoneal.** Absorption, blood levels, and urinary excretion are comparable to those with IM injection. Usual dose with normal renal function is 250–500 mg q6–8h in a saline solution of 2.5 mg/ml.

F. Side effects

1. **Toxic effects**
   a. **Ototoxicity** (both cochlear and vestibular) is the most serious side effect. This is related to total dosage (> 15 gm), impaired renal function, previous hearing loss, age (older patients), and concurrent administration of other ototoxic drugs or potent diuretics. The primary deficit is auditory and is often irreversible. Early evidence of ototoxicity includes dizziness, tinnitus, and "fullness" in the ear; high frequency hearing loss is the first detectable abnormality measured by audiogram.
   b. **Nephrotoxicity** is seen in 3–6% of patients receiving the usual dosages. Manifestations are similar to those described for gentamicin and are usually reversible with prompt cessation of treatment.
   c. **Neuromusular blockage with respiratory paralysis** is most commonly seen with rapid intravenous infusion or intraperitoneal instillation.
2. **Irritative effects.** GI distress, stomatitis, and proctitis with oral therapy; pain or sterile abscesses at IM injection sites.
3. **Malabsorption.** Dose-related with oral administration owing to villous cell damage and binding of bile salts or micelle-dependent substances. Impaired absorption includes fat, protein, cholesterol, iron, and some medications such as digitalis.
4. **Hypersensitivity.** Eosinophilia, fever, rash, pruritus (1–3%); anaphylaxis (rare).
5. **Disadvantage.** Resistance of *Ps. aeruginosa* and other hospital-acquired organisms. This has resulted in limited use of kanamycin.

IV. Amikacin (Amikan)

A. Spectrum. Active against most gram-negative bacilli, including most strains resistant to gentamicin and other aminoglycosides. Most bacterial resistance to aminoglycosides is due to inactivation by enzymes to which amikacin is not susceptible. The major mechanism of resistance to amikacin is by a barrier to bacterial cell penetration; amikacin-resistant strains are usually resistant to all aminoglycosides.

B. Indications. Preferred agent for susceptible gram-negative bacilli resistant to other aminoglycosides and alternative, less potentially toxic, agents. Amikacin is also preferred as the initial agent for empiric treatment of serious, hospital-acquired infections at institutions where there is a high incidence of gram-negative bacilli resistant to gentamicin and tobramycin.

C. Pharmacokinetics. Identical to those of kanamycin.

D. Preparations and dosages. Dosing regimens for parenteral administration are identical to those described for kanamycin.

E. Toxicity. Similar to that of kanamycin.

V. Streptomycin

A. Spectrum. Active against *Brucella, Pasteurella, Francisella,* mycobacteria, and many coliforms. Most strains of *Ps. aeruginosa* and 30–50% of *E. coli, Klebsiella, Serratia, Enterobacter,* and indole-positive *Proteus* are resistant. Gram-positive bacteria, including pneumococci and streptococci, are usually resistant. Active against 50% or more of enterococci when combined with penicillin.

B. Resistance. Exposure of the drug may result in conversion of sensitive strains to highly resistant forms within 48 hours. Some strains of bacteria actually become streptomycin-dependent. Streptomycin-resistant bacteria are often sensitive to kanamycin, neomycin, and gentamicin, but strains resistant to these other aminoglycosides are usually resistant to streptomycin.

C. Indications. Clinical usefulness of streptomycin is limited because of rapid emergence of resistance and availability of other effective antibiotics for most gram-negative infections. Best established uses are

1. In combination with penicillin for infections caused by enterococci, especially endocarditis
2. In combination with other antituberculous agents for mycobacterial infections
3. For brucellosis, tularemia, and plague

D. Mechanism of action. Interferes with protein synthesis, bactericidal. Activity is highly pH-dependent, and optimal antibacterial effect is noted in a slightly alkaline medium.

E. Pharmacokinetics

1. **Absorption.** Not absorbed by the oral route.
2. **Distribution.** Peak blood levels of 20–40 μg/ml are achieved with the usual IM dosage. Volume distribution is similar to that of gentamicin.
3. **Excretion.** 30–90% is excreted unchanged in the urine. Half-life of 2.5 hours increases to 100 hours in anuric patients.

F. Preparations and dosages

1. **IM.** 0.5–1.0 gm q12h (15 mg/kg/day). One gram daily may be given safely to patients with normal renal function for 30–45 days. For tuberculosis therapy, 1 gm 3 times weekly is often used.
2. **Pediatric dosage.** 20–30 mg/kg/day.
3. **Dose modification in renal failure.** 7.5 mg/kg/day in mild renal failure (creatinine 1.5–3); 7.5 mg/kg q24–72h with creatinine 3–5; 7.5 mg/kg q72–96h for creatinine > 5.
4. **Dose modification in hepatic failure.** None.

G. Toxicity and side effects

1. **Toxic effects**
   a. **Ototoxicity.** Primarily vestibular, resulting in vertigo, although hearing loss may also occur. This effect is related to both total dosage (prolonged therapy) and excessive blood levels (short-term therapy with large doses). Additional factors in toxicity are renal impairment and age > 40 years. Recovery of vestibular function may take 12–18 months. Nerve deafness is often irreversible, Tinnitus, dizziness, or headache is frequently the first sign of ototoxicity.
   b. **Nephrotoxicity.** Rare, except with excessive doses.
   c. **Neuromuscular.** Circumoral paresthesias, vertigo, ataxia, and headaches may occur a few hours after IM injection. Scotomas, peripheral neuritis, and encephalopathy have been reported. Intraperitoneal or rapid intravenous administration may cause respiratory paralysis, particularly among patients who have received muscle relaxants. Antidotes are neostigmine and calcium gluconate.
2. **Hypersensitivity.** Skin rash or eosinophilia occurs in 2–5% of patients. Angioedema, exfoliative dermatitis, drug fever, and anaphylaxis are rare.

3. **Pain** at injection site (can be relieved by giving with procaine). Sterile abscesses with fever are relatively common.
4. **Hematologic.** Agranulocytosis and aplastic anemia (rare).

VI. **Neomycin**

A. **Spectrum.** Similar to that of kanamycin—good activity against most gram-negative bacteria other than *Ps. aeruginosa* and poor activity against most gram-positive bacteria with the exception of *Staph. aureus.*

B. **Indications.** Strains that have natural or induced resistance to kanamycin are usually resistant to neomycin. Kanamycin is less toxic and therefore preferred for systemic infections. Neomycin is principally used orally for control of hepatic coma in severe cirrhosis and for preoperative bowel preparation in elective colon surgical procedures. The efficacy of topical use is poorly established, and the drug is often inappropriately prescribed for minor wounds and skin infections that would heal satisfactorily with local care. When skin infections are serious or extensive, systemic antibiotic treatment is preferred. Excessive use of topical neomycin may result in contact dermatitis, emergence of resistant bacteria, sensitization to other aminoglycosides, or systemic absorption that can produce neuromuscular blockade, nephrotoxicity, or ototoxicity.

C. **Mechanism of action.** Binds bacterial ribosomes and causes misreading of the genetic code; bactericidal.

D. **Pharmacokinetics.** Oral absorption is poor. Peak serum level with 4 gm PO is approximately 4 μg/ml. Higher and potentially toxic levels may follow oral or topical use in patients with renal insufficiency.

E. **Preparations and dosages**

1. **Oral.** 1–2 gm q4–6h (for hepatic coma) (see p. 290 for use as bowel preparation).
2. **Topical.** Available for dilution in isotonic saline and as an ointment (alone or in combination with polymyxin B, bacitracin, corticosteroids, etc.). The concentration of neomycin should be 5 mg/ml. It should not be used to irrigate body cavities, as it is significantly absorbed by them.

F. **Side effects**

1. **Toxicity.** Ototoxicity, particularly with parenteral therapy. This complication may also follow oral therapy, aerosol application for pulmonary infection, rectal and colonic irrigation of granulating wounds, or application to large inflamed surfaces. The effect is more pronounced in patients with renal failure and in those receiving other ototoxic drugs or potent diuretics. Hearing loss may progress after therapy has been discontinued and is usually irreversible. Neomycin is nephrotoxic when administered parenterally or when excessive quantities are absorbed following topical usage. This drug has the greatest potential of the aminoglycosides for causing neuromuscular blockade with respiratory paralysis.
2. **Hypersensitivity.** Contact dermatitis may occur with topical administration and is most common with repeated use. Sensitivity to neomycin may result in cross-allergy with other aminoglycosides, such as gentamicin, kanamycin, and streptomycin.
3. **Superinfection.** Colonization or superinfection, especially with *Staph. aureus, Ps. aeruginosa,* or *Candida* following topical usage.
4. **Malabsorption.** Dose-related and seen only with oral administration. Mechanisms are villous cell damage and binding of bile acids.

Tetracyclines

I. **Tetracycline HCl** (Achromycin, etc.)

A. **Spectrum.** Effective against a variety of gram-positive and gram-negative bacteria as well as rickettsiae, mycoplasma, and chlamydia. Antibacterial spectrum, although broad, is often unpredictable. Resistant gram-positive organisms include many *Staph. aureus,* most enterococci, 20–30% of group A β-hemolytic streptococci, and occasional pneumococci. *H. influenzae* and *Neisseria* (including gonococci and meningococci) are usually susceptible. Other gram-negative organisms that are less predictably sensitive include *E. coli, Pr. mirabilis, Klebsiella, Citrobacter, Enterobacter, Shigella,* and *Salmonella.* Most strains of indole-positive *Proteus, Serratia, Pseudomonas,* and *Providencia* are resistant. Activity against anaerobes is erratic: As many as 40% of *Peptostreptococcus* and 30–60% of *B. fragilis* are resistant. Cross-resistance among tetracyclines is usually complete, except for some tetracycline-resistant *Staph. aureus* that are sensitive to minocycline.

B. Indications. Tetracyclines are considered antimicrobials of choice for nonspecific urethritis, acne, cholera, chancroid, granuloma inguinale, psittacosis, lymphogranuloma venereum, trachoma, inclusion conjunctivitis, brucellosis, Whipple's disease, tropical sprue, typhus, Q fever, Rocky Mountain spotted fever, and blind loop syndrome. Tetracyclines are also considered first-line agents in *Mycoplasma* infections (along with erythromycin), infections involving *Chlamydia trachomatis,* exacerbations of chronic bronchitis (along with ampicillin), and uncomplicated urinary tract infections (along with several other drugs). Usage in other infections should be based on a lack of suitable alternative agents or antibiotic susceptibility data indicating efficacy. Tetracyclines may be given to penicillin-sensitive patients for syphilis, gonorrhea, relapsing fever, actinomycosis, anaerobic lung abscesses, orodental infections, sinusitis, and other common upper respiratory tract infections other than streptococcal pharyngitis. (Note that age younger than 8 years is a contraindication.)

C. Disadvantages

1. Unpredictable activity against many common bacterial pathogens.
2. Difficulty with parenteral administration.
3. Risk of superinfection, especially thrush and vaginal candidiasis.

D. Mechanism of action. Inhibition of protein synthesis by blockage of binding of transfer RNA–amino acid complex to the ribosome; bacteriostatic.

E. Pharmacokinetics

1. **Absorption.** Approximately 50% absorbed after oral administration, although this is highly variable. Oral absorption is improved if it is taken in the fasting state. Absorption is decreased by chelation with multivalent metallic ions, such as calcium, magnesium, and aluminum. Therefore dairy products and antacids should not be given concurrently.
2. **Serum levels.** Peak serum levels are 1–3 μg/ml at 1–2 hours after oral administration of 250 mg, and up to 4 μg/ml with a 500-mg dose. Intravenous therapy gives levels of 8–10 μg/ml and should not exceed 15 μg/ml. (Toxicity at serum concentrations of 15 μg/ml is true of all tetracyclines.)
3. **Distribution.** Widely distributed in tissues and diffuses well across the blood-brain barrier, even with noninflamed meninges. High concentrations are found in liver, bile, bones, and neoplastic tissue.
4. **Excretion.** Concentrated in the liver and excreted via bile into the intestine, where some is reabsorbed and some is eliminated in the feces. Fifty to sixty percent of parenterally administered drug is excreted in the urine. Serum half-life of 8 hours in normal persons is increased to 100 hours in anuric patients.

F. Preparations and dosages

1. **Oral.** 250–500 mg 4 times daily.
2. **IM.** 100 mg q8–12h. This route of administration should be avoided because of poor absorption from the injected site and severe pain even with the addition of local anesthetics. Peak plasma levels are only 0.15–0.3 μg/ml.
3. **IV.** 0.5 gm bid in solution containing 5 mg/ml infused at < 2 ml/min. Because of complications associated with IV administration, this route should be reserved for serious infections or for patients who cannot take oral drugs.
4. **Pediatric dosage.** 20–50 mg/kg/day PO; 10–20 mg/kg/day IV. This drug should be avoided in children under 8 years.
5. **Dose modification in renal failure.** A relative contraindication; when required with mild renal impairment (creatinine 1.5–5), give 0.5 gm PO every

1–2 days; with creatinine >5, give 0.5 gm PO every 2–4 days. (Doxycycline is the preferred tetracycline in renal failure.)

6. **Dose modification in hepatic failure.** A relative contraindication to tetracycline. Avoid doses > 2 gm/day PO or > 1 gm/day IV.
7. **Pregnancy.** Contraindicated due to potential renal damage and hepatotoxicity in mother and fetal abnormalities (teeth and bones). If less toxic agents are not available, maximum dose is 1 gm/day PO.
8. **Topical.** Should be avoided due to frequent hypersensitization.

G. Toxicity and side effects

1. Nausea, vomiting, anorexia, diarrhea, and epigastric distress occur in approximately 10% of patients receiving 2 gm or more orally. Gastrointestinal distress can be reduced by administration with meals. (Do not use milk products or antacids, since they prevent drug absorption.)
2. Stomatitis, glossitis, vaginitis, proctitis, pruritus ani, and black hairy tongue.
3. Deposition in teeth during early stages of calcification, causing a yellow to brown discoloration. The intensity of pigmentation is dose-related. The drug may also cause disturbances in fetal bone growth. These complications contraindicate the use of tetracycline in children under 8 years old and in pregnant females beyond 5 months' gestation, i.e., during the formation of deciduous and permanent teeth.
4. Hypersensitivity reactions are rare and include rashes (morbilliform, urticaria, or exfoliative dermatitis), fever, angioneurotic edema, eosinophilia, and anaphylaxis. Cross-hypersensitivity reactions between tetracyclines have been noted.
5. IV administration frequently causes thrombophlebitis; IM administration causes severe pain, even when local anesthetics are added, and can cause suppurative myositis.
6. Superinfection, particularly with *Candida, Proteus, Pseudomonas,* and *Staph. aureus.*
7. Pseudomembranous enterocolitis may follow oral or parenteral tetracyclines, but this is rare.
8. Prolonged blood coagulation and increased prothrombin time.
9. **Hepatotoxicity.** The spectrum of liver disease ranges from mildly abnormal results of hepatic function tests to severe liver disease with jaundice, followed by azotemia, acidosis, shock, and death. Liver biopsy in the latter cases shows fatty degeneration with little necrosis or biliary stasis. Hepatotoxicity is usually related to excessive dosage (especially with > 2 gm/day IV), pregnancy, renal disease, or previous hepatic disease.
10. **Antianabolic effect and nephrotoxicity.** Increased BUN due to inhibition of hepatic protein synthesis while catabolism continues, resulting in an increased urea load. Creatinine more reliably indicates nephrotoxicity. In the presence of impaired renal function there may be increasing acidosis, hyperphosphatemia, anorexia, nausea and vomiting, weight loss, and severe electrolyte disturbances. This effect is related to dose, duration of therapy, and extent of previous renal impairment. Nephrotoxicity appears to be potentiated by concurrent administration of diuretics and by previous methoxyflurane anesthesia. Doxycycline does not share this toxicity.
11. **Diabetes insipidus** (demeclocycline), probably due to tetracycline binding of membrane receptors for antidiuretic hormone.
12. Increased intracranial pressure with bulging fontanel in infants.

II. Other tetracyclines. Antibacterial spectrum, toxicity, and contraindications are generally similar to those of tetracycline HCl. Dose and frequency of administration are largely dependent on excretion patterns (Table 12-5).

A. Chlortetracycline (Aureomycin). Metabolized more completely by the liver, and only about 20% recovered in the urine. Half-life is 6 hours. Usual oral and parenteral doses are the same as those for tetracycline. Therapeutic doses cause elevated BUN in patients with renal failure. Should be avoided in pregnancy, hepatic disease, and advanced renal insufficiency.

Table 12-5. Tetracyclines

Agent	Dosage		Oral absorption (%)	Half-life (hr)	Peak serum level (μg/ml)	Excretion		Toxicity		Accumulated renal failure	Vestibular toxicity	Pediatric tooth discoloration
	Oral	Intravenous				Renal (%)	Other	Photo-toxicity	Anti-anabolic			
Tetracycline	250–500 mg qid	250–500 mg q12h	80	10	2–4	60	—	++	+++	+++	0	+++
Chlortetracycline	250–500 mg qid	250–500 mg q12h	30	7	2–7	20	Biliary tract	++	+++	0	0	++
Oxytetracycline	250–500 mg qid	250–500 mg q12h	60	9	1–3	70	—	++	+++	+++	0	+
Demeclocycline	150–300 mg qid or bid	—	70	15	2–4	40	—	++++	+++	+++	0	+++
Doxycycline	100 mg qd or bid	200 mg, then 100 mg bid	90	15	2–6	20	Intestinal lumen	+++	0	0	0	+
Minocycline	100 mg bid	200 mg, then 100 mg bid	100	17	2–4	10	Metabolized	+	+++	0	++++	++

B. **Oxytetracycline** (Terramycin). Somewhat superior to tetracycline in its activity against *Pseudomonas* and may prove effective in occasional urinary tract infections caused by that organism. Half-life is 10 hours. Oral and parenteral doses and precautions are the same as those for tetracycline.

C. **Demeclocycline** (Declomycin). More complete oral absorption and slow renal clearance (half-life 12–17 hours); provides more prolonged blood levels than tetracycline. Usual oral dose is 600–1200 mg/day in 2–4 divided doses. No parenteral form is available. Photosensitivity reactions are more common with this agent, and patients should avoid prolonged exposure to sunlight.

D. **Doxycycline** (Vibramycin). Well absorbed and very slowly excreted in the urine. Half-life is 15–20 hours, compared with 8 hours for tetracycline. The result is sustained plasma levels with infrequent administration. Recommended oral and intravenous dosage is 200 mg initially followed by 100 mg once or twice daily. This provides plasma levels of 1.5–3 μg/ml. For intravenous use the drug should be diluted to 0.5 mg/ml or less and given over at least 2 hours to reduce thrombophlebitis. Usual dose is recommended in renal failure. Principal advantages are ease of oral administration and relative safety in renal failure.

E. **Minocycline** (Minocin). Well absorbed and provides prolonged blood levels due to slow renal excretion. Half-life is 17 hours. Principal advantage is ease of oral administration and activity against some tetracycline-resistant strains of *Staphylococcus*. Recommended oral (or intravenous) dose is 200 mg followed by 100 mg twice daily. Vertigo is a common complaint, and this side effect is unique to minocycline among the tetracyclines, possibly reflecting superior penetration across lipid membranes such as the blood-brain barrier.

Erythromycins

I. **Spectrum.** Active against many gram-positive organisms, including pneumococci, group A β-hemolytic streptococci, and enterococci. Susceptibility of *Staph. aureus* is variable; most are susceptible, but up to 50% of strains are resistant in institutions where the erythromycins are used extensively. *H. influenzae, Neisseria, C. diphtheriae, Pasteurella, Mycoplasma, Listeria, Legionella, Brucella, Rickettsia* and treponemes are usually sensitive. Activity against anaerobic bacteria is erratic at levels achieved with usual oral doses. Coliforms and *Ps. aeruginosa* are highly resistant.

II. **Indications.** Commonly used orally for the treatment of respiratory tract infections (such as pharyngitis, otitis, sinusitis, dental infections, and pneumonitis) and of skin and soft tissue infections, and, in combination with neomycin, for prophylaxis in elective colon surgical procedures. Parenteral use is limited because of a high incidence of phlebitis.

III. **Mechanism of action.** Inhibits bacterial growth by binding with the 50S ribosomal subunit. The site of action is similar to that of chloramphenicol and clindamycin, although these compounds are distinctly different structurally. Resistance of gram-negative bacteria to erythromycin probably results from a barrier to cell-wall penetration.

IV. **Pharmacokinetics**

A. **Absorption.** 40–70% is absorbed in the upper small bowel. Peak levels of 0.5–3.0 μg/ml occur at 1–4 hours following oral administration. Levels of free erythromycin are similar with different oral preparations.

B. **Distribution.** Diffuses readily into body fluids and tissues. Bile levels are high—up to 200 μg/ml. CSF levels are low except in the presence of inflammation.

C. **Excretion.** Concentrated in the liver and primarily excreted as an active drug in the bile. Only 2–15% appears in the urine.

V. **Preparations and dosages**

A. **Oral.** Available as erythromycin enteric-coated base, erythromycin stearate, and erythromycin estolate. Dose is 250 mg–1 gm 4 times daily, usually 500 mg q6h. Erythromycin base and stearate should be taken ½ hour before meals or 2–3 hours after meals. Usual regimen for bowel preparation is 1 gm of the enteric-coated base preparation combined with 1 gm of neomycin at 19, 18, and 11 hours preoperatively.

B. IM. Erythromycin ethylsuccinate, maximum dose 100 mg q8–12h. Injections are extremely painful, may cause myositis, and should be avoided.

C. IV. Erythromycin gluceptate or erythromycin lactobionate, 0.5–1.0 gm q6h given over a 20–60-minute period. High incidence of thrombophlebitis may be reduced with use of central venous line.

D. Pediatric dosage. 30–50 mg/kg/day PO or by suppository; 40–70 mg/kg/day erythromycin lactobionate IV.

E. Dose modification in renal failure. None.

F. Hepatic disease. Usual dose.

VI. Toxicity and side effects

A. GI. Nausea, vomiting, epigastric distress, stomatitis, and diarrhea. GI side effects are common and are dose related. Pseudomembranous colitis is rare.

B. Hepatic. Cholestatic jaundice is noted with erythromycin estolate when used for more than 10 days or with repeated courses. Patients with allergies are particularly susceptible. Liver biopsy shows periportal infiltration with eosinophils. Findings include fever, leukocytosis, eosinophilia, jaundice, abdominal pain, and liver function abnormalities. These usually clear rapidly when the drug is discontinued. Erythromycins other than the estolate have occasionally been reported to be hepatotoxic.

C. Hypersensitivity. Skin rashes, angioneurotic edema, fever, serum sickness, and anaphylaxis (all are rare).

D. Thrombophlebitis with intravenous administration (common).

E. Superinfection (uncommon due to relatively narrow spectrum).

Clindamycin (Cleocin)

I. Spectrum. Effective against most gram-positive bacteria, including streptococci (other than enterococci), pneumococci, and 90–95% of *Staph. aureus*. Active against most anaerobes, including *B. fragilis*. Resistance is noted in some clostridial species (principally *C. tertium, C. ramosum, C. sporogenes,* and *C. difficile*), *Fusobacterium varium,* and occasional peptococci. Approximately 6% of *B. fragilis* strains are resistant, but this incidence shows considerable variation between institutions. All coliforms, *Ps. aeruginosa, Neisseria,* and enterococci are resistant.

II. Indications. Infections in which *B. fragilis* or other penicillin-resistant anaerobes are established or suspected pathogens; intraabdominal sepsis, female pelvic infections and serious anaerobic soft tissue infections are the major indications. Also indicated for infections in penicillin-sensitive patients involving aerobic gram-positive cocci (other than enterococci) or anaerobic bacteria. Clindamycin should not be used for CNS infections. Because of side effects (see below), this drug **should not be prescribed** for mild infections involving organisms sensitive to other drugs, i.e., upper respiratory infections, pharyngitis, bronchitis, otitis media, and acne.

III. Mechanism of action. Binds 50S subunit ribosome, thus causing interference with protein synthesis. The site of action is identical to that of chloramphenicol and erythromycin, although the mechanism of action is different.

IV. Pharmacokinetics

A. Absorption. 90% absorbed with oral administration. Peak serum levels are 2–6 μg/ml with 300 mg PO, 4–10 μg/ml with 600 mg IM, and 8–15 μg/ml with 600 mg IV.

B. Distribution. Diffuses extremely well into tissues, body fluids, and bone. CNS penetration is poor.

C. Excretion. Approximately 10% of the active drug is excreted in the urine, and some appears in stool following enterohepatic circulation; the rest is excreted as inactive metabolites. Serum half-life of 2–3 hours is not prolonged with renal dysfunction but is slightly prolonged with severe hepatic disease.

V. Preparations and dosages

A. Oral. 150–450 mg q6h, usually 300 mg q6h.

B. **IM.** 150–600 mg q8h.
C. **IV.** 150–1200 mg q8h; usually 600–750 mg q8h.
D. **Pediatric dose.** 8–20 mg/kg/day PO; 20–40 mg/kg/day parenterally.
E. **Dose modification in renal failure.** None.
F. **Dose modification in hepatic failure.** Usual parenteral dose is 300 mg q8h.

VI. **Side effects**

A. **Gastrointestinal**

1. **Pseudomembranous colitis** is the most serious side effect.

a. **Symptoms and diagnosis.** Virtually all patients with this condition have diarrhea, which may be noted during treatment or up to 4 weeks after the drug has been discontinued. The diarrhea is usually watery and may lead to severe fluid loss, electrolyte imbalance, or hypoalbuminemia. Abdominal cramps, lower quadrant tenderness, fever, and leukocytosis are common, but none is invariable.

The anatomic diagnosis is generally established by endoscopy, which shows gross or microscopic evidence of pseudomembranes. These are punctate, white or grayish exudative lesions measuring 2–5 cm in diameter; in late stages they may be confluent over several feet of colon. In some instances the mucus must be carefully wiped away to permit detection. Biopsies will confirm the diagnosis, but the endoscopist must be certain to biopsy the entire punctate lesion and carefully transfer the specimen to fixative. Most cases involve the distal colon and can be detected with sigmoidoscopy to 20 cm; 10–30% involve only the proximal colon and require colonoscopy. Pseudomembranous colitis is usually caused by toxic-producing strains of *C. difficile.* A tissue culture assay is able to identify the cytopathic toxin. Stool cultures are less useful because of the sophisticated technology required to recover this microbe, and because some persons harbor *C. difficile* without deleterious effects; the best correlation with enteric disease is toxic detection rather than recovery of the organism.

Note: Pseudomembranous colitis has been noted with numerous antimicrobial agents, the most commonly implicated ones being ampicillin, cephalosporins, and clindamycin. The diagnosis is suspected in any patient with diarrhea that occurs either during or up to 4 weeks after antimicrobial therapy. *C. difficile* is responsible for about 15–20% of cases of "simple" diarrheas associated with antibiotic usage and over 90% of antibiotic-associated cases of pseudomembranous colitis.

b. **Treatment.** (See management algorithm, Fig. 2).

(1) Discontinue implicated antimicrobial drug. Many patients respond well if the diagnosis is detected early and the drug is stopped promptly.
(2) Initiate supportive measures: fluid and electrolyte replacement; in some cases, colloid replacement for hypoalbuminemia.
(3) The role of steroids is not established.
(4) Lomotil and other antiperistaltic agents should be avoided.
(5) Occasional patients require colectomy for toxic megacolon or colonic perforation.
(6) Patients with moderate to severe symptoms or protracted diarrhea should receive specific treatment directed against *C. difficile.* The preferred drugs are oral vancomycin in a dose of 125–500 mg 4 times daily for 7–14 days and oral metronidazole in a dose of 500 mg 3 times daily for 7–14 days. An option for the less seriously ill is cholestyramine (4 gm 3 times daily for 5–10 days), which binds *C. difficile* toxin.

2. **Colitis** and **proctitis** that resemble ulcerative colitis by symptomatology and sigmoidoscopy are less frequent but may also be due to *C. difficile.* Recommendations for evaluation and treatment are the same as those described for pseudomembranous colitis.

3. **Uncomplicated diarrhea** is noted in 10–25% of patients given clindamycin regardless of the route of administration. Approximately 20% of these pa-

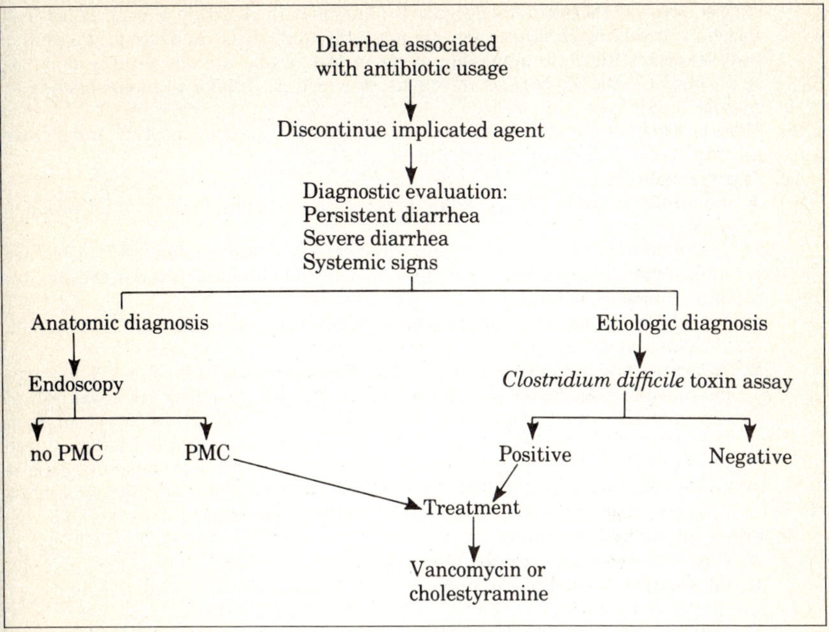

Fig. 2. Management strategy in antibiotic-associated diarrhea.

tients will have *C. difficile* toxin in stool and will respond to oral vancomycin. In other cases the diarrhea may be dose-related and will usually respond to discontinuation or reduced doses.

4. **Nausea, vomiting, and epigastric distress**

B. **Elevated SGOT.** Returns to normal when drug is discontinued or even during therapy. Liver toxicity is seen with high doses but is reversible.

C. Possible **hypotension** or **cardiac arrhythmias** with rapid IV infusion

D. **Neutropenia** (rare)

E. **Morbilliform rash** (3–5% of patients). Other forms of hypersensitivity reactions, including urticaria, Stevens-Johnson syndrome, exfoliative dermatitis, angioedema, and anaphylaxis, are rare.

F. **Thrombophlebitis** (with intravenous therapy).

Chloramphenicol

I. **Spectrum.** Wide spectrum of activity against many gram-positive and gram-negative bacteria, all rickettsiae, and most chlamydiae and mycoplasmas. Pneumococci, *H. influenzae, Strep. pyogenes, Neisseria* (gonococci and meningococci), and anaerobic bacteria (including *B. fragilis*) are almost universally sensitive. Enterococci, *E. coli, Pr. mirabilis,* and *Salmonella* are usually susceptible. *Staph. aureus* is often sensitive, but this varies; as many as 50% of strains are resistant in some hospitals. Activity against *Klebsiella, Citrobacter,* indole-positive *Proteus, Providencia,* and *Serratia* is variable. *Ps. aeruginosa* is almost always resistant, although non*aeruginosa* strains of *Pseudomonas* may be sensitive.

II. **Indications.** The principal advantages of chloramphenicol are its wide spectrum of activity and excellent penetration into tissue. Owing to the rare but serious complication of aplastic anemia, usage should be reserved for **severe infections** for which alternative drugs are not readily available. The best established indications are (1) typhoid fever; (2) bacterial meningitis in patients with penicillin allergy; (3) serious infections involving *H. influenzae* (meningitis or epiglottitis), in which susceptibility tests show resistance to ampicillin or when test results are not yet available; (4) brain abscess; and (5) serious infections in which *B. fragilis* is an established or suspected pathogen.

III. Mechanism of action. Inhibits protein synthesis by suppressing peptidyl transferase activity on the 50S ribosomal subunit; it is bacteriostatic.

IV. Pharmacokinetics

- **A. Absorption.** Good with oral administration, but unpredictable from IM injection sites.
- **B. Distribution.** Excellent penetration in tissue and body fluids. CSF levels are higher than for any other antibiotic—30–50% of blood levels, even in the absence of meningeal inflammation.
- **C. Peak blood levels.** Oral administration of 500 mg: 3–6 μg/ml; 1 gm: 8–15 μg/ml. IV administration of 500 mg–1 gm: 10–20 μg/ml.
- **D. Excretion and metabolism.** Most of the chloramphenicol is inactivated by conjugation with glucuronide in the liver. Bile levels of active drug are about 50% of serum levels. Ninety percent is excreted in the urine, but only 5–10% of this is in the active form. Half-life is 2–3 hours. In the presence of renal failure, large amounts of nontoxic metabolites accumulate, but half–life of the active drug is only modestly increased (3–4 hours). Severe liver disease (jaundice or ascites) may result in high levels of the potentially toxic free drug.

V. Preparations and dosages

- **A. Oral.** 0.25–1 gm q6h, usually 500 mg q6h.
- **B. IM.** Contraindicated due to unpredictable absorption.
- **C. IV.** 0.5–1.0 gm q6h.
- **D. Pediatric dosage.** 25–50 mg/kg/day PO, 100 mg/kg/day IV. Maximum dose for infants < 2 weeks is 25 mg/kg/day PO.
- **E. Dose modification in renal insufficiency.** Usual dose. Maximum daily dose of 2 gm is suggested in severe renal disease.
- **F. Dose modification in hepatic failure.** Maximum daily dose with ascites or jaundice is 2 gm/day; severe liver disease is regarded as a relative contraindication.

VI. Adverse effects

- **A. Hematopoietic effects.** Two distinct types of toxic bone marrow effects occur:
  1. **Dose-related reversible.** Suppression characterized by anemia, low reticulocyte count, increased serum iron, and a cellular marrow showing vacuolization of erythroid elements. Leukopenia and/or granulocytopenia may also occur. These are pharmacologic effects of the drug, caused by mitochondrial injury, which occur during therapy and have a correlation with high blood levels of free drug or extended courses of therapy. Monitoring of blood counts, reticulocyte counts, and serum iron (2–5 times/week) permits early detection of this type of toxicity. Discontinuation of the drug is followed by recovery in 1–3 weeks.
  2. The most dreaded complication is a **non-dose-related idiosyncratic aplastic anemia.** The peripheral blood shows pancytopenia, and marrow may be aplastic or hyperplastic. This complication is often first noted several weeks after the drug has been discontinued. Consequently, monitoring of blood counts may fail to interrupt the disastrous course of events. The incidence is 1/25,000–50,000 courses and appears to be somewhat more common in white female children or with repeated use. The vast majority of cases have followed oral administration of chloramphenicol for trivial infections, usually viral. Aplastic anemia is not exclusively associated with oral administration and has been observed in patients who received only the intravenous form or topical application in the eye. The first manifestations are usually purpura, pallor, or sore throat. Most cases are eventually fatal owing to hemorrhage or infection.
- **B. "Gray syndrome"** (abdominal distention, cyanosis, and circulatory failure) is seen in premature infants, neonates, and occasionally toddlers (≤ 4 months) who are unable to conjugate and excrete chloramphenicol.

C. Nausea, vomiting, unpleasant taste, diarrhea, glossitis, or stomatitis with oral therapy.
D. **Superinfection,** especially with *Candida, Staph. aureus,* or *Ps. aeruginosa.*
E. **Hypersensitivity** (uncommon): skin rashes, fever, angioedema, urticaria, or anaphylaxis.
F. **Optic neuritis,** peripheral neuritis, or delirium, particularly with prolonged therapy (rare).
G. **Pseudomembranous enterocolitis** (rare).

Vancomycin

I. **Spectrum.** Active against gram-positive bacteria, such as streptococci (including enterococci), *Staph. aureus, Staph. epidermidis, pneumococci, Listeria,* diphtheroids, *Actinomyces,* clostridia, and anaerobic gram-positive cocci. Gram-negative organisms are almost uniformly resistant.

II. **Indications.** Vancomycin commonly causes thrombophlebitis and is potentially ototoxic and nephrotoxic. Less hazardous antibiotics are preferred for most infections. Principal uses are (1) in endocarditis and other serious infections involving gram-positive cocci in patients with contraindications to penicillins; (2) as prophylaxis against penicillin endocarditis in patients allergic to penicillin; (3) in *Staph. aureus* shunt infections in renal dialysis patients; (4) in infections involving methicillin-resistant *Staph. aureus* or *Staph. epidermidis*; and (5) as the preferred (oral) drug for *C. difficile* induced enteric disease, especially pseudomembranous colitis.

III. **Mechanism of action.** Inhibits cell wall synthesis by interfering with biosynthesis of peptidoglycan; bactericidal. Activity against staphylococci and streptococci is enhanced by concurrent use of aminoglycosides; activity against *Staph. aureus* is enhanced when combined with rifampin.

IV. **Pharmacokinetics**
   A. **Absorption.** Not absorbed orally, even in the presence of an inflamed bowel. IM injection is very painful. Usual route of administration is IV for systemic infections.
   B. **Distribution.** Intravenous administration of 1.0 gm yields peak plasma concentrations of 25–40 μg/ml and trough levels of 3–10 μg/ml. Distributed well in tissues and body fluids except for low levels in CSF and bile.
   C. **Excretion.** 80–90% of active drug is excreted in the urine. Usual half-life of 6 hours increases to 9 days in the presence of anuria.

V. **Preparations and dosages**
   A. **Oral.** Usual dose for pseudomembranous colitis or antibiotic-associated diarrhea due to *C. difficile* is 125–500 mg qid. Lower doses (125–250 mg) are advocated for patients with severe renal failure.
   B. **IV.** 1.0 gm (15 mg/kg) diluted in 100–200 ml of D5W or saline and infused over 20–30 min q12h. Somewhat lower doses (1.5 gm/day) are recommended when given with an aminoglycoside.
   C. **Pediatric dosage.** 25–40 mg/kg/day IV.
   D. **Dose modification in renal failure**

Creatinine < 1.5	30 mg/kg/day
Creatinine 1.5–3	15 mg/kg/day
Creatinine 3–5	6 mg/kg/day or 30 mg/kg every 4–6 days
Creatinine > 5	1.5–3 mg/kg/day or 15 mg/kg every 7–10 days
Alternative formula:	(Creatinine clearance × 15) mg/day + 150 mg/day

   E. **Shunt infection in dialysis patients.** Single dose of 1 gm IV. (Vancomycin is not significantly eliminated with dialysis.)
   F. **Dose modification in hepatic failure.** None.

VI. **Side effects**
   A. **Ototoxicity.** Deafness is the most significant untoward reaction to intravenous administration. It may be progressive following discontinuation of therapy and is often permanent. It is related to high dosage, extended courses (> 10 days),

improper dose modification in renal insufficiency, concurrent use of loop-inhibiting diuretics or other ototoxic drugs, old age, and previous hearing loss. Ototoxicity is most common with serum levels > 80 μg/ml and is rare with serum levels of < 30 μg/ml.

B. **Nephrotoxicity.** Clinical studies have shown equivocal evidence of nephrotoxicity; studies in animals show a dose-dependent increase in creatinine, which is more severe with concurrent use of aminoglycosides in doses that are not nephrotoxic.

C. **Chills and fever**

D. **Thrombophlebitis.** This may be minimized if the drug is administered in a volume of at least 200 ml, and injected sites are rotated.

E. **Hypersensitivity.** Skin rashes (4–5% of patients); urticaria, eosinophilia, and anaphylaxis.

F. **Peripheral neuropathy** (rare)

G. **Transient hypotension** lasting 2–3 minutes with rapid infusion (over 10 min), owing to depression of cardiac function

H. **Neutropenia.** Has been described.

Sulfonamides

I. **Spectrum.** Wide spectrum of activity against many gram-positive and gram-negative bacteria. Common urinary tract pathogens such as *E. coli* and *P. mirabilis* are usually sensitive. However, *P. aeruginosa,* indole-positive *Proteus,* and *Enterobacter* are often resistant even to the high concentrations achieved in the urine. Respiratory tract pathogens, such as pneumococci, *H. influenzae, Strep. pyogenes,* and *Nocardia,* are usually sensitive.

II. **Indications.** Use of sulfonamides **for systemic infection is limited by** difficulties in maintaining effective blood levels, potential toxicity, bacterial resistance, and availability of alternative drugs. Due to emergence of resistance, these agents are no longer recommended for infections caused by gonococci, meningococci, staphylococci, and *Shigella.* Principal uses are

A. In urinary tract infections caused by susceptible pathogens, particularly *E. coli* and *P. mirabilis.*

B. As antimicrobials of choice for nocardiosis and chancroid; dermatitis herpetiformis (especially sulfapyridine); toxoplasmosis (with pyrimethamine); and trachoma (topical)

C. For rheumatic fever prophylaxis in penicillin-allergic patients

D. In prevention of burn sepsis with topical mafenide acetate (Sulfamylon)

III. **Mechanism of action.** Inhibits folic acid production by competitive antagonism with para-aminobenzoic acid (PABA). Resistant bacteria, like animal cells, use preformed folic acid.

IV. **Pharmacokinetics**

A. **Absorption.** Except for preparations designed for local bowel effects, 70–90% absorbed after oral administration.

B. **Distribution.** Blood levels with usual oral doses are 6–15 μg/ml. Distributed throughout tissues and body fluids; relatively high CSF levels.

C. **Excretion.** Inactivated primarily in the liver by acetylation or conjugation with glucuronic acid. Short-acting sulfonamides are rapidly excreted by the kidney, giving high urine levels of active drug. Excretion is facilitated by increased ouput and urine alkalinization. In renal failure, inactive metabolites accumulate, and the *N*-acetyl derivative contributes to toxicity, including urinary crystallization.

V. **Preparations and dosages**

A. **Oral**

1. **Short-acting.** Sulfadiazine, sulfisoxazole (Gantrisin), sulfachlorpyridazine (Sonilyn), trisulfapyrimidine (triple sulfa—combination of sulfadiazine, sulfamerazine, and sulfamethazine). For urinary tract infections oral dosage is 2–4 gm (loading dose), followed by 0.5–1.0 gm q4–6h. Systemic infections

should be treated with sulfadiazine, 3–4 gm followed by 1 gm q4h, or sulfisoxazole, 3–4 gm followed by 1–2 gm q4h. For children > 2 months: one-half the daily dose initially, followed by 150 mg/kg/day in 4–6 doses. In mild renal insufficiency the usual dose is used, provided that good urinary output can be maintained. With severe renal disease (creatinine > 5) or oliguria, potentially toxic metabolites accumulate and sulfas should be avoided. Severe hepatic disease is also a relative contraindication to systemic sulfas.

2. **Intermediate-acting.** Sulfamethoxazole (Gantanol). Absorbed and excreted more slowly, therefore permitting less frequent administration. Oral dosage is 1.0 gm q12h.
3. **Long-acting.** Offer no advantage over short-acting sulfonamides and are more likely to cause serious toxic reactions.

B. IV. Sulfadiazine sodium and sulfisoxazole diolamine. Dosage is 3–5 gm initially, followed by 30–50 mg/kg q6–8h. Must be diluted and infused slowly and carefully to avoid extravasation.

C. Poorly absorbed

1. **Succinylsulfathiazole** (Sulfasuxidine). This drug is used for preoperative preparation of the large bowel. Coliform bacteria are irregularly reduced by the high concentrations achieved in the colon, but this effect usually requires 5 days. Some patients exhibit a paradoxic increase in coliforms. Usual dose is 3.0 gm q4h for 5 days preoperatively. Efficacy of this preparation for prevention of postoperative sepsis has not been established.
2. **Phthalylsulfathiazole** (Sulfathalidine). Properties and uses are similar to those of succinylsulfathiazole, except that the dose is lower: 1.5 gm q4h.
3. **Salicylazosulfapyridine** (Azulfidine). The sulfa is linked by an azo bond to a salicylate. Efficacy is established for ulcerative colitis and Crohn's disease; this is owing to the antiinflammatory effect of the 5-aminosalicylate moiety rather than to the antibacterial action of sulfapyridine. Usual oral dose is 4 gm/day in 4 divided doses initially; 0.5 gm q6h for maintenance.

D. Topical

1. **Mafenide acetate** (Sulfamylon). In contrast to other sulfonamides this agent is effective against *Ps. aeruginosa* and is not inhibited by pus. Principal use is to prevent burn sepsis. Apply cream to burn once or twice daily, 1/16-inch thick, with sterile gloves. Adverse effects are pain, allergic skin reactions, and acid-base disturbances.
2. Other topical sulfonamides are generally not indicated because of inactivation by pus and cellular debris and because of their propensity to cause allergic reactions.

E. Sulfamethoxazole-trimethoprim (Co-trimoxazole, Bactrim, Septra). A fixed combination of sulfamethoxazole and the methotrexate analogue, trimethoprim. These two antimicrobials block sequential steps in the pathway of folic acid production. Their combined effect is **synergistic** against *H. influenzae, Pneumocystis carinii,* many gram-positive bacteria, coliforms, *Salmonella,* and *Shigella.* Clinical studies have shown efficacy in urinary tract infections, exacerbations of chronic bronchitis, otitis media, pneumocystis, shigellosis and salmonellosis. Trimethoprim achieves good levels in prostatic tissue and is recommended for chronic bacterial infection at this site. Most urinary tract pathogens other than *P. aeruginosa* are susceptible.

1. **Preparations**
   a. **Oral**
      (1) Tablets containing sulfamethoxazole (400 mg) and trimethoprim (80 mg).
      (2) Double-strength tablets (DS) containing sulfamethoxazole (800 mg) and trimethoprim (160 mg).
      (3) Oral suspension with sulfamethoxazole (200 mg/5 ml) and trimethoprim (40 mg/5 ml).
   b. **IV.** Solution containing sulfamethoxazole (80 mg/ml) and trimethoprim (16 mg/ml).

2. **Usual dosages** (normal renal function)
   a. Prophylaxis for urinary tract infection (UTI). ½ tablet/day or 3 times/wk
   b. UTI. 2 tablets or 1 double strength (DS) tablet q12h
   c. Shigellosis. 2 tablets or 1 DS tablet q12h for 5 days
   d. Children with otitis media. Trimethoprim, 8 mg/kg/day, and sulfamethoxazole, 40 mg/kg/day, in 2 divided doses q12h for 10 days
   e. Severe UTI treated with intravenous preparation. Trimethoprim, 8–10 mg/kg/day, and sulfamethoxazole, 40–50 mg/kg/day, given in 2–4 divided doses
   f. **Pneumocystis**
      (1) **Oral.** Trimethoprim, 20 mg/kg/day, and sulfamethoxazole, 100 mg/kg/day, in 4 divided doses for 14 days.
      (2) **IV.** Trimethoprim, 10–20 mg/kg/day, usually 15 mg/kg/day, and sulfamethoxazole. Serum levels should be monitored when using large doses or in presence of renal failure, with the objective of obtaining a 20-minute post-dose level of 5 μg/ml for trimethoprim or 100 μg/ml for sulfamethoxazole.
3. **Pediatric dose** (children > 2 mos)

Weight		Dose (ml oral suspension)	Tablets (q12h)
lb	kg		
22	10	5	½
44	20	10	1
66	30	15	1½
88	40	20	2 or 1 DS

4. **Dose modification in renal failure.** Usual dose for creatinine clearance over 30 ml/min; one-half usual dose for creatinine clearance of 10–30 ml/min; creatinine clearance <10 ml/min (serum creatinine >5) represents a relative contraindication.
5. **Side effects.** Those noted for sulfonamides are the added toxicity ascribed to trimethoprim: dose-related megaloblastic anemia, leukopenia, and thrombocytopenia. The intravenous preparation may be complicated by local irritation and inflammation with extravascular infiltration.
6. **Contraindication.** Megaloblastic anemia due to folate deficiency, pregnancy at term and during the nursing period, infants < 2 months of age, and severe renal failure.

VI. Side effects

A. **Hypersensitivity.** Rash (morbilliform, urticaria, petechiae, purpura, erythema nodosum, exofoliative dermatitis, and Stevens-Johnson syndrome); serum sickness; drug fever; anaphylaxis; eosinophilia; and nephritis. Cross-sensitivity between different sulfonamides (including thiazide diuretics) and sulfonylurea hypoglycemia agents) occurs but is not universal.

B. **GI.** Anorexia, nausea, vomiting (common); pseudomembranous colitis has been noted with sulfamethoxazole-trimethoprim.

C. **Nephropathy.** Crystalline aggregates of the drug may be deposited in the urinary tract, resulting in hematuria, elevated creatinine, renal colic, and irreversible tubular damage. Risk is decreased with high urinary flow rates (> 1 liter/day), urine alkalinization, and use of the more soluble forms such as sulfisoxazole or the trisulfapyrimidine combination. Risk increases in patients with renal failure. Sulfonamide crystalluria is early evidence of this type of reaction. Toxic nephrosis without crystalluria may also occur.

D. **Hematologic.** Acute hemolytic anemia due to hypersensitivity or to glucose-6-phosphate dehydrogenase deficiency; leukopenia, thrombocytopenia, agranulocytosis, aplastic anemia.

E. **Hepatitis.** Unrelated to dose (rare)

F. **Kernicterus** due to release of bilirubin from serum proteins (avoid sulfas in the case of infants and nursing mothers)
G. Enhanced action of **oral hypoglycemics** and **Coumadin anticoagulants**
H. **Vasculitis** due to Schwartzman reaction; precipitation of erythema nodosum or lupus erythematosus.

Polymyxins (polymyxin B and polymyxin E [colistin])

I. **Spectrum.** Active against nearly all gram-negative bacteria except *Proteus, Providencia, Neisseria,* and *Serratia.* Virually all gram-positive bacteria and anaerobes are resistant. Susceptibility patterns of polymyxin B and colistin are identical.
II. **Indications.** Despite excellent in vitro activity against gram-negative bacilli, including *P. aeruginosa,* these agents are seldom indicated for systemic infections. Tissue penetration is poor, and the incidence of serious reactions is high. Principal use of polymyxin B or colistin is for topical therapy.
III. **Mechanism of action.** Interference with lipoprotein in cell membrane, causing permeability changes in bacterial cell walls; bactericidal.
IV. **Pharmacokinetics.** Absorption after oral and topical administration is minimal, even with application to large inflamed surfaces. With parenteral therapy, levels achieved in tissue and body fluids other than urine are generally poor. CNS penetration is nil, even in the presence of meningeal inflammation. Excretion is by the kidneys, and 60–75% is recovered in the urine. Half-lives of 1.5–3 hours (colistin) and 4–7 hours (polymyxin B) increase to 3 days in anuric patients.
V. **Preparations and dosages**
   A. **Polymyxin B** (Aerosporin) (1 mg = 10,000 units)
      1. **Oral.** 75–100 mg q6–8h (10–20 mg/kg/day)
      2. **IM.** 2–2.5 mg/kg/day in 3–4 doses, not to exceed 200 mg/day (Not recommended owing to severe pain; colistin, which contains dibucaine, is usually preferred.)
      3. **IV.** 2.5 mg/kg/day in 2–4 doses by infusion in at least 200 ml over 60 minutes
      4. **Dose modification in renal failure.** 100 mg parenterally every 2–4 days in mild renal insufficiency (creatinine 1.5–5), 50 mg every 2–4 days in uremia
      5. **Dose modification in hepatic failure.** None
      6. **Topical.** 0.1–0.25% as ointment, spray, irrigating solutions, wet dressings, or ophthalmic drops
      7. **Intrathecal.** 5 mg (in 10 ml of 0.9% NaCl)/day 3 times, followed by this dose every other day
   B. **Colistin** (Colymycin)
      1. **Oral.** 100–300 mg q8h (5–10 mg/kg/day)
      2. **IM.** 2.5–5 mg/kg/day in 4 divided doses. In renal disease, use twice the dose recommended for polymyxin B.
      3. **Intrathecal.** Contraindicated due to presence of dibucaine
VI. **Toxicity**
   A. **Nephrotoxicity.** Hematuria, proteinuria, casts, and rising creatinine are common and should signal immediate cessation. Nephrotoxicity often progresses for 1–2 weeks after therapy is discontinued but usually is reversible. Acute tubular necrosis may occur.
   B. **Neurotoxicity**
      1. Facial and peripheral paresthesias, nausea and vomiting, dizziness, ataxia, drowsiness, weakness, visual disturbances, slurred speech, or areflexia. These findings are relatively common and usually reversible.
      2. Neuromuscular blockade, resulting in respiratory muscular weakness. This reaction is not reversed with neostigmine but may respond to calcium gluconate.
      3. With intrathecal polymyxin B, meningeal irritation, headache, fever, and increased cells and protein in CSF.

C. **Pain** with IM injection. Colistin is less painful, since it contains dibucaine.
D. **Hypersensitivity.** Rash, fever, and eosinophilia. Cross-sensitivity between polymyxin B and colistin has been noted.
E. **Superinfections,** particularly with *Proteus,* gram-positive bacteria, and *Candida.*
F. **Nausea, vomiting, and diarrhea** with large oral doses.

Metronidazole (Flagyl)

I. **Spectrum.** Found active against some **protozoa** such as *Trichomonas vaginalis, Entamoeba histolytica,* and *Giardia lamblia.* Also active against **anaerobic bacteria** including nearly all strains of *B. fragilis,* other *Bacteroides* species, *Fusobacterium,* clostridia, anaerobic spirochetes, and strictly anaerobic gram-positive cocci. Microaerophilic streptococci, *Propionibacterium acnes*, and the agents of actinomycosis are resistant. Metronidazole is the only available antimicrobial drug that is consistently bactericidal against *B. fragilis.* Aerobic bacteria and microaerophilic bacteria, other than *Campylobacter fetus* and *Gardnerella vaginalis,* are resistant.

II. **Indications**

A. **Protozoan infections.** Trichomoniasis (only available agent); giardiasis (acceptable alternative to quinacrine); and amebiasis (most effective agent for both colitis and hepatic form).

B. **Anaerobic bacterial infections.** Efficacy established in anaerobic infections with results comparable to those obtained with clindamycin and cefoxitin in genital tract infections or intraabdominal sepsis. Activity is restricted to obligate anaerobes, so metronidazole must be combined with another agent (usually an aminoglycoside) for mixed infections in which coliforms or pseudomonads are considered important. Penicillin is generally preferred for infections involving penicillin-sensitive anaerobes, and metronidazole appears inferior to penicillin or clindamycin in anaerobic pulmonary infections. Special considerations include

1. **Cerebral abscess.** Metronidazole is probably the most effective agent available when anaerobic bacteria are involved; penicillin is sometimes added empirically due to concurrent aerobic bacteria such as *Strep. milleri.*
2. ***B. fragilis* endocarditis.** Preferred agent.
3. **Recurrent or persistent sepsis** owing to *B. fragilis* or other anaerobes, which fails to respond to traditional agents.
4. **Nonspecific vaginitis.** Appears superior to ampicillin and may be used as the primary agent or for ampicillin failures (1.5 gm/day for 7 days).
5. **Crohn's disease** with draining fistulae. Anecdotal reports are favorable.
6. ***C. difficile*–**induced colitis. The efficacy of metronidazole is established, and this drug is considerably cheaper than vancomycin. However, experience with metronidazole is less extensive, and occasional cases of *C. difficile*-induced colitis caused by this agent are a theoretical concern.
7. **Prophylaxis** for gynecologic surgery or elective colon surgery. Reported results are no better than those noted with the neomycin-erythromycin oral preparation for elective colon surgical procedures nor with ampicillin for gynecologic procedures.

III. **Mechanism of action.** Incorporation into microbes requires a low oxidation-reduction potential. Sensitive cells reduce the nitro group on the imidazole ring; the reduced metabolite, which appears to be responsible for both antimicrobial activity and mutagenicity, is only transiently present.

IV. **Pharmacokinetics**

A. **Absorption** with oral administration is generally good; somewhat better in the fasting state.

B. **Serum levels** after a single oral dose of 250 mg and 500 mg are 5–6 mg/ml and 10–12 mg/ml, respectively. A single 2-gm oral dose produces peak levels of 40–50 mg/ml and levels of 5–10 mg/ml 24 hours after administration. Continued administration of 500 mg qid for 3 days gives predose levels of 15–20 mg/ml and peak levels of 25–35 mg/ml. There is no further drug accumulation after the 3rd day. Blood levels with oral, rectal, or vaginal administration approximate those achieved with intravenous administration.

C. **Excretion.** It is excreted primarily in the urine as unchanged metronidazole (15–20%) and as biologically inactive metabolites (20–50%). The drug is extensively metabolized in the liver to products with reduced biologic activity due to oxidation and conjugation. Renal clearance is slow, and the drug has a half-life of 6–10 hours.

D. **Distribution.** Metronidazole diffuses well into tissue and body fluids, including bile, bone, breast milk, placenta, abscesses, and the central nervous system.

V. **Administration and dosages**

A. **Oral.** Usual dose is 250 mg–750 mg bid or tid depending on infection. Recommended dose for (1) trichomoniasis: 250 mg tid for 7–10 days, or a 2-gm single dose; (2) amebiasis: 750 mg tid for 5–10 days; (3) giardiasis: 250–500 mg tid 7 days, or 2 gm/day for 3 days; (4) anaerobic bacterial infection: usual dose is 500 mg qid; (5) *C. difficile*-induced colitis: 250 mg tid for 7–14 days.

B. **Pediatric.** 35–50 mg/kg/day in 3 divided doses.

C. **Topical.** 500-mg vaginal suppositories daily for 10 days for trichomoniasis. These suppositories produce effective serum levels of metronidazole; before the intravenous formulation was available, rectal or vaginal insertion was advocated for nontrichomonal infections in patients unable to take oral medications.

D. **Parenteral.** 15 mg/kg (approximately 1 gm for a 70-kg patient) infused over 1 hour followed by maintenance doses of 7.5 mg/kg (500 mg for a 70-kg patient).

E. **Dose modification in hepatic failure.** Reduced dosage is commonly advocated, but precise recommendations are not available.

F. **Dose modification in renal failure.** None.

VI. **Side effects and toxicity**

A. **GI.** Nausea, metallic taste (very common), anorexia, vomiting, diarrhea, epigastric distress, abdominal cramping, glossitis, stomatitis, furry tongue. Rare patients develop *C. difficile*–induced colitis.

B. **CNS.** Headache, vertigo, ataxia, seizures, and peripheral neuropathy. Peripheral neuropathy is most common and is usually reversible. CNS toxicity is dose-related and caution is advised when the drug is used in high doses, prolonged courses, or in patients with serious hepatic disease.

C. **Hematologic.** Metronidazole is a nitroimidazole and may cause neutropenia. The peripheral white count returns to normal, and treatment need not be discontinued unless neutropenia is severe. Monitoring of WBC and differential is suggested with repeated courses or large doses.

D. **Antabuse-like reaction** owing to accumulation of acetaldehyde by interference with oxidation of alcohol. Ingestion of alcoholic beverages may cause abdominal pain, vomiting, headache, flushing, and hypotension. Patients must be warned of this possible side effect.

E. Oral or vaginal **moniliasis.**

F. **Urine** of some patients receiving large doses will be dark or reddish brown. This has no established significance.

G. **Hypersensitivity** reactions are rare.

H. **Mutagenicity and tumorigenicity.** The reduced product of metronidazole, which is responsible for antimicrobial activity, is also mutagenic in the Ames test and may be carcinogenic in experimental animals. The clinical application of these findings is unclear, since carcinogenesis in animals was observed only with lifetime administration and the metronidazole recipients actually lived longer than untreated controls. No increased incidence of cancer was noted in a 10-year follow-up of women treated for trichomoniasis.

Nitrofurantoin (Furadantin)

I. **Spectrum.** Active against many urinary tract pathogens, including most *E. coli* and enterococci. Approximately 50–75% of *Klebsiella* and *Enterobacter* are sensitive; 30–40% of *Proteus* species are sensitive; but *P. aeruginosa* is resistant.

II. Indications. Restricted to urinary tract infections, due to low tissue levels with systemic therapy. This drug is usually a second-line choice because of its high incidence of side effects. Topical nitrofuran (nitrofurazone) is widely used, but its efficacy is poorly established and it may cause allergic reactions.

III. Mechanism of action. Interference with bacterial enzyme systems, bactericidal.

IV. Pharmacokinetics

- **A. Absorption.** Rapidly and completely absorbed from the GI tract; absorption decreased when administered with antacids.
- **B. Distribution.** Blood levels are low (< 2.5 μg/ml), and therapeutic levels are achieved only in the urine.
- **C. Excretion.** Approximately 40% is excreted in the urine, giving urine concentrations of 15–50 μg/ml. The rest is rapidly inactivated. In renal failure most of the drug is rapidly inactivated. Serum half-life is 20 minutes.

V. Preparations and dosages

- **A. Oral.** 50–100 mg q6h. Nitrofurantoin macrocrystals (Macrodantin) have comparable activity and fewer gastrointestinal side effects.
- **B. IM.** 180 mg bid.
- **C. IV.** 180 mg diluted in at least 500 ml of 5% dextrose in water and administered at a rate of 60 drops/min. Dilute just before use. Usual dose is 180 mg q12h.
- **D. Pediatric dosage.** 5–7 mg/kg/day PO (contraindicated in infants < 1 month). Dosage should be reduced by one-half if treatment is continued beyond 10 days. Parenteral dose is 6.5 mg/kg/day for children over 12 years; no parenteral dose has been established for children under 12.
- **E. Dose modification in renal failure.** Contraindicated due to low levels achieved in urine.
- **F. Dose modification in hepatic failure.** None.

V. Side effects

- **A. GI.** Nausea and vomiting are common with oral therapy. This may be minimized by use of Macrodantin, administration with food or milk, and reduction in dosage.
- **B. Peripheral neuropathy** due to degenerative changes in the anterior horn cells. It may be severe and irreversible, occurring most commonly in patients receiving prolonged therapy and those with impaired renal function. Additional neurologic reactions include headache, dizziness, nystagmus, and drowsiness.
- **C. Hypersensitivity reactions.** Rash, urticaria, and anaphylaxis. Pulmonary sensitivity reactions may be acute or chronic. Acute reactions usually begin within 1 week of treatment, with fever, chills, dyspnea, pulmonary infiltrate with consolidation or pleural effusion, and eosinophilia. Subacute and chronic pulmonary reactions usually occur during prolonged treatment and are characterized by malaise, dyspnea, cough, altered pulmonary function tests, and chest x-rays showing interstitial infiltrates or fibrosis.
- **D. Hematuria** when used for bladder irrigation.
- **E. Intrahepatic cholestasis and toxic hepatitis.**
- **F. Hemolytic anemia** in patients with glucose-6-phosphate dehydrogenase deficiency.

Methenamine

I. Spectrum. Active against common gram-positive and gram-negative urinary tract pathogens. Sensitivity testing is not required, since the antibacterial effect is predictable, provided that the urinary pH is maintained at 6.0 or less. Urea-splitting organisms such as *Proteus* and some *P. aeruginosa* are usually refractory due to their effect of alkalinizing the urine.

II. Mechanism of action. Methenamine is available alone and as the mandelate or hippurate salt. In an acid medium, methenamine releases formaldehyde, which acts as a urinary antiseptic. The organic acids (mandelic and hippuric acid) are also antibacterial in acidic urine.

III. **Indications.** Antibacterial effect is restricted to the urine, and methenamine and its salts should not be used to treat pyelonephritis. Their main use is for prophylaxis or suppressive treatment of urinary tract infections. The urinary pH must be maintained at 6 or less. Generally methenamine is well tolerated, and bacterial resistance does not develop, even with prolonged courses. However, the urinary pH must be continually monitored, and large doses of these urine-acidifying agents are often required. For this reason methenamine is usually restricted to patients who prove refractory to other agents.

IV. **Pharmacokinetics.** Well absorbed after oral administration. Eliminated almost entirely in the urine by glomerular filtration and tubular excretion. The drug is inactive until hydrolyzed in an acid urine.

V. **Dosages and administration**

A. **Methenamine and methenamine mandelate.** Adults, 1 gm PO qid; children 6–12 years, 500 mg qid; children < 6 years, 50 mg/kg in 3 divided doses.

B. **Methenamine hippurate.** Adults, 1 gm PO bid; children 6–12 years, 500 mg bid.

C. **Note.** Urinary pH must be monitored to ensure antibacterial activity. This is usually accomplished by the patient when treatment is on an outpatient basis. The pH should be 6 or less, and supplementary urine-acidifying agents are given accordingly:

1. **Ammonium chloride,** 8–12 gm/day (effective only for a few days, because of renal compensatory mechanism).
2. **Methionine** 8–12 gm/day (disagreeable odor may be disguised by taking with meals; effective in acidifying the urine over prolonged periods).

D. **Dose modification in hepatic failure.** Contraindicated in severe hepatic disease.

E. **Dose modification in renal failure.** The drug (and the acidifying agents) are contraindicated.

VI. **Toxicity**

A. **Gastric distress** due to the release of some formaldehyde in the stomach. Enteric-coated preparations have been only partially effective in reducing this effect.

B. **Hypersensitivity reaction,** usually rash.

C. **Bladder irritation** with dysuria and frequently albuminuria and hematuria. Usually results from large doses for 3–4 weeks. The drug should be discontinued and, if severe, the patient should receive an alkalizing salt such as sodium bicarbonate.

D. **Incompatibilities.** Methenamine should not be given concurrently with sulfas, since the acid urine necessary for activity for methenamine may cause sulfa crystalluria.

Nalidixic Acid (NegGram)

I. **Spectrum.** Active against many urinary tract pathogens, including most *E. coli* and *Proteus*. Less active against *Klebsiella* and *Enterobacter*. Most *Ps. aeruginosa* and gram-positive bacteria, including enterococci, are resistant.

II. **Indications.** Serum levels are relatively low, and use is generally restricted to treatment of urinary tract infections. The principal indication is for lower urinary tract infections involving susceptible pathogens, especially certain *Proteus* strains. Because of the restricted spectrum, it is often necessary to repeat urine cultures during the course of treatment.

III. **Pharmacokinetics.** Well absorbed following oral administration, giving peak levels of 3–65 μg/ml (mean: 25 μg/ml) following a 1-gm dose. Virtually all the drug is eliminated in the urine—15–20% in a microbiologically active form and the rest as inactive glucuronides. Concurrent administration of alkali improves oral absorption and increases urine levels of active drug by increasing dissolution and decreasing renal tubular reabsorption. Half-life is approximately 1½ hours. In renal failure there is delayed excretion of active drug and accumulation of useless metabolites.

IV. **Dosages**

A. **Adults.** Usual dose is 1 gm PO qid. If treatment is continued for > 10–14 days, the dose should be reduced to 2 gm/day. **Children.** Usual dose is 55 mg/kg initially and 33 mg/kg for prolonged treatment.

B. **Dose modification in hepatic failure.** None.

C. **Dose modification in renal failure.** The drug is contraindicated due to low urinary levels of the active form and accumulation of possibly toxic metabolites.

V. **Toxicity and side effects**

A. **GI effects.** Nausea and vomiting are relatively common; diarrhea is infrequent.

B. **CNS toxicity.** Visual disturbances are most frequent. Less common are hallucinations, disorders of sensory perception, convulsions (especially in patients with a predisposition to seizures), and intracranial hypertension in children.

C. **Skin rash.** Photosensitivity urticaria, erythematous or maculopapular.

D. **Cholestatic jaundice** (rare).

E. **Blood dyscrasias** (rare).

F. **Arthralgias or arthritis** (rare).

Antituberculous agents

I. **Isoniazid** (INH)

A. **Spectrum.** Activity restricted to mycobacteria. 1–5% of *Mycobacterium tuberculosis* are resistant. Atypical mycobacteria may be relatively resistant.

B. **Indications**

1. **Active disease.** Disease is considered **active** when (1) AFB smears of cultures are positive, (2) symptoms are ascribed to tuberculosis, or (3) laboratory findings (urinalysis, CSF, serial changes on x-ray, etc.) indicate infection. **All patients with active disease should receive a second antituberculosis agent,** and treatment should be continued for at least 6 months. Interrupted therapy or use of INH as a single agent encourages the emergence of resistant strains.

2. **Preventive therapy** (chemoprophylaxis): Recommended for patients who are at particular risk for developing active disease.

   a. **Dosage** for preventive treatment is 300 mg/day for adults and 10 mg/kg/day up to 300 mg/day for children. The drug is given in a single daily dose and continued for 12 months.

   b. **Indications** for preventive therapy.

      (1) Household members of recently diagnosed cases of active pulmonary tuberculosis should be skin-tested and treated with INH immediately. If the skin test is negative initially and again at 2–3 months after contact is broken, INH is discontinued. If the initial skin test is positive, the person should have a chest x-ray, and if there is no evidence of active disease, prophylaxis is continued for at least 6 months.

      (2) Persons with less extensive exposure should be skin-tested immediately and again at 2–3 months. Chemoprophylaxis is restricted to those with a skin test conversion. This applies to the usual types of exposure by hospital personnel caring for patients with unrecognized TB.

      (3) Skin test conversion within past 2 years. A skin test conversion is defined as a reaction that has increased by at least 6 mm from < 10 mm induration to > 10 mm.

      (4) Positive skin test in persons < 35 years. Chemoprophylaxis recommendations for persons with skin test reactions of unknown duration are based on increased risk of active disease in infancy, adolescence, and early adulthood, and increased risk of INH-associated hepatitis with older age. Preventive treatment is considered mandatory for children < 6 years and is generally advocated for persons 6–35 years. It is not routinely recommended for persons > 35 years of age in the absence of additional risk factors (see **c.**).

      (5) Positive skin test in persons without previous adequate treatment who have chest x-ray changes consistent with inactive tuberculosis.

(6) Positive skin test with additional conditions associated with increased risk factors for TB: prolonged corticosteroid therapy, immunosuppressive therapy, leukemia or lymphoproliferative diseases, unstable diabetes, alcoholism, silicosis, or following gastrectomy.

c. Precautions and contraindications

(1) Pregnant females should have preventive treatment delayed until after delivery.

(2) Acute liver disease is a contraindication, although mild chronic hepatic dysfunction is not.

(3) A history of INH-associated hepatitis or other hypersensitivity reaction contraindicates future use of INH; no preventive treatment is given.

(4) Patients must be highly motivated to ensure compliance.

C. Mechanism of action. Inhibits synthesis of cell wall mycolates by multiplying mycobacteria; bactericidal.

D. Pharmacokinetics

1. **Absorption.** Rapidly and almost completely absorbed from the GI tract.
2. **Distribution.** Diffuses readily into body fluids and tissues.
3. **Metabolism and excretion.** Primarily inactivated by acetylation in the liver. Compared with the parent compound, acetyl derivatives of INH are one-tenth as toxic and one-hundredth as active against mycobacteria. The rate of hepatic acetylation is genetically determined. Approximately 50% of Americans and 90% of Orientals are rapid acetylators. "Slow inactivators" have blood levels of active drug that are 2–5 times higher than those of "rapid inactivators." 50–80% of the orally administered dose is eliminated in the urine; 1–36% is eliminated as free isoniazid, this percentage being inversely proportional to the rate of hepatic acetylation. The serum half-life is more dependent on the rate of hepatic acetylation than on renal function. It is 0.5–5 hours with normal renal function, and 0.7–7 hours in renal failure.

E. Preparations and dosages

1. **Oral.** For adults: 300–600 mg daily, usually 300 mg daily in a single dose (3–5 mg/kg/day). Children: 10–20 mg/kg/day up to 300 mg/kg/day. Higher doses (10–15 mg/kg in adults, 25–30 mg/kg in children) are reserved for selected cases of particularly serious infections and those involving relatively resistant strains, including atypical mycobacteria.
2. **IM.** Same dosage.
3. **Dose modification in renal failure.** Usual dose is given to patients with serum creatinine, < 2 mg/100 ml. Patients with severe renal failure should initially receive 300 mg daily, but subsequent doses are optimally based on serum concentration. INH intoxication is usually associated with serum levels of > 30 μg/ml; the level 24 hours after dosing should be less than 1 μg/ml. Rapid acetylators will usually require no dose reduction in renal failure, while slow acetylators may require a slight reduction, i.e., to 200 mg/day.
4. **Dose modification in hepatic disease.** None.

F. Side effects

1. **Hepatitis.** INH-associated hepatitis is clinically, biochemically, and histologically indistinguishable from viral hepatitis. Transaminase levels are the most sensitive screening test and are generally elevated to 3 times normal in patients with significant disease. Liver biopsies of such individuals usually show acute hepatocellular injury; cholestasis, massive hepatocellular necrosis, and histology resembling chronic active hepatitis are less common. Fever, eosinophilia, and rash are uncommon. It is uncertain whether this liver disease represents a toxic or a hypersensitivity reaction to either INH or its metabolites.

   Mild hepatic dysfunction evidenced by slight or transient elevations in serum transaminase levels ($<$ 2–3 times normal) arises in 10–20% of persons taking INH. Liver biopsies of such individuals frequently show foci of hepatocellular necrosis. This is regarded as a mild reaction that usually occurs in the first 2–4 months of treatment. It is generally self-limited and does not necessitate discontinuation of the drug. When there is symptomatic liver disease, the drug should be discontinued. The incidence of the more severe form of liver disease has a correlation with age: for patients < 20 years it is rare; 20–34 years, 0.3%; 34–49 years, 1.2%; and > 50 years, 2.3%. **Precautions:** All patients receiving INH should be warned of the possibility of hepatitis. They should be advised to discontinue the drug and report if they develop any of the following suggestive symptoms: anorexia, nausea, and vomiting of more than 3 days' duration; fatigue or weakness of more than 3 days' duration; dark urine or icterus. Routine liver functions testing is not recommended, but liver function should be monitored in all patients with hepatitis symptoms. The drug must be discontinued in cases of symptomatic persons with biochemical evidence of hepatitis. If transaminase levels are measured for other reasons in asymptomatic persons and found to be greater than 3 times normal without an alternative explanation, the need for INH must be weighed against possible liver damage. In most instances the liver disease subsides when the drug is discontinued. Persons with persistent biochemical evidence of hepatitis after stopping INH for 2–4 weeks should have a liver biopsy.

2. **Hypersensitivity reactions** are rare and include fever, lymphadenopathy, rash, eosinophilia, agranulocytosis, hemolytic anemia, aplastic anemia, and thrombocytopenia.
3. **Neurotoxicity.** Symmetric peripheral neuritis resembling pyridoxine-deficiency neuropathy is a toxic reaction that is most likely to occur in slow inactivators, malnourished patients, and persons receiving excessive dosage. It may be prevented with pyridoxine (50–100 mg daily), which is recommended routinely for malnourished patients and those receiving over 300 mg/day.
4. Other forms of neurotoxicity include amnesia, convulsions, muscular twitching, ataxia, paresthesias, mental abnormalities, sedation, toxic encephalopathy, and optic neuritis with optic atrophy.
5. **Gastrointestinal.** Nausea, vomiting, and epigastric distress.
6. Interferes with metabolism of diphenylhydantoin (Dilantin); toxic effects of this agent may be potentiated, and the dosage of Dilantin may require reduction.
7. Large doses (15–20 gm/day) may cause metabolic acidosis, elevated blood glucose, seizures, or coma.

II. Ethambutol

A. Spectrum. Active against mycobacteria, including most strains of *M. tuberculosis,* at a 1-mg/ml level. In vitro primary drug resistance has been reported for up to 10% of *M. tuberculosis,* but criteria for susceptibility in these studies may be excessively strict, since "resistant strains" often represent subpopulations within otherwise susceptible populations. Thus, in vitro resistance does not always imply in vivo resistance.

B. Indications. First-line antimycobacterial agent for active tuberculosis. It should not be used as a single agent due to the emergence of resistant forms. Optic neuritis is a relative contraindication. Because of its bacteriostatic rather than bactericidal activity, ethambutol is **not** advocated for short-course treatment.

C. Mechanism of action. Precise mechanism of action is not well established, but it appears to inhibit one or more metabolites of actively growing mycobacteria.

D. Pharmacokinetics.

1. **Oral absorption.** Approximately 75–80% absorbed; absorption is not improved in the nonfasting state.
2. **Peak serum levels** of 2–3 mg/ml are obtained at 2–4 hours after a 15-mg/kg oral dose. Serum levels are undetectable after 24 hours. The drug does not accumulate with continued administration except with renal failure.
3. **Distribution.** Diffuses well into the body fluids and tissue; effective levels (1–2 mg/ml) can be achieved in CSF with inflamed meninges using a dose of 25 mg/kg/day.
4. **Excretion.** Most of the drug is excreted in the urine as active compound; 10–

15% is eliminated in the urine as metabolic products, and 20–25% is eliminated unchanged in the feces.

E. Administration and dosages

1. **Adults.** 15–25 mg/kg/day as a single oral dose. Usual dose is 15 mg/kg. Higher doses (25 mg/kg) may be used initially for severe infections, retreatment cases, and infections involving resistant strains for periods up to 60 days. (Use of > 15 mg/kg/day requires monthly evaluations of visual function, including ophthalmoscopy, finger perimetry, testing of color discrimination, and Snellen visual activity.)
2. **Children.** No dosage is established for children < 13 years.
3. **Parenteral.** Not available.
4. **Dose adjustment in hepatic failure.** None.
5. **Dose adjustment in renal failure.** The drug accumulates in patients with renal impairment, but dosage adjustment formulae are not well established. Recommended dose with a creatinine of 1.5–5 is 10–15 mg/kg/day; for a creatinine > 5 the dose is 5–10 mg/kg/day.

F. Toxicity and side effects

1. **Retrobulbar neuritis** is the most serious side effect and is related to both dose and duration of treatment. Findings include reduction in visual activity, red-green color discrimination, and peripheral visual fields. These changes may be unilateral or bilateral. In most instances eye toxicity is reversible over several weeks or months if the drug is promptly discontinued. Some patients have been subsequently retreated without ill effects.

   Precautions—All patients should be warned to discontinue the drug and have ophthalmologic studies if visual symptoms occur. Evaluation for eye toxicity includes ophthalmoscopy, finger perimetry, testing for color discrimination, and Snellen visual activity test. These should be performed on each eye. Testing should be routinely performed before beginning treatment and when there is any complaint related to vision. The incidence of retrobulbar neuritis is sufficiently rare with a dose of 15 mg/kg/day that most authorities no longer advocate testing at monthly intervals with this dosage; however, such testing is recommended for all persons receiving larger doses and for patients with renal impairment receiving the drug. Care must be applied in assessing visual function due to other possible eye diseases or chance variation. On the Snellen test an otherwise unexplained decrease of 2 lines or 10–20 points is considered significant.
2. **GI.** Nausea, anorexia, vomiting.
3. **CNS.** Headache, peripheral neuritis, confusion, disorientation, hallucinations (rare).
4. **Liver.** Transient elevation of transaminase. (Causal relationship to ethambutal is not established.)
5. **Hypersensitivity.** Anaphylaxis, rash, arthralgia, pruritus, fever (rare).
6. **Hyperuricemia.** Serum urate levels may increase due to decreased uric acid renal clearance. If this occurs, it should be apparent within 3 months. Precipitation of gouty arthritis has been reported.

III. Rifampin

A. Spectrum. Active against many mycobacteria, including over 97% of *M. tuberculosis*. Most strains of *M. tuberculosis* that are resistant to INH and other first-line agents are sensitive to rifampin. *M. kansasii* and *M. marinum* are usually sensitive, but other atypical mycobacteria (*M. avium-intracellulare, M. scrofulaceum,* and *M. fortuitum*) are relatively resistant to this as well as to other antituberculosis agents. Rifampin is also active against gonococci and meningococci, many anaerobic bacteria, most aerobic gram-positive cocci, some aerobic gram-negative bacilli, *Brucella, M. leprae, H. influenzae, C. trachomatis,* and *Legionella*. Most strains of *M. tuberculosis* are susceptible to 0.5–1 μg/ml; most strains of *Staph. aureus* are sensitive at 0.004 μg/ml.

B. Indications

1. **Mycobacterial infections.** Rifampin is a first-line agent for pulmonary and extrapulmonary tuberculosis when combined with other agents. Because of

rapid emergence of resistance it should not be used alone. Advantages include activity against most strains of *M. tuberculosis,* bactericidal action, and penetration into phagocytic cells.

2. **Meningococcal prophylaxis.** Home contacts and close associates of persons exposed to patients with meningococcal infections should be given rifampin. The usual dose is 600 mg/day (10–20 mg/kg/day for children) in a single daily dose 2 hours after a meal for 4 days.
3. Rifampin is not recommended for other bacterial infections as a single agent due to the rapid emergence of resistance. It is highly active against *Staph aureus* and *Staph. epidermidis,* however, and may be used in combination with other antibiotics for serious infections involving these organisms.

C. **Mechanism of action.** Complexes with DNA-dependent RNA polymerase to prevent initiation of messenger RNA formation; bactericidal.

D. **Pharmacokinetics**

1. Well absorbed when taken on an empty stomach.
2. Peak blood levels are 4–32 μg/ml (mean 7 μg/ml) at 2–4 hours after oral administration of 600 mg. Half-life is about 3 hours. Rifampin has the property of penetrating polymorphonuclear cells to provide antimicrobial activity against intracellular organisms. Penetration into bone, tissue, body fluids and CNS is good.
3. Eliminated largely as a deacetylated metabolite that is microbiologically active in the bile. Smaller amounts, predominantly as unchanged drug, are excreted in the urine.

E. **Dosages and administration**

1. **Parenteral.** Available directly from the manufacturer for unusual cases.
2. **Oral.** 600 mg/day 2 hours after a meal as a single daily dose; children > 5 years receive 10–20 mg/kg/day.
3. **Dose modification with renal failure.** None.
4. **Dose modification with hepatic disease.** Severe liver disease (jaundice or ascites) is a contraindication; less severe liver disease is a relative contraindication and requires careful monitering of liver function tests (see **F.1**).

F. **Toxicity and precautions**

1. **Liver disease.** Abnormal liver function tests (elevated transaminase, alkaline phosphatase, and bilirubin) occur in up to 10–15% of patients (usually within the 1st 6 weeks of treatment) but are sufficiently serious to require discontinuation in fewer than 1%. Liver biopsies of such patients generally show widespread degenerative changes with minimal inflammatory reaction. This histologic picture can often be distinguished from INH-associated liver disease, which resembles viral hepatitis. Both the pathologic changes and the deranged liver function tests usually return to normal despite continued use of rifampin. The drug may also interfere with hepatic uptake of bilirubin, causing an elevation of unconjugated bilirubin without hepatic necrosis. Patients with preexisting liver disease and those taking other hepatotoxic drugs are vulnerable to severe liver disease with clinical jaundice. Such patients should be monitored with periodic liver function tests. The drug should be discontinued if there is symptomatic liver disease or progressive abnormalities in liver function tests ascribed to rifampin.
2. **Gastrointestinal.** Nausea, vomiting, and diarrhea; these are infrequently severe enough to require discontinuation of the drug.
3. **Nervous system.** Confusion, lassitude, difficulty in concentration, dizziness, ataxia, painful extremities, numbness, temporary hearing defect (uncommon).
4. **Hypersensitivity.** Pruritus, rash, urticaria, fever, eosinophilia (uncommon).
5. **Hematologic.** Transient leukopenia and thrombocytopenia; positive Coombs test.
6. **Teratogenic** effects have been noted with large doses in animals. This must be considered in the case of female patients who are pregnant or may become pregnant.

7. Patients should be warned that urine, stool, saliva, tears, and sweat may be the orange-red color of the drug.

8. Suppression of both humoral and cell-mediated immunity has been reported, but the clinical significance of these observations is unknown.

9. Intermittent use can cause reactions presumed to be immunologic in origin, including flu-like symptoms, thrombocytopenia, leukopenia, renal failure, and shock. This emphasizes the importance of regular administration.

10. Drug interactions

a. The plasma half-life of rifampin is decreased in patients who take INH and are slow INH inactivators. No dosage adjustment is recommended.

b. PAS interferes with rifampin absorption, so the two agents should not be given concomitantly.

c. Induction of hepatic enzymes may cause reduced half-life of barbiturates; coumadin (prothrombin times must be carefully followed in patients receiving this anticoagulant); Dilantin (susceptibility to seizures may arise); exogenous steroids (patients receiving maintenance doses may develop adrenal insufficiency); exogenous estrogens (women receiving oral contraceptives may become pregnant); and methadone (may cause withdrawal symptoms).

Antifungal agents

I. Amphotericin B

A. Spectrum and uses. Active against most fungi, including *Histoplasma, Coccidioides, Candida, Aspergillus, Blastomyces, Cryptococcus, Sporotrichum,* and Phycomycetes. Inactive against bacteria, including *Actinomyces* and *Nocardia*. This drug is the most difficult to administer and is the most potentially toxic of all antiinfective agents.

B. Mechanism. Amphotericin B is a lactone ring with seven conjugated double bonds that confer rigidity and hydrophobic properties. The drug binds to cell-membrane sterols of fungi (principally ergosterol), resulting in altered physical properties of the membrane with increased permeability and loss of essential metabolites.

C. Pharmacokinetics

1. Absorption. Oral absorption is poor, even in the presence of intestinal ulceration.

2. Distribution. Prolonged plasma concentrations of 1–3 μg/ml are usually achieved with maintenance intravenous administration of 1.0 mg/kg 3 times weekly. Most fungi are susceptible to 0.1–0.8 μg/ml. Plasma half-life is approximately 24 hours. The drug is distributed throughout the body fluids and tissues. CSF levels are approximately one-fortieth those in plasma.

3. Excretion. Only 2–5% is recovered in the urine. Presumably, most of the drug is inactivated or stored in tissue. Good levels are demonstrable as long as 9 days after therapy is discontinued; urinary excretion continues for up to 2–4 months; tissue levels are detectable up to 1 year.

D. Preparations, dosages, and administration

1. IV. Initial dose is 1–5 mg; daily increments of 5–10 mg/day are then given until maintenance dosage is achieved. Maintenance doses vary according to the disease; the maximum is 1 mg/kg/day in adults and 1.5 mg/kg/day in children. The maintenance dose is administered daily or on alternate days, depending on the severity of the disease and the tolerance of the patient. This drug must be dissolved in 5% glucose and water and not saline; no other ingredients should be in the infusion bottle (i.e., vitamins, KCl, etc.). It should be administered by slow infusion over a period of 4–6 hours, preferably with a 22-gauge needle.

Side effects may be minimized by taking appropriate measures.

a. Heparin (20–30 mg/ml) in the IV solution reduces the incidence of thrombophlebitis.
b. Hydrocortisone, 25–50 mg or equivalent doses of another glucocorticoid, in the IV solution or injected into the tubing at the start of therapy will reduce the frequency, but not the intensity, of fever and chills.
c. Premedication with aspirin, 15–20 mg/kg one-half hour before therapy, will reduce chills, fever, and headache.
d. An antihistamine or chlorpromazine 1 hour before therapy will reduce nausea and vomiting.

During therapy, serum creatinine, serum potassium, and hematocrit should be monitored 2–3 times weekly. If serum creatinine exceeds 3.0 mg/100 ml, the dose should be reduced or the interval between administrations increased. Total dose varies with the condition being treated, ranging from 200 mg for candidemia to 2 gm for most systemic fungal infections.

The total recommended dose is not significantly altered by the presence of renal failure.

2. **Intrathecal, intracisternal,** and **intraventricular** (Ommaya reservoir). Subarachnoid injections cause arachnoiditis, and the drug does not reach the basilar meninges well. Intracisternal or Ommaya reservoir infusions are generally preferred. The drug should be dissolved in 5% glucose to give a final concentration of 0.25 mg/ml. The addition of dexamethasone, 0.25 mg/ml, may reduce the local toxic effect. A volume of cerebrospinal fluid equal to the volume to be injected should be withdrawn before injection. The 1st dose is 0.025 mg (0.1 ml), the 2nd is 0.05 mg, and the 3rd is 0.10 mg. Subsequent doses are increased by 0.1 mg until maintenance levels of 0.5–0.7 mg are reached. Injections are given every 2 days until maintenance levels are reached; then they are given twice weekly.
3. **Topical** amphotericin B may be used for lesions localized in the pleural space, urinary tract, joints, superficial lesions, or draining sinus tracts.

E. **Side effects**

1. **Chills and fever, headache, and nausea and vomiting.** These occur in 50–80% of patients receiving full therapeutic doses.
2. **Nephrotoxicity.** A direct pharmacologic effect of the drug, which is dose-related. When renal function is normal before treatment, a total dose of 2 gm or less seldom causes permanent renal disease, less than half of patients receiving 4 gm will have residual disease, and more than 80% receiving over 5 gm will have irreversible nephrotoxicity. Histopathologic studies show necrosis and calcification of convoluted tubules. This is manifested by rising creatinine, potassium wasting (hypokalemia), and defective renal excretion of acid (renal tubular acidosis). Nephrotoxic effects do not progress after therapy has been discontinued.
3. **Thrombophlebitis** is common with intravenous therapy and often requires rotation of injection sites. This complication is minimized by using concentrations of < 0.1 mg/ml in slow infusion, i.e., over 4–6 hours, and by adding heparin or corticosteroids to the infusion fluid.
4. **Anemia** may arise because of direct suppression of erythropoiesis (and sometimes platelet formation). This effect is related to dose and renal status. Anemia and thrombocytopenia are reversible after discontinuation of therapy and do not necessarily represent a contraindication to continued use but may require transfusions during therapy.
5. **Hypersensitivity.** Rash, anaphylaxis.
6. **Arachnoiditis** with intrathecal therapy, indicated by pain, paresthesias, impaired vision, paresis (usually transient), and urinary retention.
7. **Auditory neurotoxicity** is occasionally noted with intracisternal injections.
8. Ommaya reservoirs are often complicated by **blockage** or **bacterial infection.**

II. **Flucytosine** (Ancobon)

A. **Spectrum.** The susceptibility of *Candida* and *Torulopsis* in vitro varies widely between laboratories due to the simultaneous presence of resistant and susceptible forms within a single population of fungi. When detection of resistant subpopulations is minimized, 80–90% of strains are sensitive. *Cryptococcus neoformans* is usually sensitive, but resistance tends to develop during treatment. Secondary drug resistance is less common with *Candida* and *Torulopsis*. Partial resistance of *Aspergillus* has been noted at all concentrations tested. *Histoplasma capsulatum, Blastomyces dermatitidis,* and *Coccidioides immitis* are resistant.

B. Indications. Advantages are relatively low toxicity and good absorption with oral administration. Favorable results have been reported with septicemia and urinary tract infections involving *Candida* and *Torulopsis glabrata*. Ambiguities in the natural course of such infections make these studies difficult to assess, however. Flucytosine has been used as a single agent for cryptococcal meningitis with good initial results, but relapse rates are high, about 50%. At present, this drug should nearly always be used with amphotericin B—a combination that is often synergistic, reduces the dose requirement of amphotericin B alone, and may delay the emergence of resistance to flucytosine. Although experience is limited, the primary indications for flucytosine plus amphotericin B are cryptococcal meningitis, *Candida* endophthalmitis, *Candida* meningitis and (possibly) other forms of disseminated candidiasis. Use in infections caused by other fungi (*Histoplasma, Coccidioides, Blastomyces,* Phycomycetes, *Aspergillus,* and *Sporothrix*) is not advocated.

C. Mechanism of action. Incorporated into susceptible fungi and deaminated to 5-fluorouridine, which acts as a metabolic antagonist by blocking methylation of deoxyuridylic acid by thymidine synthetase. Cytosine arabinoside is a competitive inhibitor of flucytosine. Flucytosine is fungicidal with prolonged contact.

D. Pharmacokinetics

1. **Absorption.** 80–90% of the orally administered dose.
2. **Peak serum levels.** 50–75 μg/ml with 150 mg/kg/day.
3. **Distribution.** Protein binding is minimal, and molecular weight is low. Excellent penetration into tissues and body fluids, including aqueous humor and CNS. CSF levels are 8–15 mg/ml with the usual oral doses.
4. **Elimination.** Eliminated almost entirely by the kidney as unchanged drug in the urine. Half-life with normal renal function is 3–5 hours.

E. Administration and dosages

1. **Oral.** Adults and children: 150 mg/kg/day in 4 divided doses.
2. **Parenteral.** No form available.
3. **Dose modification in hepatic failure.** None.
4. **Dose modification in renal failure.** For creatinine 1.5–3, give 50 mg/kg bid; creatinine 3–5, give 50 mg/kg qid. Dose schedule for creatinine > 5 or rapidly changing creatinine is not established.

F. Toxicity and side effects

1. **Leukopenia, thrombocytopenia, or anemia** especially in patients with renal failure or with serum levels > 100 μg/ml.
2. Hepatic dysfunction, with elevated transaminase as the earliest sign. This is usually asymptomatic and reversible.
3. **Diarrhea and rash** (rare).
4. **Teratogenic** in animals—caution advised in treating females of childbearing age.

III. Miconazole (Monistat)

A. Spectrum and use. Second-line antifungal agent, generally reserved for patients who cannot tolerate or have not responded to amphotericin B. Efficacy has been documented in coccidiodomycosis, candidiasis, paracoccidiodomycosis, and cryptococcal meningitis.

B. Mechanism. Broad spectrum of antifungal and antibacterial activity. Postulated mechanism is interaction with cell membranes to cause leakage of cytoplasmic contents. Effectiveness is decreased with concurrent use of amphotericin B, and the two drugs should not be used together.

C. Pharmacokinetics.

1. **Absorption.** Well absorbed when given orally.
2. **Distribution.** Widely distributed in tissue, although CNS penetration is poor,

necessitating intrathecal administration for fungal meningitis. Peak serum levels with 600–1,000-mg doses are 6–8 μg/ml.

3. **Elimination.** Metabolized in the liver to an inactive form that is excreted in urine, bile, and stool.

D. Dosage. 400–1200 mg q8h.

E. Side effects.

1. **Most common.** Pruritus (25%), anemia (40%), nausea (40%), hyponatremia (50%), and phlebitis. Hyponatremia is the most serious common side effect, is ascribed to inappropriate ADH secretion, and may require voluminous IV infusions.
2. **Occasional or rare.** Fever, chills, tachycardia, arrhythmias, thrombocytosis, thrombocytopenia, leukopenia, elevated liver enzymes, and anaphylaxis. Cardiac toxicity may be related to rapid infusion.

IV. Ketoconazole (Nizoral)

A. Spectrum. Active against most strains of *Candida, Coccidioides, Histoplasma, Blastomyces, Paracoccidioides,* and dermatophytes; less active against *Cryptococcus, Sporothrix,* and *Aspergillus;* inactive against Phycomycetes.

B. Mechanism. Ketoconazole is an imidazole that is structurally similar to miconazole. Like miconazole, the drug inhibits ergosterol synthesis.

C. Indications and dosages. Major advantage over miconazole and amphotericin B is availability in oral form. Efficacy has been demonstrated in chronic mucocutaneous candidiasis, superficial *Candida* infections, dermatomycosis, and paracoccidioidomycosis. Experience with coccidioidomycosis and histoplasmosis is variable; experience with disseminated candidiasis and other deep mycotic infections is too limited for a recommendation. Recommended therapeutic regimens vary considerably depending on the fungus and the site of infection:

1. **Superficial mycosis**
   - a. **Chronic mucocutaneous candidiasis.** 100–400 mg/day for 6–12 months (or indefinitely).
   - b. **Vaginal candidiasis.** 400 mg/day for 5 days.
   - c. **Oral candidiasis.** 200 mg/day for 1–2 weeks.
   - d. **Dermatomycosis.** 200 mg/day for 4–8 weeks.
   - e. **Pityriasis versicola.** 200–400 mg/day for 3–6 weeks.
   - f. **Onchomycosis.** 200 mg/day for 1–12 months.
2. **Deep mycosis**
   - a. **Coccidioidomycosis.** 200–400 mg/day for at least 12 months (or indefinitely).
   - b. **Paracoccidioidomycosis.** 200–400 mg/day for 3–12 months.
   - c. **Histoplasmosis.** 200–400 mg/day for 2–4 months.
3. **Pediatric dosage.** 50 mg/day for children < 20 kg, 100 mg/day for children 20–40 kg, and 200 mg/day for children > 40 kg.

D. Pharmacokinetics

1. **Dosage.** Oral dose is usually one or two 200-mg tablets daily but may be as high as 600–1000 mg/day in some infections. Peak serum level with a 200-mg dose is 2–4 μg/ml at 2–4 hours and 1 μg/ml at 8 hours. Gastric acidity is required for dissolution and absorption. Antacids, anticholinergic drugs, and H_2 blocking agents should be avoided or given at least 2 hours after ketoconazole. Patients with achlorhydria should dissolve the drug in 4 ml of 0.2 N HCl prior to ingestion.
2. **Distribution.** Widely distributed in tissue and body fluid, but penetration into the CNS is poor, should not be used in fungal meningitis. Binding to serum albumin is 99%.
3. **Elimination.** Metabolized primarily by the liver to inactive metabolites, which are eliminated in the urine (10–15%) and bile (50–60%). Only 2–4% of the active form is found in the urine, and 20–65% is present in stool. No adjustment in dosage is necessary for patients with renal failure. Guidelines for patients with severe hepatic disease are not established.

E. Side effects

1. **Hepatotoxicity,** including massive hepatic necrosis

2. **GI.** Nausea, vomiting, and/or abdominal pain in 3%; this is dose related and usually does not require discontinuation of the drug
3. **Skin.** Pruritus in 1–2%, rash in 1%
4. **CNS.** Dizziness, somnolence, and/or headache (rare)

V. Griseofulvin (Fulvicin-U/F, Grifulvin, Grisactin)

A. Spectrum. Active against dermatophytic fungi—*Microsporum, Trichophyton,* and *Epidermophyton floccosum.* Other fungi and other microorganisms are resistant.

B. Indications. Indicated for dermatophytosis, including tinea capitis (scalp), tinea corporis (body), tinea cruris (groin), tinea barbae (beard area), tinea pedis (feet), and tinea unguium (nails). These are the forms of mycotic infection of superficial keratinized tissue caused by dermatophytes. Superficial infections caused by other organisms are not sensitive to the drug; this emphasizes the importance of identifying the responsible agent. Resistant fungi include those causing otomycosis, tinea versicolor (caused by *Pityrosporon orbiculare*), and superficial candidiasis (including nail and intertriginous infections). Treatment is most effective with infections of the feet, palms, and nails. Contraindications include acute intermittent porphyria and hepatic failure.

C. Mechanism of action. Alters orientation of newly deposited chitin in fungal hyphae, affects mitosis, and may compete with synthesis of nucleic acids.

D. Pharmacokinetics

1. **Oral absorption** is variable due to insolubility of the drug in aqueous media of the upper GI tract. Absorption is improved if taken with a fatty meal.
2. Peak **serum levels** following oral administration of 500 mg to fasting adults are 0.5–2 mg/ml at 3–5 hours.
3. The drug is rapidly taken up by living **epidermis,** and the cells contain tightly bound griseofulvin as they mature into horny cells of hair, nails, and keratinized skin.
4. **Excretion.** Eliminated largely as unchanged drug in feces. Only 0.6% of the oral dose is recovered in the urine.

E. Administration and dosages

1. **Oral.** Available in microcrystalline form (larger crystals are outmoded). Adult dose is 500 mg–1 gm/day in a single or divided oral dose after meals. Absorption is increased with high-fat meals.
2. **Pediatric.** 10 mg/kg/day.
3. **Duration of treatment.** Depends on the time required for infected keratinous tissue to be replaced with noninfected tissue. This is usually 4–6 weeks for infections of the body and hair, 6–8 weeks for tinea pedis, and 4–6 months for nail lesions. Refractory infections may require treatment for 1 year or longer.
4. **Dose modification in hepatic failure.** Contraindicated.
5. **Dose modification in renal failure.** None.

F. Toxicity and side effects

1. **GI.** Nausea, vomiting, diarrhea, dry mouth.
2. **Hypersensitivity.** Griseofulvin is prepared from a species of *Penicillium,* but hypersensitivity reactions in pencillin-sensitive persons are unusual. Hypersensitivity reactions include rash, urticaria, arthralgias, serum sickness, angioneurotic edema, and photosensitivity reactions.
3. **CNS.** Headache (often subsides even when drug is continued), confusion, syncope, blurred vision, impaired performance, insomnia.
4. **Leukopenia** (rare).
5. **Proteinuria** (rare).
6. **Interactions.** Decreases activity of coumadin; barbiturates decrease activity of griseofulvin.

13 Prophylactic Antibiotics

I. **General principles.** Antibiotics are considered **prophylactic** when they are used in **clean** or **potentially contaminated** operations with the expectation of preventing infections in the postoperative period. The term **prophylaxis** is not applicable to antibiotics employed for established contamination, since this situation requires actual **therapy**. For example, antibiotic **prophylaxis** can be used in an elective colon operation, but antibiotic **treatment** is used for a perforated appendix.

II. **Guidelines for use of prophylactic antibiotics**

A. **The operation should carry significant risk of contamination or postoperative infection.** Clean procedures such as thyroidectomy, mastectomy, and hernia repair have a low incidence (1–3%) of wound sepsis, and prophylactic antibiotics should not be considered for them. On the other hand, relatively high-risk procedures such as colon or gastric resection or hysterectomy are appropriate settings for prophylactic antibiotics.

B. **The suspected pathogens should be defined, and the antibiotics should be active against them.** This criterion is best satisfied in cardiac and vascular surgical procedures, in which gram-positive cocci, i.e., staphylococci, pneumococci, and streptococci, are the usual pathogens. An antibiotic with a limited spectrum, such as a semisynthetic penicillin and cephalosporin, can be used in this situation.

C. **The antibiotics should be present in effective tissue concentrations at the time of incision.** Experimental studies have shown that antibiotics should be initiated 1–2 hours prior to operation in order to achieve adequate tissue levels in the incision. If the drugs are started during the procedure, there may be a delay in delivery of the drug to the critical site. The drug should be administered approximately 1 hour before the incision is made. Rather than ordering the drug "on call" to the operating room, which could produce unpredictable timing, it is best to have the antibiotic given by anesthesia personnel just before induction.

D. **The drug should be short term and primarily intraoperative.** The rationale for prophylactic antibiotics is protection during operation and in the immediate postoperative period. Extended use of such drugs merely increases the risk of superinfection and does not reduce the subsequent incidence of septic complications. A regimen appropriate for hysterectomy and for cardiovascular and orthopedic procedures is a cephalosporin antibiotic, such as cefazolin or cephalothin, given 1 gm per dose for **three doses,** once 1–2 hours before operation, once during the procedure, and once 6 hours postoperatively.

E. **Potent antibiotics used for resistant microorganisms should not be used prophylactically.** The widespread use of such agents encourages resistance within the hospital flora and thereby renders the antibiotics ineffective. Drugs with a narrow spectrum are preferred, reserving the more potent agents for life-threatening infections that may develop. Thus, aminoglycoside drugs are interdicted, whereas penicillins and cephalosporins are appropriate.

F. **The benefits of antibiotic prophylaxis should outweigh the dangers.** There is a fine line between benefits and risks, particularly when antibiotics are used extensively within a hospital.

III. **Dangers in the use of prophylactic antibiotics**

A. **Untoward effects of drug.** Side effects are either **allergic** or **directly toxic.** For example, patients treated with penicillin may develop rash or fever as a manifestation of allergy; and patients receiving tetracycline can experience direct toxicity to the liver, kidney, or GI tract.

B. Induction of resistant microorganisms in the host's microflora. Sites at greatest risk for changes in the flora are the oropharynx and GI tract. Overgrowth is most commonly seen with

1. Resistant gram-negative bacilli, such as *Pseudomonas, Proteus,* and *Serratia*
2. Staphylococci
3. Fungi

C. Impact on the hospital flora, with the emergence of multiply resistant bacteria. An entire hospital, or specific units within a hospital, can become colonized with highly resistant strains of bacteria that have evolved in response to antibiotic usage. In the present era, gram-negative bacilli have developed resistance to penicillins and to aminoglycosides such as kanamycin and, to a lesser extent, gentamicin. This resistance is mediated by plasmids or R factors that are passed from bacterium to bacterium. Since these extrachromosomal genetic elements code for multiple antibiotic resistances, the use of one antibiotic can select for resistance to as many as three or four others.

D. Delays in diagnosis of occult infection. Intraabdominal abscesses, especially in subdiaphragmatic spaces or in the pelvis, simmer for weeks to months following the use of prophylactic antibiotics. Indolent and often atypical presentations of these infections occur. By the time the infection is obvious, the patient is so weak and debilitated that the prognosis is often grave.

IV. Indications for prophylactic antibiotics

Few controlled, prospective studies are available that precisely define the indications for prophylactic antibiotics. Common usage and custom, rather than scientific judgment, are often the major reasons for use of these drugs. In the following procedures antibiotics are felt to play an important role in protecting the patient against infection in the postoperative period.

V. Cardiac surgical procedures

Valve replacements and procedures requiring cardiopulmonary bypass carry a risk of postoperative infection in the untreated patient of approximately 15%. When a bypass is not used, the risk of infection is approximately 5%. The most common organisms causing infection are staphylococci, particularly *Staphylococcus epidermidis,* and gram-negative bacilli; streptococci, pneumococci, and diphtheroids are also encountered. Prophylactic antibiotics appear to reduce the risk of these infections. Gram-negative bacilli may cause postoperative endocarditis and wound infection, even when prophylactic antibiotics are used.

A rational regimen employs a semisynthetic penicillin, such as oxacillin or nafcillin, or a cephalosporin, such as cephalothin or cefazolin. These agents should be given 1–2 gm per dose, 1–2 hours before the surgical procedure, and continued every 6 hours for a total of three doses (or a maximum of five doses).

Prophylaxis is **not** recommended for cardiac catheterization, angiography, or insertion of pacemakers.

VI. Vascular surgical procedures involving grafts. The risk of infection owing to gram-positive cocci, particularly staphylococci, has been amply documented in vascular surgical procedures. The highest risk is associated with procedures involving a groin incision; gram-negative bacilli can be the source of infection at this site. A cephalosporin regimen, as noted for cardiac procedures (**V**) should be employed.

VII. Orthopedic surgical procedures. Prophylactic antibiotics should be used for total joint replacements involving the hip, knee, or elbow. An antistaphylococcal drug is preferred for such procedures, i.e., a cephalosporin or oxacillin or nafcillin, in the intraoperative period. Similarly, prophylaxis should be used for the placement of pins and other hardware. The most critical determinants in postoperative wound sepsis are the extent of environmental contamination, the length of the procedure, and the skill of the surgeon. (Most authorities recommend prophylactic antibiotics for open fractures. This is more in the way of **treatment,** since contamination is already present. A cephalosporin antibiotic is used in this setting.) There is no indication for prophylactic antibiotics in other forms of elective orthopedic procedures.

VIII. Gynecologic procedures

A. Vaginal hysterectomy in premenopausal women carries a high risk of vaginal cuff infections. Several studies have shown that such infections are reduced by the use of intraoperative antibiotics, such as cefazolin or another cephalosporin. The three-dose regimen of 1–2 gm prior to, during, and just following the procedure is used. Septic complications are less common in abdominal hysterectomies or in procedures involving postmenopausal women, but it appears that prophylactic antibiotics can reduce postoperative endomyometritis and febrile morbidity even in these settings.

B. Cesarean sections, particularly those performed under emergency circumstances, have a high incidence of postoperative wound sepsis. Some clinical trials, although not all, show a reduction with intraoperative cephalosporins used in the same manner as for other gynecologic procedures (**A**). Recent studies have shown that the first dose of the drug can be given after clamping the cord. In elective cesarean sections the septic morbidity is considerably lower, and it is doubtful that prophylactic antibiotics add anything to this already low infection rate.

IX. Elective colon operations

A. Mechanical preparation of the bowel, with the removal of gross fecal material, is an essential part of preoperative readiness for colon operations. However, even with effective mechanical bowel preparation, the wound infection rate in patients **not** receiving prophylactic antibiotics has ranged from 22% to 62%, with an average of about 40%.

B. Risk factors. The major risk factor in a surgical procedure on the colon is the character of the procedure itself, since it requires an incision through an area of bowel heavily colonized by the normal microflora. Other risk factors include

1. Type of operation; low anterior resection appears to be at greatest risk for postoperative wound infection
2. Prolonged procedure
3. Severe blood loss
4. Preexisting stomas
5. Drain left in the wound
6. Underlying disease, especially inflammatory bowel disease
7. Poor nutrition and hypoalbuminemia
8. Extensive preoperative radiotherapy
9. Obstructing cancer
10. Other sites of infection, such as urinary tract infection, pneumonia, and skin infections

C. Tissue levels of antibiotics vs. intraluminal levels. There are two general approaches to antibiotic prophylaxis in a colon procedure: (1) obtaining high tissue levels of antimicrobial drugs and (2) using poorly absorbed antibiotics to achieve high intraluminal concentrations.

1. **Tissue levels.** Current notions of antibiotic prophylaxis owe a great deal to the experimental work of Burke with local staphylococcal infections in guinea pigs. These classic studies demonstrated maximum protection against infection when therapeutic levels of antibiotics were present in tissues at the time of contamination, with rapidly decreasing protection when the drugs were given later. This provides the rationale for administering drugs at least 1 hour prior to the operative procedure. It should be noted, however, that these experiments were performed with a single organism, *Staph. aureus,* which possessed high virulence, using a fixed inoculum. These conditions do not pertain to the mixed aerobic/anaerobic infections associated with colorectal surgery.
2. **Intraluminal levels.** Another approach to prevention of postoperative wound sepsis in colon procedures is **reducing the inoculum of microorganisms** below the critical number for initiating infection. Since the origin of the pathogens in postoperative wound sepsis is the colonic microflora, suppression of this flora in the intraoperative period should reduce the number of bacteria that make their way extraluminally. Small numbers of microbial contaminants can be handled by normal host defense mechanisms, whereas

a large inoculum will very likely cause wound sepsis. This provides the rationale for oral antibiotic bowel preparation.

3. Since certain drugs administered by mouth also produce systemic levels of antibiotics, it is difficult in practice to determine whether protection is based on local suppression of bowel flora or on tissue levels of drug. For example, erythromycin is absorbed by the oral route, although the serum and tissue levels with the dose used in bowel preparations would not be expected to offer a protective barrier. However, oral metronidazole is efficiently absorbed, achieving excellent serum and tissue levels after oral administration.

D. Oral neomycin-erythromycin bowel preparation. A bowel preparation widely used in the United States since 1972 employs neomycin sulfate and an erythromycin base, administered as follows:

Day 1	Low-residue diet. Bisacodyl, 1 capsule PO at 6 P.M.	
Day 2	Continue low-residue diet. Magnesium sulfate, 30 ml 50% solution (15 gm) PO at 10:00 A.M., 2:00 P.M., and 6:00 P.M. Saline enemas in evening until return clear.	
Day 3	Clear liquid diet; supplemental IV fluids as needed. Magnesium sulfate, in dose above, at 10:00 A.M. and 2:00 P.M. No enemas. Neomycin, 1 gm Erythromycin base, 1 gm	PO at 1:00 P.M., 2:00 P.M. and 11:00 P.M.
Day 4	Operation scheduled at 8:00 A.M.	

The neomycin-erythromycin preparation incorporates several desirable features:

1. These drugs achieve very high intraluminal concentrations in the bowel since only 50% of erythromycin and virtually no neomycin is absorbed. Calculating on a basis of 1 liter of colonic contents and 3 gm of each drug, the concentration of erythromycin in the colon should be 0.5–1.5 mg/ml, and that of neomycin, 1.0–3.0 mg/ml. At these concentrations there is excellent suppression of the bowel flora. In the microgram concentrations achieved in the bloodstream, erythromycin has only modest activity against anaerobes, but it is highly effective at the milligram levels found in the bowel lumen.
2. Neither drug of this combination is used clinically in the treatment of postoperative wound infections. Cephalosporins and metronidazole, on the other hand, are possible therapeutic agents.
3. The three-dose schedule of neomycin and erythromycin is meant to permit a high oral dose while avoiding the inconvenience and possible discomfort of taking all the drugs at one moment. Administration at 1:00 P.M., 2:00 P.M., and 11:00 P.M. allows for mixing of the drugs as the bowel contents move down the gastrointestinal tract in wavelike motions. After 11:00 P.M. it is unlikely that any medications would reach the colon, especially with the use of preoperative anticholinergic drugs. It should be emphasized that lengthy 3- or 5-day preoperative antibiotic bowel preparations are not necessary, since the goal of intraoperative suppression of bowel flora can be achieved by the shorter regimen.
4. This short regimen discourages the emergence of resistant bacteria or yeast in the intestinal flora. Prospective studies have shown that these resistant forms do not emerge when this short oral preparation is used.
5. Studies using a placebo comparison have shown no side effects associated with the neomycin-erythromycin bowel preparation.
6. The choice of drugs and the route of administration provide an inexpensive way to achieve adequate preparation of the bowel. At present it is estimated that this oral regimen has a total cost of approximately $5–$10. In comparison, parenteral preparations of cephalosporins can cost $50–$200, depending on the drug, number of doses, and route of administration.

   On the basis of prospective trials, the expected rate of postoperative wound infections is 6–9% when the neomycin-erythromycin bowel preparation is used for elective colon operations. Thus, this bowel preparation is an inexpensive, convenient, safe, and effective method of reducing postoperative wound infections. Any alternative regimen would have to be measured by this standard.

E. Alternative oral preparations. Instead of erythromycin base, alternative regimens have employed tetracycline or metronidazole, along with neomycin or kanamycin. Tetracycline is administered by the oral route. Metronidazole can be given orally, intravenously or intrarectally. Postoperative wound infection rates are approximately 6–10% with either of these regimens, in the same order of magnitude as those achieved with the neomycin-erythromcyin preparation.

F. Parenteral antibiotics

1. Parenteral cephalosporins have been administered prophylactically for elective colonic surgical procedures in lieu of oral drugs. Mechanical bowel preparation is included with all such regimens. Thus far, experience with parenteral agents as the only prophylaxis has been disappointing. Clinical trials with cephalothin and cefamandole produced postoperative wound infection rates in elective colonic procedures of approximately 35%, not statistically different from untreated controls. At the time of this writing, the findings are incomplete for cefoxitin and the third-generation cephalosporins, but the burden of proof remains with the advocates of parenteral regimens.
2. Parenteral cephalosporins have been added to oral bowel preparations in the hope of improving protection against inadvertently introduced organisms. In a clinical trial recently reported, the addition of parenteral cephalothin to the neomycin-erythromycin oral preparation had no impact on the incidence of wound infections. Indeed, there is no evidence at present that parenteral antibiotics add anything to the protection afforded by the various oral preparations such as neomycin-erythromcyin, metronidazole-neomycin, and tetracycline-neomycin. However, should there be a strong feeling in favor of using a parenteral drug, we would recommend the use of cefoxitin, 1 gm before, 1 gm during, and 1 gm 6 hours after the operative incision.

G. Prophylaxis for colon operations performed under emergency conditions or in obstructed patients. Mechanical preparation of the bowel requires a fairly leisurely 2–3-day schedule and cannot be employed in emergency colon procedures. Antibiotics administered by mouth are also inappropriate in such circumstances, since there is not sufficient time for peristalsis to deliver the drugs to the colon. The same problem applies to patients with colonic obstruction, and they should be handled very gently with regard to mechanical cleansing. In cases of severe obstruction, it would be ill advised to attempt any manipulation before operation. Since there is a high risk of postoperative infection in these settings, parenteral antibiotic administration should be employed.

Cefoxitin	2 gm just before surgery, during operation, and q6h/postoperatively for a total of five doses
Metronidazole	500 mg (can be started PO) q8h for five doses

The use of metronidazole alone in this situation is controversial. Most authorities would add a 2nd drug to cover the aerobic flora, such as an aminoglycoside (gentamicin, tobramycin, or amikacin).

X. Operations on the small bowel

A. Because small-bowel contents are liquid and transit time is rapid, extensive preoperative mechanical preparation is unnecessary. Nothing should be administered by mouth for 8–12 hours prior to operation, in order to reduce the volume of intestinal contents. In the upper small bowel, the bacterial flora is sparse, so antibiotics are not required for routine procedures.

B. For surgical procedures on the distal ileum, it seems reasonable to recommend the neomycin-erythromycin oral bowel preparation, since this level of bowel has an intestinal flora similar to, although less complex than, that of the colon.

XI. Abdominal surgery not involving the intestine. If an elective laparotomy is performed it is advisable to evacuate the colon by the use of enemas on the day and evening before procedures not involving the **intestine.** An empty colon can aid in exposure and, most importantly, averts contamination by uncontrolled defecation during the operation. Antibiotic prophylaxis is not indicated in this setting.

XII. Operations on the stomach and duodenum

A. Gastric acid and motility provide effective barriers to contamination of the stomach and duodenum, and the microflora at these sites is remarkably sparse. Elective surgical procedures for peptic ulcer disease are associated with a low rate of wound sepsis, probably as a result of the relatively uncontaminated surgical field. For this reason, prophylactic antibiotics are not recommended in these procedures.

B. Certain disease states alter the control mechanisms of the flora, leading to bacterial overgrowth in the stomach and duodenum:

1. Gastric atrophy and hypochlorhydria
2. Gastric carcinoma or ulcer
3. Bleeding gastric or duodenal ulcer
4. Obstruction at the level of the duodenum or stomach

Wound infection rates in these settings are approximately 30%. This high rate is related to the frequent necessity for emergency intervention and to the high bacterial contamination of gastric and duodenal contents in these disease states.

C. The **bacteriology** of such infections is related to the oropharyngeal flora, along with some coliforms. It is uncommon to find *Bacteroides fragilis* in this situation.

Aerobes	**Anaerobes**
Escherichia coli	*Fusobacterium*
Klebsiella	*Peptostreptoccus*
	B. melaninogenicus

D. A conventional cephalosporin can be used, since the coverage is adequate for the types of bacteria encountered.

Cefazolin **or** cephalothin	1 gm before, during, and q6h after operation, for three to five doses

Alternative drugs include cefamandole and cefoxitin.

XIII. Operations to correct a blind-loop syndrome. A blind loop is associated with heavy bacterial contamination of the small intestine, and a corrective procedure should be done with antimicrobial prophylaxis. It would be best to use the oral preparation, along with a parenteral cephalosporin (such as cefoxitin), since an orally administered drug may not reach the sites of bacterial overgrowth.

XIV. Ischemic bowel disease or vascular catastrophes. In these situations, **treatment** is a more appropriate term, and a broad-spectrum coverage, which in our estimation would include either clindamycin, metronidazole, cefoxitin, or chloramphenicol plus an aminoglycoside (see p. 18–19), should be used.

XV. Biliary tract procedures

Uncomplicated cholecystectomy in a healthy patient with gallstones is associated with a low risk of infection; hence, prophylactic antibiotics are not needed. The major factor in the risk of postoperative wound sepsis is **bactibilia,** colonization of the bile with bacteria from the intestinal tract. Patients with bactibilia at the time of procedure have a 30–40% incidence of postoperative infection; prophylactic cephalosporin can reduce this figure to 5–10%. The following conditions are associated with bactibilia, and indicate a potential need for prophylaxis:

A. Age >70 years
B. Obstruction of the common duct
C. Recent history (within 3–4 weeks) of cholecystitis with fever and/or chills
D. Previous biliary tract surgical procedure

Perioperative cephalosporin has proved successful in such cases. The first dose should be timed approximately 1–2 hours prior to operation and followed by 1–2-gm doses for a total of three to five doses.

Cefazolin	1 gm q8h for three to five doses

This antibiotic achieves high levels in the serum and in the bile, and it covers most of the potential pathogens.

It has been recommended that a Gram's stain of bile be obtained intraoperatively, in order to decide whether prophylactic antibiotics should be started. Any bacteria seen in the gram's stain would constitute "positive" bactibilia. This procedure, however, has proved rather cumbersome, and the risk factors already listed provide sufficient guidelines for preoperative assessment.

An operation for acute cholecystitis or cholangitis obviously requires antibiotics, but these settings are more properly considered **therapy** (see p. 46).

XVI. Urology. The criterion for using prophylactic antibiotics is **bacilluria,** a urine contaminated with $>10^5$ bacteria/ml on an early morning, clean-catch specimen. If the urine is not infected, prophylaxis is **not** recommended. On the other hand, the presence of infected urine indicates that appropriate drugs, chosen according to the sensitivities determined prior to operation, should be employed for procedures done by the transurethral route, such as endoscopy, prostatic resection, and retrograde catheterization. The principle of intraoperative antimicrobial usage applies to this situation as well.

Prophylactic antibiotics have no place in the prevention of urinary tract infections associated with **indwelling catheters.** Use of an antimicrobial agent in this situation serves to select for more resistant organisms to colonize the urine. Urinary tract colonization owing to indwelling catheters is delayed best with a closed drainage system (see p. 312).

XVII. Neurosurgical intervention. The only procedure for which prophylaxis is indicated is insertion of an intraventricular shunt. There is recent evidence that a short course of an intraoperative cephalosporin reduces the risk of infection with staphylococci, particularly *Staph. epidermidis* and diphtheroids. Other neurosurgical procedures are considered "clean" and do not involve prophylaxis. (See Sec. **XXI** for traumatic head injuries.)

XVIII. Pulmonary procedures. There are no controlled studies to test the efficacy of prophylactic antibiotics in pulmonary surgical intervention. It would seem reasonable to use a brief intraoperative prophylactic course for procedures involving transection of the bronchial tree, such as segmental resections, lobectomy, and pneumonectomy. The rationale is that the normal flora may be contaminating the mainstem and initial bronchial branches, particularly when intubation has been performed. Transection of the esophagus during mediastinal surgical intervention also is a situation in which it is reasonable to use prophylactic drugs.

XIX. Elective operations for tuberculosis or coccidioidomycosis. If time permits, and the diagnosis is available in advance, these infections should be treated before operation. For tuberculosis, it is recommended that at least 3 weeks of chemotherapy with INH and rifampin be instituted. Prior to operations for coccidioidomycosis, it is desirable to administer approximately 500 mg of amphotericin B. It should be emphasized, however, that there have been many exploratory operations in which unsuspected tuberculosis or fungal lesions have been entered without chemotherapeutic cover. Prompt institution of antimicrobial agents after operation will usually prevent seeding of the infection into the wound. The feared complications of poor wound healing and draining sinuses were generally seen in the prechemotherapeutic area.

XX. Burns. In their initial period, second- and third-degree burns are vulnerable to infection with group A *Streptococcus pyogenes,* an organism that can normally colonize the skin and nasopharynx. This is the rationale for using penicillin G, in relatively low doses (1.2 million units/day), during the first 3–5 days. There is divided opinion on this point; some authorities recommend penicillin G or a semisynthetic penicillin (oxacillin or nafcillin) or a cephalosporin to add antistaphylococcal cover, while others do not use any prophylaxis in this initial period. As discussed in Chap. 9, topical application of antiseptics is strongly recommended to reduce the colonization of burned tissue by gram-negative and gram-positive organisms.

XXI. Trauma. Traumatic injuries are heavily contaminated by environmental microorganisms, the exogenous flora, as well as those from the host's skin or mucocutaneous surfaces, the endogenous flora. During wartime, it was found that the uniforms and skin of soldiers were covered with a patina of feces, so that soft-tissue injuries could be infected by intestinal bacteria when there had been no damage to the bowel itself.

A. **Serious trauma to a mucosal surface** that harbors a normal flora should be treated with antibiotics. (Since contamination of healthy tissues has already taken place, the use of antibiotics in this setting should be considered **treatment** rather than prophylaxis.) The two major sites at risk are the intestinal tract and the respiratory tract.

B. **Penetrating wounds to the abdomen** should be treated with an antibiotic regimen that encompasses both aerobic and anaerobic bacteria. Since *B. fragilis* is an important pathogen in this situation, an appropriate drug must be included for this organism. Recommended regimens are

clindamycin, chloramphenicol, or metronidazole plus an aminoglycoside
or cefoxitin as a single agent (see pp. 18–19)

Antibiotic therapy should be started as soon as the diagnosis of bowel perforation has been established. Delay increases the risk of serious peritonitis and abscess formation.

C. **Penetrating wounds of the chest** carry a high risk of empyema, lung abscess, or pneumonia. Such injuries should be treated with a cephalosporin that will cover the major pathogens associated with the respiratory tract and some gram-negative contaminants as well.

D. **Human bites** should be treated with penicillin or ampicillin because of the frequency of serious infection associated with such injuries. Multiple organisms can be cultured from these wounds, all from the normal flora of the mouth: group A streptococci, *Hemophilus,* and numerous anaerobes such as *Fusobacterium, B. melaninogenicus,* and anaerobic streptococci (see pp. 197–198).

E. **Animal bites** may also become infected, and the pathogen can be an unusual one, *Pasteurella multocida,* a part of the normal mouth flora of many animals. In general, animal bites are treated with antibiotics only when there is extensive tissue destruction. Cat bites are the most frequently infected, whereas dog bites are only rarely followed by sepsis.
Primary closure and repair should not be attempted with a human bite because of the risk of sepsis. Dog bites, however, can be repaired, even when they involve the face and mucous membranes.
Appropriate consideration should be paid to the prevention of **rabies** (see pp. 198–200 for guidelines).

F. **Major soft-tissue injuries,** especially when there is gross contamination of the wound, should be treated with antibiotics. Although the specific pathogen is unknown at onset, a prudent choice is a cephalosporin. It should be emphasized that the most important means of preventing infection in this setting are judicious debridement and careful wound management.
Antibiotic treatment is usually recommended when adequate debridement is delayed. Such delay may be instituted in order to save important structures, such as tendons, nerves, and fascial spaces; or to attend to the patient's poor underlying condition before undertaking surgical management. Delays may also be caused by logistic problems. In general, a wound that has remained relatively healthy despite delay does not require antibiotics. On the other hand, if delay in debridement manifests itself by local signs of sepsis, including pain, erythema, lymphangitic spread, and formation of a purulent exudate, antibiotic treatment is called for. Systemic signs such as fever, chills, reduced renal function, and jaundice suggest serious sepsis, which is often associated with bacteremia.

G. **Basilar skull fractures** may involve the sinuses or mucous membranes of the nasopharynx. The great risk in this setting is **purulent meningitis,** caused usually by the pneumococcus and occasionally by *Hemophilus,* streptococci, or coliforms. Fractures at other sites on the skull or facial bones also can enter the sinuses and bring the threat of meningitis. Penicillin G in large doses (2–3 million units q4h) has been recommended to avert such serious infections. Some authorities prefer to await the early signs of meningeal irritation and then to initiate treatment for the likely pathogens, all of which are susceptible to conventional antibiotics. The argument against prophylaxis is that antibiotics change the flora of the nasopharynx and sinuses, thereby permitting more resistant organisms to enter the meninges. The most important point to be emphasized is that such injuries carry the **risk of meningitis,** and the patient should be carefully observed during the initial few days for this complication.

XXII. Prophylactic antibiotics to prevent endocarditis in the susceptible host (recommendations based on guidelines from the Committee on Prevention of Rheumatic Fever and Bacterial Endocarditis of the American Heart Association* and Medical Letter consultants†)

A. Conditions appropriate for prophylaxis

1. Valvular heart disease

a. Prosthetic valve

b. Rheumatic valve disease (history of rheumatic fever without valve disease is *not* an indication)

c. Congenital valve disease; an exception is an uncomplicated atrial septal defect

d. Prior history of **endocarditis**

2. Mitral valve prolapse if associated with a mitral insufficiency murmur

3. Idiopathic hypertrophic subaortic stenosis

B. Procedures with established or suspected risk

1. Respiratory tract

a. All dental procedures likely to cause gingival bleeding

b. Surgical procedure or instrumentation of the respiratory tract (use of prophylaxis with fiberoptic bronchoscopy fits this broad recommendation, although the patients do not have bacteremia and we do not advocate prophylaxis in this setting)

2. Gastrointestinal and genitourinary tract

a. Surgical procedure or instrumentation of the genitourinary tract, colon, and gallbladder (use of prophylaxis for colonic endoscopy fits this broad recommendation, although the incidence of bacteremia is low, the risk is not established, and we do not advocate routine prophylaxis in this setting)

b. Obstetric infections, but **not** for routine deliveries

c. Surgical procedure on infected or contaminated tissue

d. The risk appears to be enhanced for patients with prosthetic valves. Some authorities recommend more liberal use of prophylaxis for these patients as, for example, with upper or lower gastrointestinal endoscopy, barium enema, liver biopsy, vaginal delivery, D&C, or IUD insertion.

C. Regimens

1. Procedures involving the respiratory tract

Preprocedure	**Subsequent doses (total 4–8 doses)**
Parenteral	
Penicillin-aminoglycoside regimen (30–60 min preprocedure) Aqueous penicillin G, 1–2 million units IM or IV **plus** procaine penicillin, 600,000 units IM **plus** streptomycin, 1 gm IM	Penicillin V, 500 mg PO q6h
Vancomycin regimen (penicillin-allergic patients) Vancomycin, 1 gm IV over 30 min, starting 60 min prior to procedure	Erythromycin, 500 mg PO q6h
Oral (not recommended for patients with prosthetic valves)	

**Circulation* 56:139A, 1977.

†*Medical Letter on Drugs and Therapeutics* 23:91, 1981.

Penicillin V, 2 gm PO 30–120 min preprocedure	Penicillin V, 500 mg PO q6h
Erythromycin, 500 mg–1 gm PO, 30–120 min preprocedure	Erythromycin, 500 mg PO q6h

2. **Procedures involving the GI or GU tract (parenteral regimens only)**

Preprocedure	Two later doses
Penicillin-aminoglycoside regimen (30–60 min preprocedure)	Same dose q8h twice
Aqueous penicillin G, 2 million units IM or IV **or** ampicillin, 1–2 gm IM or IV	Same dose q8h twice
plus	
Gentamicin, 1.5 mg/kg IM	Same dose q8h twice
or streptomycin, 1 gm IM	Same dose q12h twice
Vancomycin-aminoglycoside regimen	
Vancomycin, 1 gm IV over 30 min, starting 60 min pre-procedure	Same dose q8h twice
plus	
Gentamicin, 1.5 mg/kg IM, 30–60 min preprocedure	Same dose q8h twice
or streptomycin, 1 gm IM, 30–60 min preprocedure	Same dose q12h twice

XXIII. Prophylaxis with other implanted prostheses. There is an ever-growing population of patients with implanted artificial joints or vascular prostheses. Late infections of these devices occur, of unknown pathogenesis, raising the question of whether such patients should be given antibiotic prophylaxis for dental and genitourinary tract procedures, as are patients with valvular heart disease, in an effort to prevent infection. There are no data to demonstrate a salutary effect of prophylactic antibiotics in this situation, so the physician must use clinical judgment in each case. If the consequences of infection would be devasting, it is reasonable to administer a prophylactic penicillin or cephalosporin with the knowledge that its efficacy is presently unproved.

14 Epidemiology and Prevention

Hospital Epidemiology

The hospital ward is the surgeon's workshop. Any break in infection control threatens the patient with the dire complications of sepsis which can undermine the surgical wound and potentially cause greater risk to the patient's life than the original operation.

I. **Rates of infection.** Approximately 20–30% of hospitalized surgical patients have infection, either developing before admission or occurring during hospitalization. A **hospital-acquired** infection is defined as one that manifests itself 72 hours after an admission or after surgery, or is related to a hospital procedure. Medical services tend to have higher rates of **community-acquired** infection, whereas surgical wards have more hospital-acquired ones. Indeed, approximately 70% of all hospital-acquired infections occur in patients who have undergone a surgical procedure.

The incidence of hospital-acquired infection, according to hospital type, is shown below:

University hospitals	6–8%
Community hospitals	6–8%
City hospitals	10–15%

It is estimated that a nosocomial infection increases the length of hospital stay by an **average of 1 week.** The additional cost for each infection is reckoned to be $6,000–$9,000 per patient (as of 1979). The expenses for a nosocomial infection depend on the site. Wound infections are the most expensive and urinary tract infections the least, perhaps less than $1,000 per episode. The annual cost in the United States for hospital-acquired infections is 1 billion dollars, as a low estimate, and up to 10 billion dollars, as a high estimate. These economic factors tell a small part of the story, for each hospital-acquired infection has its own tale of sorrow, disappointment, and tragedy.

II. **Risk factors in hospital**

A. The hospitalized patient is an **altered host.** Impaired immune status may be caused by diseases such as carcinoma, lymphoma, and diabetes, or it may arise from treatment with immunosuppressive drugs.

B. **Compromise of physical barriers** against infection is produced in all hospitalized patients by

Surgical procedures
Urinary bladder instrumentation and catheterization
Indwelling venous and arterial catheters
Respiratory tract procedures, such as nebulization, respirators, endotracheal tubes, and tracheostomies

C. The **hospital environment** tends to breed its own **microflora,** usually comprising highly resistant microorganisms. Antimicrobial usage and semiefficient chemical disinfecting procedures, combined with convenient reservoirs for microbial proliferation, promote the growth of these potentially dangerous pathogens.

D. The **technology of modern surgical practice** has produced the high-intensity support unit, which houses, within a small area, many sick patients all attended by the same staff moving frequently from person to person. Not surprisingly, surgical intensive care units and burn units have the highest incidences of nosocomial infection and present the greatest risk of contact spread of pathogens within the hospital environment.

III. Nosocomial pathogens. With the development of more potent antimicrobial agents, the types of hospital-bred pathogens are increasing in number and variety. Organisms that were not mentioned in microbiology textbooks 20 years ago are now causing epidemics within hospitals. The following findings are based on several surveys; specific percentages vary from hospital to hospital.

A. Gram-negative bacilli. This group, causing 75% of hospital-acquired infections, includes

	Percent*
Escherichia coli	37
Klebsiella	16
Enterobacter	9
Proteus-Providencia	13
Pseudomonas aeruginosa	17
Pseudomonas (other)	2
Serratia	4

The organisms that breed in hospitals tend to be resistant to many antibiotics, and may flourish in epidemic patterns throughout an institution. The antibiotic resistance patterns can be used as epidemiologic markers for the spread of these organisms.

B. *Staphylococcus aureus* currently accounts for 20% of nosocomial infections. The highest incidence of this organism is found in orthopedic, neurosurgical, and cardiovascular units. Although formerly the major culprit in all types of surgical wounds, it is now considerably less frequent with the advent of the gram-negative pathogens. Methicillin-resistant *Staph. aureus* is on the rise nationally, raising the possibility of such a scourge of resistant staphylococcal infections as was seen in the 1950s.

C. Fungi. The commonest pathogens are *Candida* and *Aspergillus*. *Candida* usually causes superficial oral and vaginal infections. The more deep-seated problems arising from it, however, are associated with serious alterations in the immune status of the host. In recent years *Candida* has become a frequent pathogen in general surgical patients, not restricting itself to those with cancer or diabetes.

D. Viruses. Hepatitis is surely the most common hospital-acquired viral infection, especially within hemodialysis units (see pp. 55–59). There is also potential danger of spreading herpes simplex virus, varicella/zoster, and cytomegalovirus within the hospital, especially to patients who are immunosuppressed by underlying disease or chemotherapy.

E. Protozoa. *Pneumocystis carinii* is known to be transmitted within the hospital, primarily among patients with lymphoma and leukemia or other immunodeficiency diseases.

IV. Superinfection. Superinfection is a form of hospital-acquired infection characterized both clinically and microbiologically as a new infection occurring during the course of antimicrobial therapy. It may involve the site of the original infection or may occur at a remote location. Usually an initial response to antibiotics is followed by the recurrence of sepsis with a new resistant pathogen. It is important to establish **clinical evidence** of infection, since cultures of exudates often yield new resistant pathogens during antimicrobial therapy. If the patient is responding to the initial drug, the appearance of a new organism may constitute colonization rather than superinfection, and no changes in the treatment are indicated.

*Incidence based on analysis of approximately 22,000 nosocomial infections involving gram-negative bacteria in 82 United States hospitals in 1979 (from National Nosocomial Infections Study report, CDC, US Dept. Health and Human Services, Annual Summary for 1979).

A. The **incidence** of true superinfection is related to host factors such as age or compromised defenses and to the spectrum of the antimicrobial regimen. Most cases occur in patients who are receiving broad-spectrum antibiotics. Prolonged duration of treatment is an additional predisposing factor.

B. Mechanism. The superinfecting organism may be initially part of the host's own microflora or may be acquired from environmental sources. Antimicrobial drugs encourage these resistant forms by suppressing competing susceptible bacteria. There is an alteration in the host's ecologic balance, and new organisms are acquired to fill the void.

C. Microbiology. Superinfection pathogens are resistant to the antimicrobial(s) being given. Common isolates in these infections are *Staph. aureus, Candida, Ps. aeruginosa, Serratia,* and resistant strains of *E. coli, Proteus,* and *Klebsiella.*

D. Management

1. Prevention is obviously the optimal method of controlling superinfection. It is best accomplished by selecting narrow-spectrum antimicrobial agents that produce minimal changes in the host's microflora. Antimicrobial prophylaxis and extended courses of treatment should be avoided whenever their efficacy has not been established.
2. Mild superinfections can often be eliminated by discontinuing all antimicrobial drugs.
3. Serious superinfections generally require new antimicrobial drugs directed at the new pathogen. An exception is cases involving *Candida;* many patients with localized infections with this organism respond when predisposing drugs are discontinued and intravenous lines are changed. More persistent *Candida* infections need therapy with amphotericin B (pp. 281–282).

V. Types of nosocomial infections. The anatomic site associated with hospital-acquired infections is fairly consistent among various institutions. This repetitive pattern reflects common problems within our hospitals and also suggests that control measures can be applied with an equal chance of success in most institutions.

Site	Percent of nosocomial infections on surgical wards
Urinary tract	45
Wound	30
Respiratory tract	20
Intravascular	5

A. Requirements for nosocomial infection. For infection to spread within a hospital, there must be

1. A source of the infecting pathogen
2. Susceptible hosts
3. A means of transmission

Our modern hospitals have multiple sources—patients, personnel, and environmental reservoirs. The susceptible hosts are always present, since they are the population of patients within the institution. The major factor susceptible to control measures is the means of transmission.

B. Source of pathogens

The sources of infecting organisms are **sick patients** with active disease, **others who are incubating** the disease, and **carriers.** Visitors are only rarely implicated in nosocomial infections. Inanimate objects in the environment become important sources when they are in direct contact with patients, e.g., nebulizers, wound dressings, and intravascular lines. Patients may acquire organisms from their own **microflora,** an endogenous source, although the temporal relationship indicates a hospital-acquired infection.

C. Routes of transmission

Infecting organisms can be transmitted to a susceptible host by **contact** or by a **vehicle,** or they may be **air-** or **vectorborne.** Certain pathogens, particularly the more hardy ones, can employ more than one means of transmission, depending on the available conditions. Others are relatively restricted by their biologic properties. Principles of control within a given hospital depend on knowledge of how each organism is transmitted.

1. **By contact**
   a. **Direct contact** is the most common method within the hospital, since it involves person-to-person transmission.
   b. **Indirect contact** is transmission to the susceptible patient by an inanimate object, such as dressings, bed linens, and contaminated instruments.
   c. **Droplet contact** occurs only at close range, generally less than 3 feet, when a patient is exposed to nasopharyngeal discharges through coughing, sneezing, or talking. The droplets are usually large ones that do not survive well in the air but may be propelled directly to the susceptible host.
2. **By vehicle.** Infecting organisms can be carried by food, water, drugs, blood products, or intravenous infusions.
3. **Airborne.** Certain organisms can remain in suspended small droplets or dust particles for relatively long periods. These pathogens tend to be highly invasive and are transmitted from the air to the respiratory tract or directly through the skin of the susceptible host. For an organism to be capable of airborne transmission, it must have the ability to survive environmental pressures and thereby exist in droplet or dust form; it must also possess a high order of virulence in order to cause disease with a relatively small inoculum through mucous membranes or skin.
4. **Vectorborne.** Arthropod-borne disease is rarely seen within hospitals in developed countries. Such conditions as malaria, carried by mosquitoes, or rickettsial diseases, carried by lice and ticks, are responsible for hospital-acquired infections in the developing countries.

VI. Principles of isolation

A. Prevention. The overriding principle for isolation procedures is the need to protect patients, hospital personnel, and visitors from contact with an infectious agent. As already noted above, the emphasis is on interrupting the chain of transmission. It should be possible to define appropriate barriers for each pathogen without exhausting the limited resources of the hospital staff. **It is poor policy to write a blanket order for "isolation" of all infected cases.** Patients with simple wound infections do not require elaborate glove, mask, and gown techniques to contain the infectious agents.

Handwashing before and after attending to each patient is the major dictum in prevention. Person-to-person spread via contaminated hands is the most important mechanism of transmission in hospitals. Sir William Osler's aphorism is still relevant: "Soap and water and common sense are the best disinfectants."

B. A classification into **five levels of isolation** has been designed that should provide maximum protection against intrahospital spread and at the same time husband hospital resources:

1. **Strict isolation,** to prevent spread of pathogenic agents by both contact and airborne routes.
2. **Respiratory isolation,** to prevent spread of pathogens by direct contact or droplets that are coughed, sneezed, or breathed into the environment.
3. **Protective isolation,** to protect patients with serious impairment of host defenses from acquiring pathogenic and even relatively avirulent organisms. Because of their compromised immune status, such patients are highly susceptible to a variety of microorganisms.
4. **Enteric precautions,** to prevent spread of organisms that are transmitted through direct or indirect contact with feces, urine, or environmental sources within the room. The mode of transmission is generally the fecal-oral route.
5. **Wound and skin precautions,** to prevent transmission of pathogens by direct contact with infected wounds and heavily contaminated articles.

Table 14-1 indicates recommended isolation for several diseases.

Wound Infections

A most frustrating event in surgical practice is the breakdown of a wound by infection. All the careful planning and execution of an operative procedure is totally vitiated by the appearance of infection, which may destroy primary healing, undermine tissue planes, and even invade healthy surrounding tissues.

I. **Rates of infection.** A surgical wound infection can dramatically increase the length and expense of hospitalization. A wound infection at a single site prolongs hospitalization an average of **13 days.** If the wound infection is associated with sepsis at another, often remote, site (a situation encountered in 60% of patients with wound infections), the normal course of hospitalization is increased by approximately **30 days.**

The risk of wound sepsis varies according to the type of operation. As noted in Table 14-2, overall rates from several institutions range from 4.8% to 7.4%.

Approximately 75% of all surgical procedures performed in a general hospital are in the **clean** category. As a guideline to determining whether a problem exists regarding wound sepsis, an institution should estimate its incidence of infection in clean operations and compare it to the published figures of 1.8–5.1%. Occurrences higher than these established rates should be investigated for possible breaks in technique.

The interval between operation and diagnosis of wound infection is rather variable. Fifty percent of wound infections are apparent in the 1st week. There is a late-onset form, representing 5% of wound infections, that occurs 4 weeks or more after the operation. This category comprises mostly patients with implanted devices, such as prostheses, artificial joints, and vascular grafts.

II. **Definitions**

A. A wound is considered **infected** when pus is discharging from it. In terms of classification, it is not essential that the specific microbial pathogen be identified, although this information often is crucial to therapeutic decisions. In actual surgical practice, between 25% and 50% of wound infections are not cultured; if these bacteriologically neglected wounds were deleted from consideration, the statistics would obviously be skewed. Pathogenic bacteria can be recovered with equal frequency from wounds which appear to be healing well, however. Thus, the diagnosis of **infected** vs. **noninfected** is based on clinical grounds—specifically the presence of a purulent discharge.

B. A wound is considered **possibly infected** when there are mild signs of inflammation with a serous discharge, in the absence of true purulent exudate. Tender, erythematous, and indurated areas often can be palpated at suture sites; such "stitch abscesses" are not considered infected unless they drain pus. Possibly infected wounds should be followed on a daily basis for an ultimate decision concerning their status. In some situations it is wise to remove a few sutures and to probe the subcutaneous tissues superficially for pockets of pus.

C. A wound infection is **incisional** when the infection is limited to the superficial wound. Approximately 60–80% of wound infections are in this category.

D. A wound infection is **deep** when there is involvement of structures adjacent to the wound; for example, intraabdominal, retroperitoneal, or deep, soft tissues.

III. **Classification of surgical procedures.** The determinants of wound infection include

Type of operation
Surgical exposure of a mucosal surface harboring a normal microflora
Presence of gross contamination at the operative site

A standard classification has been recommended by the Committee on Control of Surgical Infections of the American College of Surgeons:*

*Adapted from American College of Surgeons, Committee on Control of Surgical Infections of the Committee on Pre- and Post-operative Care, *Manual on Control of Infection in Surgical Patients.* Philadelphia: Lippincott, 1976.

Table 14-1. Infectious diseases grouped according to degree of recommended isolation

Disease	Private room	Mask	Gown	Gloves	Excreta	Blood	Secreta
Strict isolation							
Smallpox	X	X	X	X	X	X	X
Anthrax, inhalation; plague, pneumonic; vaccinia, generalized and progressive, and eczema vaccinatum	X	X	X	X			X
Burn, skin, or wound infection, major, with *Staphylococcus aureus* or group A *Streptococcus* that is not covered by a dressing or that has copious purulent drainage	X	X	(X)	(X)			X
Lassa fever, Marburg virus disease	X	X	(X)	(X)		X	X
Pneumonia, *Staph. aureus,* group A *Streptococcus*	X	X	(X)	(X)			
Diphtheria, pharyngeal or cutaneous	X	X	(X)				X
Varicella (chickenpox); herpes zoster, disseminated	X	X*	X	X			X
Congenital rubella syndrome; disseminated neonatal Herpesvirus hominis (herpex simplex)	X		(X)		X	X	X
Rabies	X			(X)			X
Respiratory isolation							
Tuberculosis, pulmonary (including tuberculosis of the respiratory tract), suspected or sputum-positive (smear)	X	X*					X
Meningococcal meningitis; meningococcemia	X	X					
Measles (rubeola); mumps; rubella (German measles); pertussis (whooping cough)	X	X*					X
Enteric precautions	D		(X)	(X)	X		
Cholera; colitis, *Clostridium difficile;* Gastroenteritis, enteropathogenic or enterotoxigenic *Escherichia coli; Salmonella; Shigella; Yersinia enterocolitica;* typhoid fever							
Diarrhea, acute, with suspected infectious etiology	D		(X)	(X)	X		X
Hepatitis, viral types A, B, or unspecified	D				X	X	X
Wound and skin precautions							
Gas gangrene (due to *C. perfringens*)	D			(X)			X
Herpes zoster, localized	D	X	X	X			X
Burn, skin, or wound infections, limited, including infections with *Staph. aureus* or group A *Streptococcus,* that are covered and the discharge adequately contained by a dressing; plague, bubonic	D	(X)	(X)	(X)			X
Burn, skin, or wound infections, major (**except** *Staph. aureus* and group A *streptococcus,* see Strict Isolation), that are not covered by a dressing or that have copious purulent drainage; Melioidosis, extrapulmonary, with draining sinuses	D		X	X			X

Table 14-1 (continued)

Disease	Private room	Mask	Gown	Gloves	Excreta	Blood	Secreta
Discharge precautions—oral and lesion secretions							X
Actinomycosis, draining lesions; anthrax (cutaneous); brucellosis, draining lesions; burn infection, minor; Candidiasis, mucocutaneous; coccidioidomycosis, draining lesions; conjunctivitis, acute bacterial (including gonococcal); conjunctivitis, viral; gonococcal ophthalmia neonatorum; gonorrhea; granuloma inguinale; herpangina; herpes oralis; *Herpesvirus hominis* (herpes simplex), except disseminated neonatal disease; infectious mononucleosis; keratoconjunctivitis, infectious; listeriosis; lymphogranuloma venereum; melioidosis, pulmonary; *Mycoplasma pneumoniae* pneumonia; nocardiasis, draining lesions; orf; pneumonia, bacterial, if not covered elsewhere; psittacosis; Q fever; respiratory infectious disease, acute (if not covered elsewhere); scarlet fever; skin lesion, minor; streptococcal pharyngitis; syphilis, mucocutaneous; trachoma, acute; tuberculosis, extrapulmonary, draining lesions; tularemia, draining lesion; wound infections, minor.							
Discharge precautions—excretions					X		
Amebiasis (amebic dysentery); *C. perfringens* (*C. welchii*) food poisoning; enterobiasis; giardiasis; hand, foot, and mouth disease; herpangina; infectious lymphocytosis; leptospirosis (urine only); meningitis, aseptic; pleurodynia; poliomyelitis; staphylococcal food poisoning; tapeworm disease (only with *Hymenolepis nana* and *Taenia solium* [pork]); viral diseases, other (ECHO or Coxsackie gastroenteritis, pericarditis, myocarditis, meningitis)							
Blood precautions						X	
Arthropod-borne viral fevers (dengue, yellow fever, Colorado tick fever); hepatitis, viral type A, B, or unspecified; malaria							

X = recommended at all times; Ⓧ = with direct contact; X* = for susceptibles; D = desirable, but optional.

Source: U.S. Department of Health and Human Services, Centers for Disease Control, Center for Infectious Disease, Atlanta, Georgia, *Guidelines for Prevention and Control of Nosocomial Infections*. July 1982, 1–9.

Table 14-2. Incidence of wound sepsis according to type of operation

	Percentage of wound sepsis		
Type of operation	Five hospitals (UV light study)	Foothills Hospital, Calgary	Presbyterian-St. Luke's Hospital, Chicago
Clean (75%)*	5.1	1.8	4.2
Clean-contaminated (15%)*	10.8	8.9	not given
Contaminated (5%)*	16.3	21.5	6.0
Dirty (5%)*	28.5	38.3	10.1
Overall	7.4	4.8	4.8

*Percent of total operations.

A. A **clean operation** is a nontraumatic, uninfected operative procedure in which neither the respiratory, alimentary, nor genitourinary (GU) tract nor the oropharyngeal cavities are entered. Clean wounds are elective, primarily closed, and undrained.

Clean operations
Nontraumatic
No inflammation encountered
No break in technique
Respiratory, alimentary, and GU tracts not entered

B. A **clean-contaminated operation** is a procedure in which the respiratory, alimentary, or genitourinary tract is entered without unusual contamination, or a wound is mechanically drained.

Clean-contaminated operations
Gastrointestinal or respiratory tract entered without significant spillage
Appendectomy
Oropharynx entered
Vagina entered
Genitourinary tract entered in absence of infected urine
Biliary tract entered in absence of infected bile
Minor break in technique

C. A **contaminated operation** includes open, fresh traumatic wounds, operations with a major break in sterile technique (e.g., open cardiac massage), and incisions encountering acute, nonpurulent inflammation.

Contaminated operations
Major break in technique
Gross spillage from gastrointestinal tract
Traumatic wound, fresh
Entrance of genitourinary or biliary tracts in presence of infected urine or bile

D. A **dirty and infected operation** includes old traumatic wounds and those involving clinical infection or perforated viscera. This definition suggests that the organisms causing postoperative infection are present in the operative field **before** operation.

Dirty and infected operations
Acute bacterial inflammation encountered, with pus
Transection of "clean" tissue for the purpose of surgical access to a collection of pus
Perforated viscus encountered

Traumatic wound with retained devitalized tissue, foreign bodies, fecal contamination, and/or delayed treatment, or from dirty source

IV. Risk factors. Risk factors play a major role in determining whether a wound infection develops in the postoperative course.

A. Microbial contamination. The type of pathogen and the amount of contamination (inoculum size) is determined by the type of surgical procedure. More virulent organisms, such as *Staph. aureus,* have a higher likelihood of producing infection than less virulent strains, such as *Streptococcus viridans.* A larger inoculum size predisposes to infection.

B. Host factors

1. The extremes of age
2. Marked obesity
3. Presence of perioperative infection, even at a distant site
4. Use of corticosteroids or immunosuppressive drugs
5. Diabetes
6. Malnutrition

C. Local wound factors

1. Devitalized tissue
2. Foreign bodies
3. Poor blood supply
4. Location of wound (wounds situated in the groin or anal regions have a higher risk of infection)

D. Operative technique

1. Inadvertent contamination, such as spillage from the bowel
2. Operative procedure of excessive length
3. Rough handling of tissues
4. Bleeding in the operative site, with hematoma formation
5. Formation of dead spaces in the wound
6. Excessive foreign bodies, e.g., use of thick or braided suture material instead of fine and monofilament sutures, or too many sutures
7. The use of a cautery, which produces devitalized tissues

E. Wound drainage

1. Inadequate drainage of blood, pus, body fluids, and necrotic materials
2. Excessive use of open (Penrose) drains
3. Placement of a drain in the primary incision rather than in an adjacent, separate, stab wound.
4. Primary closure of a "dirty" wound (delayed wound closure should be employed whenever possible in this setting)

V. Complications. Wound infections can be **benign,** managed successfully by local care, or **serious,** with either local or systemic complications.

A. Local

1. Destruction of tissues
2. Separation of wound
3. Failure of the operation
4. Incisional or deep hernia
5. Septic thrombophlebitis
6. Recurrent pain
7. Disfiguring or disabling scar

B. Systemic

1. Fever
2. Increased catabolism, leading to malnutrition
3. Bacteremia and septic shock
4. Metastatic infection
5. Failure of vital organ systems, such as kidneys, liver, and lungs

VI. Microbiology

A. Pathogens that infect surgical wounds are classified as **exogenous** or **endogenous.**

1. **Exogenous** contamination comes from personnel or environmental sources, such as respiratory equipment, intravenous catheters, and urinary catheters.

Table 14-3. Incidence of microbial pathogens in wound infections*

Type of pathogen	Infections with single pathogen (%)	Infections with multiple pathogens (%)
Gram-positive		
Staphylococcus aureus	54	17
Enterococci	3	25
Other gram-positive cocci	8	18
Total	65	60
Gram-negative bacilli		
Klebsiella-Enterobacter	11	22
Escherichia coli	9	27
Pseudomonas	4	14
Proteus mirabilis	3	15
Other gram-negative bacilli	6	20
Total	33	98
Fungi		
Candida	1.5	2
Asperigillus	0.5	1
Total	2	3

*Anaerobes not cultured.

In many circumstances, direct contact with the wound by the surgical team is the final pathway for spread of these organisms. Exogenous contamination is responsible for most infections in clean wounds.

2. **Endogenous** contamination is from the patient him- or herself. Endogenous sources include the gastrointestinal tract, genitourinary tract, skin, anterior nares, and sites of active infection remote from the wound, such as a urinary tract infection. With the exception of clean wound infections, endogenous microorganisms are responsible for most infections in the other categories of surgical operations.

B. The specific type of microorganism in an infected wound depends on the location of the wound, the extent of the procedure, and whether a mucosal surface has been transected, as well as on technical factors such as collection of specimens, transport to the laboratory, and degree of expertise of the laboratory in culturing conventional and fastidious organisms such as anaerobes, fungi, and viruses. Approximately one-third of wound infections are caused by a single pathogen and two-thirds by multiple organisms. The most prevalent organisms are listed in Table 14-3.

When a single pathogen is involved, *Staph. aureus* is the most common isolate, causing 54% of infections. Gram-negative bacilli as the only pathogens are present in one-third of wounds. The majority of wound infections involve multiple pathogens, however, among which gram-negative bacilli are the predominant forms. The enterococcus is only rarely isolated as a single pathogen (3%).

A somewhat different view of wound bacteriology is perceived when the setting is elective colon operations and the laboratory uses techniques that permit optimal recovery of aerobic and anaerobic bacteria (pp. 16–17). Mixed infections account for 90% or more of wound infections, and anaerobic bacteria are the major pathogens.

VII. Guidelines for preventing surgical wound infections. The Centers for Disease Control (CDC) published in 1982 a series of guidelines for infection control. Composed by a working group of experts, these guidelines are ranked into three categories:

Category I. Strongly recommended for adoption. These measures are strongly supported by well-designed and controlled clinical studies that show their effectiveness in reducing the risk of nosocomial infections, or are viewed as useful by the majority of experts in the field. Measures in this category are judged to be applicable to the majority of hospitals, regardless of size, patient population, or endemic nosocomial infection rate, and are considered practical to implement.

Category II. Moderately recommended for adoption. These measures are supported by highly suggestive clinical studies or by definitive studies in institutions that might not be representative of other hospitals. Measures that have not been adequately studied but that have a strong theoretical rationale, indicating that they might be very effective, are included in this category. Category II measures are judged to be practical to implement. They are not to be considered a standard of practice for every hospital.

Category III. Weakly recommended for adoption. These measures have been proposed by some investigators, authorities, or organizations but, to date, lack both supporting data and a strong theoretical rationale. Thus, they might be considered as important issues that require further evaluation; or they might be considered by some hospitals for implementation, especially if such hospitals have specific nosocomial infection problems or sufficient resources.

VIII. Recommendations for prevention of surgical wound infections*

A. Surveillance and classification

1. a. At the time of operation or shortly thereafter, all operations should be classified and recorded as **clean, clean-contaminated, contaminated,** or **dirty and infected** (see sec. **III**). **Category I.**
   b. The classification should be recorded as such in the medical record. **Category II.**
2. The person in charge of surveillance of surgical patients should gather the information necessary to compute the classification-specific wound infection rates for all operations in the hospital. These rates should be computed at least every 6–12 months, entered into the records of the infection control committee, and made available to the department of surgery. **Category I.**
3. Every 6–12 months, procedure-specific clean wound infection rates should be computed for the hospital and all active surgeons. These rates should be given to all surgeons, so that they can compare their own rate with that of others; the rates can be coded so that names do not appear. **Category II.**
4. An effort should be made to contact discharged patients to determine their infection rate for the 1st 30 days after operation. **Category III.**

B. Preparation of the patient before operation

1. If the operation is elective, all bacterial infections that are identified, excluding ones for which the operation is performed, should be treated and controlled before the operation. **Category I.**
2. The hospital stay before the operation should be as short as possible; in particular, tests and therapeutic measures that will prolong the preoperative stay beyond 1 day should be performed as outpatient services, if possible. **Category III.**
3. If the operation is elective and the patient is grossly malnourished, the patient should receive oral or parenteral hyperalimentation before the operation. **Category II.**
4. If the operation is elective, the patient should bathe (or be bathed) the night before with an antiseptic soap. **Category III.**
5. a. Unless hair near the operative site is so thick that it will interfere with the surgical procedure, it should not be removed. **Category II.**
   b. If hair removal is necessary, it should be done as near the time of operation as possible, preferably immediately before. **Category II.**
6. a. The area around and including the operative site should be scrubbed with a detergent solution followed by application of an antiseptic solution. This

*U.S. Department of Health and Human Services, Centers for Disease Control, Center for Infectious Diseases, Atlanta, Georgia, *Guidelines for Prevention and Control of Surgical Wounds.* March 1982, pp 1–8.

area should be large enough to include the entire incision and an adjacent area large enough for the surgeon to work during the operation without contacting unprepared skin. **Category I.**

b. Tincture of chlorhexidine, iodophors, and tincture of iodine are the recommended antiseptic products for preparing the operative site. Plain soap, alcohol, or hexachlorophene are not recommended as single agents for operative site preparation, unless the patient's skin is sensitive to the recommended antiseptic products. Aqueous quaternary ammonium compounds should not be used. **Category I.**

7. For major operations involving an incision and requiring use of the operating room (OR), the patient should be covered with sterile drapes in such a manner that no part of the patient is uncovered except the operative field and those parts necessary for anesthesia to be administered and maintained. **Category I.**

C. Preparation of the surgical team

1. Everyone who enters the OR should wear at all times (1) a high-efficiency mask to cover the mouth and nose fully; (2) a cap or hood to cover head hair fully; and (3) shoe covers. A beard should be fully covered by the mask and hood. **Category I.**

2. a. The surgical team (those who will touch the sterile surgical field, sterile instruments, or an incisional wound) should scrub their hands and arms to the elbows with an antiseptic before each operation. Scrubbing should be done before every procedure and take at least 5 minutes before the first procedure of the day. **Category I.**

b. Between consecutive operations, scrubbing times of 2–5 minutes may be acceptable. **Category III.**

c. Chlorohexidine, iodophors, and hexachlorophene are the recommended active antimicrobial ingredients for the surgical hand scrub. Aqueous quaternary ammonium compounds, for example, benzalkonium chloride, should not be used. **Category I.**

d. Hexachlorophene should not be used by pregnant women. **Category II.**

3. a. After scrubbing their hands with an antiseptic and drying them with a sterile towel, the surgical team should don sterile gowns. **Category I.**

b. Gowns used in the OR should be made of reusable or disposable fabrics that have been shown to be nearly impermeable to bacteria, even when wet. **Category II.**

4. a. The surgical team should wear sterile gloves. If a glove is punctured during the operation, it should be promptly changed. **Category I.**

b. For open bone operations and orthopedic implant operations, two pairs of sterile gloves should be worn. **Category II.**

D. Ventilation and air quality in the operating room

1. All OR doors should be kept closed except as needed for passage of equipment, personnel, and the patient; personnel allowed to enter the OR, especially after an operation has started, should be kept to a minimum. **Category I.**

2. For new construction, OR ventilation should include a minimum of 25 air changes per hour. All inlets for outside air should be located as high above ground as possible and remote from exhaust outlets of all types. All air, recirculated or fresh, should be filtered before entering the OR. **Category I.**

E. Cleaning and culturing in the OR and culturing personnel

1. The OR should be cleaned between surgical operations, daily, and weekly, according to established procedures for each scheduled cleaning. **Category I.**

2. Routine culturing of the OR environment or personnel who use the OR should not be done. **Category I.**

3. Use of tacky or antiseptic mats at the entrance to the OR is not recommended for infection control. **Category I.**

F. Operative technique. The surgical team should work as far as possible with an efficiency that permits them to handle tissues gently, prevent bleeding, eradicate dead space, and minimize devitalized tissue and foreign material in the wound. **Category I.**

G. Wound care

1. Incisional wounds classified as **dirty and infected** should not ordinarily have skin closed over them at the end of an operation, that is, they should not ordinarily be closed primarily. **Category I.** (If an operation is performed as part of the treatment of a low-grade infection involving an implanted device, it is sometimes better to close the wound after operation to prevent superinfection with microorganisms more virulent than those already causing infection.)
2. If drainage is necessary for an uninfected wound, a closed suction drainage system should be used, and it should be placed in an adjacent stab wound rather than in the main incisional wound. **Category I.**
3. Personnel should wash their hands before and after taking care of a surgical wound. **Category I.**
4. Personnel should not touch an open wound directly, unless they are wearing sterile gloves. When the wound is sealed, dressings may be changed without gloves. **Category I.**
5. Dressings over closed wounds should be removed if they are wet or if the patient has signs or symptoms suggestive of infection, for example, fever or unusual wound pain. When the dressing is removed, the wound should be inspected for signs of infection. Any drainage from a wound that is suspected of being infected should be cultured and smeared for Gram's stain. **Category I.**

Urinary Catheters

Catheterization of the urinary tract is the major source of hospital-acquired infections on surgical wards. It is also a necessary adjunct to the modern practice of surgery. Defining its indications and controlling its risks should be the goals of all members of the surgical team.

I. Rates of infection. Urinary tract infections are responsible for 40% of all hospital-acquired infections, affecting approximately 600,000 patients per year in the United States. Three-fourths of urinary tract infections acquired in the hospital are related to catheterization. At any given time, 10–15% of all patients in a general hospital are being managed with an indwelling urinary catheter. The prevalence of infection is approximately 25%.

The infected urinary tract is the most common portal of entry for significant bacteremia, a significant cause of death in postoperative patients. An infected urinary tract also increases the risk of postoperative infection at other sites. It is not uncommon to find the urinary pathogen in purulent sputum or wound discharges following an operation. An additional problem is that bacteria acquired by catheterization are multiply resistant to antimicrobial agents.

II. Risk factors. Certain groups of patients are at particularly high risk for developing urinary tract infections from catheters:

A. Women before or following delivery
B. Elderly patients
C. Debilitated patients
D. Diabetics
E. Patients with significant residual urine in the bladder

III. Single "straight" catheterization

A. Indications

This procedure carries a lower risk than an indwelling catheter; it is indicated in the following circumstances:

1. Acute urinary retention or inability to void
2. Removal of clots, stones, or concretions
3. For urologic studies such as cystography, localization of stricture, renal function tests, and determination of residual urine
4. To obtain urine samples for culture from patients who are unable to provide a "clean catch" or whose urine cultures have yielded conflicting results

Table 14-4. Incidence of bacilluria following single catheterization of the bladder

Patients	Incidence of bacilluria (%)
Ambulatory males	0.5
Hospitalized males	5.0
Ambulatory females	1.0
Hospitalized, nonpregnant females	4.0
Bedridden, nonpregnant females	13.0
Pregnant females in uncomplicated labor	10.0
Pregnant females in complicated labor	23.0

B. Incidence of infection. Although single catheterization is the least traumatic method of sampling the lower urinary tract, it is attended by some risk, particularly in bedridden patients and pregnant women (Table 14-4). For these reasons, the decision to perform single catheterization should not be made lightly in these special groups.

IV. Indications for indwelling (Foley) bladder catheterization. Despite the significant risks of urinary catheterization, it is common practice in some hospitals to catheterize the majority of patients undergoing major operative procedures. Certainly, indwelling catheterization is required in certain circumstances, but these should be carefully defined. Common indications are

A. To relieve temporary obstruction, either anatomic or physiologic

B. To facilitate careful measurement of urinary output in seriously ill patients with fluid management problems, renal failure, cardiac insufficiency, or shock

C. To divert the urinary stream in order to provide a dry environment for comatose and incontinent patients

D. For chronic incontinence for which no surgical procedure can be effective, e.g., spinal cord injuries and neurologic diseases such as multiple sclerosis

E. During surgical procedures involving the urethra, bladder, prostate, and surrounding structures

In reality, **most indwelling Foley catheters are inserted for convenience** of the nursing and surgical staff, a practice that should be strongly discouraged.

Many patients experience difficulty in voiding in the immediate postoperative period. This situation often can be managed by encouragement, gentle massage of the lower abdomen, or provision of the necessary privacy required by some patients to initiate urination. Another approach is to attempt two or three straight catheterizations during this early period, before taking the easy but dangerous tack of inserting an indwelling catheter.

Scrupulous measurement of urinary output usually is unnecessary in the postoperative care of uncomplicated patients. Rather than risk catheterization, approximations can be made of the urinary output in patients who are partially incontinent. Estimations can be based on amount of wetting and frequency, daily weight (which is the best guide of fluid balance), skin turgor, peripheral and presacral edema, and respiratory rales.

V. Incidence of bacilluria associated with indwelling catheterization. The original catheterization system was "open"—the drainage tube led into a bag or drainage bottle with an open top. Fifty percent of patients using this system develop bacilluria by day 1, and nearly 100% by day 4.

The "closed" urinary drainage system involves aseptic insertion techniques and maintenance of the collection system below the level of the bladder. This system reduces the incidence of bacilluria to a rate of approximately 5% of patients per day of catheterization; thus, only 50% of catheterized patients are infected between the 11th and 13th day after inserting the catheter, when the system is used properly.

VI. Microbiology. Most pathogens associated with nosocomial urinary tract infections are resistant to a variety of antimicrobial agents. Indeed, their resistance patterns are useful guidelines for epidemiologic monitoring of spread within the hospital. In large surveys, the organisms most commonly encountered, in order of frequency, are:

1. *E. coli*
2. *Proteus mirabilis*
3. *Klebsiella*
4. *Enterobacter*
5. *Pseudomonas*
6. *Proteus* (indole-positive)
7. *Serratia*
8. *Strep. faecalis*
9. Staphylococci
10. *Candida*

The relative frequency within a specific hospital is dependent upon local epidemiologic conditions. It is the task of surveillance to establish the baseline incidence and frequency for each of these organisms. Significant deviations from the usual patterns indicate the emergence of an epidemic. Such deviations can serve as an early warning system that makes it possible to initiate control measures before significant dissemination occurs.

VII. Sources of urinary tract pathogens. The microorganisms responsible for hospital-acquired urinary tract infections have four major reservoirs:

A. The bacteria that normally inhabit the urethra or perineal skin.

B. The intestinal microflora of the patient, which becomes colonized shortly after admission with the flora of the particular institution. The organisms within the feces are easily spread to the perineum and penile meatus or introitus, whence they can be disseminated to the urinary bladder.

C. Organisms spread person-to-person by contaminated hands of personnel. This is probably the major route of hospital-acquired urinary tract infections. Outbreaks of *Serratia* and *Proteus rettgeri* have been attributed to this route of transmission.

D. Extrinsic equipment, such as contaminated antiseptic solutions, improperly disinfected cystoscopes, commercial packages containing contaminated fluids and dressings, and irrigating solutions.

Microoorganisms can contaminate the lumen of the catheter or collecting bag and ascend from within to colonize the bladder. Alternatively, they can colonize the urethra-catheter mucous blanket that surrounds the catheter as it passes into the bladder.

VIII. Early complications of indwelling urinary catheterization

A. Catheter fever refers to fever and shaking chills following insertion, manipulation, or irrigation of the catheter, usually within 4 hours. The fever is a manifestation of gram-negative bacteremia and is seen most frequently in patients with an infected urinary tract. Large urinary residuals also predispose to catheter fever. A febrile episode is more common when the catheterization has been somewhat traumatic, particularly in the face of obstruction or clots. This causes an abrasion in the urethra that may be the portal of entry for bacteria. Most episodes of catheter fever pass without sequelae and do not require specific antibiotic treatment. If the fever persists for more than 4 hours, treatment with a broad-spectrum antibiotic such as an aminoglycoside is indicated. Some patients with catheter fever develop hypotension, and a few develop septic shock. These cases require more rigorous measures directed at maintaining hemodynamic status and suppressing the infecting pathogens (see Chap. 8).

B. Meatitis is a frequent complication, especially if hygiene is not maintained at an optimal level.

C. Urethritis occurs in some cases and can lead to intense pain and occasionally hemorrhage. Infection may spread to produce a periurethral abscess.

D. Prostatitis can be caused by trauma with the catheter balloon. The initial event is ischemic necrosis, which progresses to bacterial prostatitis. Ascending infection can produce epididymitis.

E. **Cystitis** can result from a bacterial infection or from trauma produced by the balloon. The infection can ascend to the kidneys to produce **pyelonephritis.** The urinary sediment shows multiple white blood cells and red blood cells, and the patient experiences pressure or pain in the pelvic region or back.

IX. Late complications of indwelling urinary catheterization

A. **Recurrent urinary tract infections and septicemia** are the most serious complications of long-term indwelling catheterization. Some patients experience chills and fever on a regular basis, as frequently as every few weeks. Gram-negative sepsis and shock can develop, a situation that in older patients may lead to their demise. The infecting pathogen usually is a resident organism, present for a long time. Thus, knowledge of the infecting strain in the asymptomatic period provides an early clue when the patient develops septicemia. In practical terms, antibiotic therapy will almost surely be a broad-spectrum drug such as an aminoglycoside, since such patients have resistant bacteria.

B. **Stone formation** is a problem of long-term catheterization. The situation is compounded in bedridden patients, who mobilize calcium from their bones, excreting it in their urine. As such individuals often have poor oral fluid intake, the urine is concentrated, adding to the propensity to form stones. Another risk factor is the presence of urea-splitting organisms, such as *Proteus*.

C. **Meatal stenosis and fibrosis,** and even **stricture of the urethra,** can occur after removal of the catheter.

X. Prophylactic antimicrobial agents in catheterized patients

A. Routine administration of potent antimicrobial agents to patients undergoing urinary catheterization produces only a transient delay in infection. The price paid for this temporary effect is selection of highly resistant organisms for the inevitable colonization. Prophylactic antimicrobial regimens that have been used include

Nalidixic acid	1 gm, 4 times daily
Nitrofurantoin	100 mg, 3–4 times daily
Sulfonamides, such as sulfisoxazole	0.5–1 gm, 4 times daily

B. Some surgeons routinely use **acidifying agents,** such as methenamine mandelate, 1 gm 4 times daily, in order to acidify the urine. Alternatively, ascorbic acid, 500 mg 2–4 times daily, has been given. Acidification is useful for controlling infections caused by urea-splitting bacteria such as *Proteus*. For other bacteria, however, there is little evidence of benefit.

XI. Urinary tract cultures.

Routine culture of the urinary tract in catheterized patients is not recommended. Even if a positive culture is obtained, it is not an indication for antimicrobial therapy. As long as the catheter is in place, such therapy would suppress the specific organism, but it may encourage a more resistant organism to emerge. Following removal of the catheter, it is advisable to obtain urine for culture. At this time, urinary tract pathogens, if present, should be treated aggressively for at least 2 weeks with an appropriate antimicrobial agent. Repeat cultures should be obtained after completion of this therapeutic course.

XII. Methods of urinary tract drainage

A. **Closed catheter drainage system.** Introduction of the closed catheter system has radically reduced the incidence of acquired bacilluria and subsequent urinary tract infections. The important elements of this system are as follows:

1. The collection bag or vessel is protected from extrinsic contamination.
2. There is no continuity between urine in the drainage tube and that within the collecting bag or vessel. It is most dangerous to have a continuous column of urine from the collecting bag straight through the drainage system and into the bladder.
3. The collecting bag or vessel is kept below the level of the bladder in order to prevent retrograde flow of urine into the bladder.
4. Sterility of the system is maintained, with particular attention to the junctions between the catheter, the collecting tube, and the container.

Adherence to these principles reduces the incidence of urinary tract infection in the catheterized patient and also reduces the spread of pathogens between patients.

B. Intermittent prophylactic irrigation. This method is used in conjunction with the closed system. An irrigating solution is instilled through a Y tube connected to the catheter. The intermittent system does not increase the safety or efficiency of the standard closed drainage system. In addition, there are several major disadvantages:

1. Considerable nursing time is required to maintain the proper schedule. If the collection tube is clamped too long, the bladder fills to unsafe volumes.
2. Continual changing of the irrigation system and clamps provides ample opportunity for breaks in sterility.
3. The system is not well adapted to use at home or under situations of custodial care or para-nursing supervision.
4. The irrigating solutions can cause irritation, producing pelvic pain. Approximately 5% of patients develop microscopic hematuria, and 1% have gross hematuria as a result of the acidic solution.

C. Constant bladder rinse with three-way catheter

1. There are several commercial three-way catheters that can be adapted for continuous bladder irrigation, using one of these solutions:
   a. Acetic acid, 0.25%, in physiologic saline. The urine pH should be maintained below 5.0. In order to achieve this, it may be necessary to infuse 1,000 ml of irrigating solution q8h. If hematuria or pelvic discomfort occurs, the concentration of acetic acid can be reduced by 50%.
   b. Neomycin sulfate, 40 mg, and polymyxin B, 200,000 units, mixed in 1–2 ml of saline, then added to 1,000 ml of saline. The system should be adjusted to deliver approximately 1,000 ml of irrigating solution q24h.
2. The continuous irrigation system has strong adherents who believe that the risk of bacilluria is considerably reduced by its strict application. This concept is not universally accepted, however, and many institutions prefer to use the closed drainage system without the adjunct of irrigation. **Disadvantages** to the continuous bladder rinse are that
   a. Skilled nursing personnel are required to maintain the time schedule and adequate sterility of the system.
   b. The method is not easily adapted for home use or for nursing home situations, in which trained personnel may not be available.
   c. The system may be ineffective once infection of the urinary tract, particularly the upper tract, is established.
   d. Culture of the urine in order to follow the acquisition of bacilluria is extremely difficult with this system.
   e. Sterility may be violated when irrigation solutions are renewed.
   f. Resistant bacteria are selected by this system.
   g. Theoretically, antimicrobial agents require a certain period of contact time in order to exert their activity against microorganisms. Continual rinsing may not provide adequate exposure at high enough concentrations.

D. Alternative methods of urinary drainage

1. **Condom catheterization (external catheter).** In male patients a condom catheter may be a satisfactory method for measuring urine output or keeping an incontinent patient dry. The technique is most advantageous when used for a limited period of time, about 1–4 weeks. The main disadvantage is trauma to the glans and penile shaft, which can lead to severe balanitis and phimosis. To prevent this occurrence, the catheter should be changed each day, with careful cleansing of the area with mild soap and water. In addition, the condom should be secured with gentle tension on the penile shaft, just enough to avoid leakage but not so much as to cause pressure necrosis of the underlying skin. The condom system is difficult to maintain in agitated patients because the patients try to manipulate the system which can lead to an increase in infection.
2. **Suprapubic catheterization.** For short-term urinary diversion, such as is required in gynecologic or urologic surgical procedures, a trochar introduced directly into the bladder through the lower abdominal wall is an efficient and

rather safe means of drainage. For placement of the suprapubic catheter, the patient should be well hydrated, so that the bladder contains at least 500 ml of urine; or this quantity of saline can be introduced by a single catheterization. A number of different catheters can be used, as well as several commercial trocar sets.

3. **Intermittent direct catheterization.** In the immediate postoperative period, when a patient may have difficulty voiding, two or three intermittent catheterizations can be used to advantage in order to circumvent usage of an indwelling catheter. Intermittent catheterization has also been used on a long-term basis by patients with spinal cord injuries and neurologic disabilities. This requires a highly motivated patient who can be trained over some period of time to perform self-catheterization. A clean, nonsterile technique can be employed in the patient's home. The daily intake of fluid is restricted to below 1,500 ml, with an overnight restriction of < 200 ml. The catheterization generally is performed at 4-hour intervals in an effort to keep the bladder volume below 400 ml. Each patient, after appropriate training, can work out her or his own schedule for intermittent self-catheterization.

XIII. Recommendations for urinary catheter care*

Category I† = strongly recommended for adoption.
Category II = moderately recommended for adoption.
Category III = weakly recommended for adoption.

A. Personnel

1. Only persons (e.g., hospital personnel, family members, and patients themselves) who know the correct techniques of aseptic insertion and maintenance of the catheter should handle catheters. **Category I.**
2. Hospital personnel and others who care for catheters should be given periodic inservice training stressing the correct techniques and potential complications of urinary catheterization. **Category II.**

B. Catheter use

1. Urinary catheters should be inserted only when necessary and left in place only for as long as necessary. They should not be used solely for the convenience of patient-care personnel. **Category I.**
2. For selected patients, other methods of urine drainage such as condom catheter drainage, suprapubic catheterization, and intermittent urethral catheterization can be useful alternatives to indwelling urethral catheterization. **Category III.**

C. Handwashing.

Handwashing should be done immediately before and after any manipulation of the catheter site or apparatus. **Category I.**

D. Catheter insertion

1. Catheters should be inserted using aseptic technique and sterile equipment. **Category I.**
2. Gloves, drape, sponges, an appropriate antiseptic solution for periurethral cleaning, and a single-use packet of lubricant jelly should be used for insertion. **Category II.**
3. As small a catheter as possible, consistent with good drainage, should be used to minimize urethral trauma. **Category II.**
4. Indwelling catheters should be properly secured after insertion to prevent movement and urethral traction. **Category I.**

E. Closed sterile drainage

1. A sterile, continuously closed drainage system should be maintained. **Category I.**
2. The catheter and drainage tube should not be disconnected, unless the catheter must be irrigated (see sec. **F. Irrigation**). **Category I.**

*U.S. Department of Health and Human Services, Centers for Disease Control, Center for Infectious Diseases, Atlanta, Georgia, *Guidelines for Urinary Catheter Care.* February 1981, pp. 1–5.

†See pages 306–307 for complete explanation of the ranking scheme.

3. If a break in aseptic technique, disconnection, or leakage occurs, the collecting system should be replaced using aseptic technique after disinfecting the catheter-tubing junction. **Category III.**

F. Irrigation

1. If irrigation is necessary to prevent obstruction due to bleeding (e.g., after prostatic or bladder surgery) or to relieve obstruction due to bleeding or other causes, an intermittent method of irrigation should be used. **Category I.**
2. The catheter-tubing junction should be disinfected before disconnection. **Category II.**
3. A large-volume sterile syringe and sterile irrigant should be used and then discarded. The person performing irrigation should use aseptic technique. **Category I.**
4. If the catheter becomes obstructed and can be kept open only by frequent irrigation, the catheter should be changed, if it is likely that the catheter itself is contributing to the obstruction (e.g., formation of concretions). **Category II.**
5. Continuous irrigation of the bladder has not been proved to be useful and should not be performed as a routine infection prevention measure. **Category II.**

G. Specimen collection

1. If small volumes of fresh urine are needed for examination, the distal end of the catheter, or preferably the sampling port, if present, should be cleansed with a disinfectant and urine, then aspirated with a sterile needle and syringe. **Category I.**
2. Larger volumes of urine for special analyses should be obtained aseptically from the drainage bag. **Category I.**

H. Urinary flow

1. Unobstructed flow should be maintained. **Category I.** Occasionally it is necessary to obstruct the catheter temporarily for specimen collection or other medical purposes.
2. To achieve free flow of urine, (1) the catheter and collecting tube should be kept from kinking; (2) the collecting bag should be emptied regularly, a separate collecting container being used for each patient (the drainage spigot and nonsterile collecting container should never come in contact); (3) a poorly functioning or obstructed catheter should be irrigated (see sec. **F.**) or, if necessary, replaced; and (4) the collecting bag should always be kept below the level of the bladder. **Category I.**

I. Meatal care. Twice-daily cleansing with povidone-iodine solution and daily cleansing with soap and water have been shown in two recent studies **not** to reduce catheter-associated urinary tract infection. Thus, at this time, daily meatal care with either of these two regimens cannot be endorsed. **Category II.**

J. Catheter change interval. Indwelling catheters should not be changed at arbitrary fixed intervals. **Category II.**

K. Spatial separation of catheterized patients. To minimize the chances of cross-infection, infected and uninfected patients with indwelling catheters should not share the same room or adjacent beds. **Category III.**

L. Bacteriologic monitoring. The value of regular bacteriologic monitoring of catheterized patients as an infection control measure has not been established, and the measure is not recommended. **Category III.**

Hospital-Acquired Pneumonia

I. General principles. Nosocomial pneumonia occurs in 0.5–5.0% of all hospitalized patients. It is second only to urinary tract infection as a cause of hospital-acquired infection. The mortality of nosocomial pneumonia is considerable: In some series one-third of patients die either as a direct or as an indirect result of this infection. When the invading pathogen is a resistant, gram-negative bacillus, mortality rates of over

50% have been reported. The areas at greatest risk within the hospital are intensive care units and burn units, due both to the sick patients found there and to the intrahospital spread of potential pathogens within these areas.

II. Pathophysiology of nosocomial pneumonia. The pathogens of pneumonia associated with hospitalization derive from two major sources: contamination of the oropharynx with gram-negative bacilli, and contamination of inhalation therapy equipment.

A. Colonization of the oropharynx by hospital-acquired microorganisms occurs most often in seriously ill patients and in those admitted to intensive care units. On a hospital-wide basis, oropharyngeal colonization by gram-negative bacilli is seen in 20% of patients by the 1st day of hospitalization and in 45% by the 4th day. Patients with underlying pulmonary disease run the highest risk of colonization; 75% of this group are colonized. By way of comparison, only 2% of normal individuals have oropharyngeal colonization by gram-negative bacilli.

1. Once colonization with gram-negative organisms occurs, the route of delivery to the bronchioles and alveoli is by aspiration. It can be assumed that all comatose patients are aspirating oropharyngeal contents into the lower respiratory tract. Even healthy individuals may aspirate during sleep, but pulmonary defenses such as the mucociliary escalator system, alveolar macrophages, surfactant, and immunoglobulins in secretions protect the lung from infection.
2. The following risk factors predispose to nosocomial pneumonia, in the setting of oropharyngeal colonization:

   Coma
   Anoxia
   Antibiotic therapy
   Cytotoxic drugs
   Acidosis
   Hypotension
   Pulmonary disease
   Corticosteroids
   Immune deficiency state
   Azotemia

3. The risk of developing nosocomial pneumonia is difficult to determine in a specific patient, since it relates to colonization, underlying diseases, length of stay in the hospital, and use of respiratory therapy equipment. The pathogen that causes pneumonia has previously colonized the oropharynx in 85% of cases. Thus, prospective cultures of sputum in high-risk patients give an early clue to the pathogen when pneumonia has become clinically apparent.

B. Contamination of inhalation therapy equipment is another source of nosocomial pneumonia. It is usual practice to employ a system that adds moisture or medication to the gas mixtures, in order to prevent desiccation of the bronchial epithelium and to deliver various drugs. The techniques for adding such fluids are humidification and nebulization. Hospital-associated bacteria colonize the breathing circuits, which include the tubing, nebulizers, humidifiers, and valves, and the organisms grow to large numbers at these sites. They are delivered to the lower respiratory tract by **aerosol.** Localization within the lung of such aerosols is dependent on droplet size.

Particle size (diameter of droplet)	**Localization in the lung**
$>10\ \mu$	Nasopharynx
$5–10\ \mu$	Trachea
$2–3\ \mu$	Bronchi and bronchioles
$1–2\ \mu$	Bronchioles and alveoli

The most dangerous droplets are $1–2\mu$ in diameter, as they can be delivered directly to the smaller bronchioles and alveoli, thereby bypassing the pulmonary defense mechanisms. In addition, large numbers of droplets can overwhelm pulmonary defense mechanisms at several levels in the tracheobronchial tree. Any piece of equipment that nebulizes to produce small particles, such as an ultrasonic nebulizer, carries a higher risk of causing pneumonia. Routine humidifiers are relatively low-risk units, since they do not produce an aerosol that conveys bacteria in the gas mixtures. Small-volume nebulizers, often used for delivering medication in an intermittent positive-pressure breathing machine, have an intermediate risk of causing pneumonia, due to their small reservoir system and the relatively large droplets that they produce. The greatest risk of infection is associated with **large-reservoir nebulizers,** especially the "mainstream nebulizers" that are attached directly to compressed air or oxygen valves. This equipment produces droplets of varying diameters, including those of 1–2 μ. In addition, the nebulizing jet and the large volume of fluid within the reservoir may become contaminated.

III. Bacteriology. The pathogens responsible for nosocomial pneumonia vary from hospital to hospital, depending on the specific bacterial flora associated with the institution. Even units within the same hospital may have different organisms. In general, gram-negative organisms are the main culprits. They tend to be resistant to many antibiotic agents. These pathogens often are well adapted for survival on moist surfaces and in decontamination solutions (such as quaternary ammonium compounds, phenolics, and hexachlorophene). *Staph. aureus* also causes hospital epidemics of pneumonia, although less frequently than in the past.

A. The common pathogens associated with nosocomial pneumonia are as follows:

1. *Ps. aeruginosa*
2. *Klebsiella*
3. *E. coli*
4. *Serratia*
5. *Enterobacter*
6. *Staph. aureus*

B. Unusual microorganisms can also cause nosocomial pneumonias. In some institutions these lesser-known pathogens become the major cause of hospital-acquired infections:

1. Other *Pseudomonas* species (*maltophilia, cepacia, fluorescens*)
2. *Flavobacterium*
3. *Acinetobacter*
4. *Achromobacter*

Since it is difficult to distinguish colonization of the respiratory tract from pneumonia, only repeated isolation of these unusual organisms from the same patient, or from a group of patients, has clinical significance.

IV. Maintenance of inhalation therapy equipment. The goal of proper maintenance of equipment being used by patients is to reduce the number of bacterial contaminants below the critical inoculum required for inducing infection. Particular attention is paid to changing equipment and water reservoirs, so that microorganisms cannot multiply to large concentrations.

A. There should be a change **q48h** in the patient breathing circuit, including tubing, nebulizing equipment, and reservoirs. (Some authorities suggest changes q8–12h for continuous respiratory therapy and q24h for intermittent therapy; this program increases costs without showing any proved benefit over the 48-hour regimen.)

B. Reservoirs should be completely emptied and refilled q8–12h. It is most important to discard all fluid in the reservoir in order to avoid buildup of bacterial growth. Fluid from the tubing should not be allowed to flow back into the clean reservoir.

C. The reservoir should be filled with sterile, or nearly sterile, water. Tap water should be used only if it has been checked and monitored for bacterial contaminants. In intensive care units it is recommended that only sterile liquids be used in nebulizers.

D. Unit-dose or small-dose medication vials should be employed. Large, multiple-dose vials may become contaminated between usages.

E. The breathing circuits, such as tubing, valves, and nebulizers, must be cleaned initially to remove particulate material and then disinfected or sterilized. Among the methods recommended are sterilization by steam or ethylene oxide and liquid disinfection by pasteurization or activated gluteraldehyde. Whichever method is selected, it is important that quality control be maintained to ensure adequate decontamination.

F. A number of practices used in some institutions have fallen into disrepute. For example, the following compounds should **not** be used for decontaminating inhalation therapy equipment: quaternary ammonium compounds (such as Zephiran), phenolics, and hexachlorophene. There was some enthusiasm for nebulized 0.25% acetic acid, but this has not been widely accepted, nor has the technique proved effective. Nebulized antibiotics have not reduced the incidence of nosocomial pneumonias; in some institutions they have been associated with emergence of resistant organisms that have caused such infections. Hence, nebulized disinfectants or antibiotics should not be used.

G. A surveillance system for nosocomial infection is the most effective means of monitoring inhalation therapy equipment. It is also recommended that systematic cultures of equipment be performed in order to maintain high efficiency in decontamination procedures. Once the equipment is attached to the patient, contamination can come from the patient's oropharynx. Therefore, in-use bacterial cultures are not particularly helpful as a means of monitoring inhalation therapy equipment.

V. Endotracheal intubation. Endotracheal intubation creates the highest risk of nosocomial pneumonia, since the pulmonary defense mechanisms in the upper respiratory tract are circumvented by the tube. Nearly all patients who are intubated become contaminated by gram-negative bacilli within 2–3 days. Some patients need intubation for this period of time and even longer. Prevention of infection in this setting is based on the same principle for all inhalation therapy: reduction of contamination by extrinsic organisms. This involves meticulous care when suctioning and handling the endotracheal tube:

A. Sterile gloves should be used during suction and handling.

B. Sterile, disposable catheters should be employed. There should be a basin of sterile water to rinse the cannula during the suctioning procedure, and both the catheter and the water must be discarded after they are used. Sterile water or medications should come from unit-dosage vials, rather than from large, multidose vials that can become contaminated.

C. Strict handwashing procedures should be practiced between attendance on different patients.

D. There are no indications for use of nebulized antimicrobial drugs or disinfectants.

Intravascular Catheters

Like so many mechanical adjuncts to modern surgical practice, intravenous infusions and intraarterial lines are necessary, albeit sometimes risky, invasions of the skin barrier. Approximately 8 million patients in the United States receive intravenous therapy each year, representing one-quarter of all hospitalized patients.

The major risk of intravascular infusion devices is infection, either local or disseminated by the bloodstream. The isolation of organisms from plastic intravenous catheters varies from 4% to 58%. The rate of septicemia is considerably less, however, reported as 1–8%. In general, septicemia, documented by positive blood cultures taken from veins at other sites, occurs in only 10% of patients from whom organisms are isolated from the infusion site or catheter tip.

I. Risk factors influencing catheter-associated sepsis

A. Phlebitis is strongly associated with subsequent infection. Indeed, many of the other factors detailed below are relevant because of their influence on formation of local fibrin thrombi. Many such thrombi are sterile, being caused by chemical or physical irritation. They manifest themselves by pain, induration, and erythema. Most patients with catheter-associated septicemia, however, have an infected thrombus as the source.

B. Underlying disease heightens the risk of sepsis. Immunocompromised conditions, associated with steroids, malignancy, or burns, are the most susceptible to such infection.

C. The **length of time** the catheter remains in place is critical. The risk increases after 48 hours and is particularly high after 72 hours of catheterization.

D. **Manipulation** of the catheter augments the risk of introduction of exogenous microorganisms. Such manipulations include measurement of central venous pressure and attempts to deal with leakage, infiltration, or occlusion of the line.

E. **The skin flora** surrounding the catheter site represents the most common source of pathogens. For this reason, catheters should be inserted with strict aseptic technique, and all subsequent handling should be done with great care.

F. **Infection at a remote site** can be disseminated to the catheter by septicemia, even with inapparent seeding of the bloodstream. Hence, patients with wound infections, urinary tract infections, and pneumonia have a higher risk of developing catheter infections, usually with the same pathogen.

G. The **type of infusion fluid** can determine catheter-related infections. In some instances, the fluid itself may become contaminated, particularly when drugs, electrolytes, or vitamins are added during the infusion. Hyptertonic infusions, such as used in hyperalimentation, cause chemical phlebitis, which predisposes to infection.

H. The **type of catheter** is related to the risk of infection. The highest incidence of infection is with cutdowns, followed in frequency by plastic indwelling catheters, steel needles, and, lowest on the list, scalp-vein needles inserted in peripheral vessels.

I. **Location of the intravenous infusion** is important. Infusions using the saphenous-femoral veins in the lower limbs have high rates of septic complications. In newborns, umbilical catheterization carries a high risk of sepsis. In the upper trunk, subclavian infusions are more frequently infected than peripheral veins in the arm.

J. **A special IV team** may lower the risk of infection, although this point has not been proved. One study, retrospective in nature, showed that only 10% of indwelling plastic catheters were placed by physicians, yet this group was responsible for 90% of catheter-associated infections. Of course, physicians tended to place catheters in sicker patients, often under emergency conditions. There has been no prospective study to test the value of an IV team in reducing infection.

II. **Microbiology.** A great variety of bacteria and fungi have been recovered from venous catheters. *Staph. epidermidis,* abundant in the normal microflora of the skin, is the organism most commonly found on the catheter tip and surrounding skin. It has relatively low virulence, however. *Staph. aureus* is the pathogen most frequently encountered in positive blood cultures. As noted in Table 14-5 the diversity of potential pathogens makes it difficult to predict in advance which one is involved in a specific infection.

III. **Complications of intravenous catheterization**

A. **Infiltration** of infusion fluid produces local pain, discomfort, and swelling of adjacent tissues.

B. **"Chemical" or uncomplicated thrombophlebitis** is a reaction of sterile inflammation and fibrin formation associated with a foreign body and chemical infusions. Skin overlying the infusion site is warm and erythematous. In autopsy studies, subclavian catheters have been found to be encased with a fibrin sleeve within 24 hours of insertion.

C. **Purulent thrombophlebitis,** an infectious process, is characterized by suppuration in the lumen of the vessel. The physical findings may be indistinguishable from those of uncomplicated phlebitis, but the presence of gross pus, draining spontaneously or by expression from the cannula site, indicates infection. This complication occurs in 0.2% of IV lines.

D. **Cellulitis** is indicated by warm, red, and indurated skin and soft tissues surrounding the site of cannula insertion.

E. **Bacteremia,** with or without **septic shock,** is caused by the same organisms as infection at the IV site.

F. **Occult IV-site infection** describes an infection that does not produce much local

Table 14-5. Microbiology of plastic catheters and associated septicemia

Organism	Isolated from catheter tip (%)	Blood isolates in associated septicemia (%)
Staphylococcus epidermidis	41	9
Staph. aureus	16	32
Klebsiella-Enterobacter	7	11
Enterococci	6	9
Herellea	4	7
Pseudomonas	3	9
Candida and other fungi	3	7
Proteus	3	5
Serratia	3	7
Streptococcus pyogenes	—	2
Miscellaneous (*Bacillus,* diphtheroids, unspecified)	14	2
Total	100	100

Source: Adapted from D. G. Maki et al., Infection control in intravenous therapy. *Ann. Intern. Med.* 79:867, 1973.

reaction. Signs of inflammation and pus are minimal or absent. The patient has signs of bacteremia, however, and may even be hypotensive. Definitive diagnosis depends on direct inspection of the vein or culture of the cannula.

G. Suppurative thrombophlebitis is an uncommon but particularly severe form of occult IV-site infection, characterized by persistent bacteremia, fever, chills, and hypotension, eventually leading to septic shock and death. The striking features of this condition are that

1. It is most often associated with cutdowns but can be seen with plastic indwelling catheters. The clinical presentation occurs 2–10 days after removal of the catheter.
2. Signs of local inflammation and drainage often are absent. Even in fatal cases, only 50% are diagnosed ante mortem on the basis of physical findings.
3. The area at highest risk is the lower limbs, especially the saphenous vein.
4. Blood cultures are persistently positive, despite appropriate antibiotics. The microbiology of this form of occult suppurative phlebitis is

Gram-negative bacilli (*Klebsiella, Enterobacter, Proteus, Providencia, Pseudomonas, Serratia,* and *E. coli,* in that order)	80%
Staphylococcus	10%
Fungi (*Candida, Torulopsis, Aspergillus*)	10%

IV. Contaminated IV infusion solutions. In recent years there have been several outbreaks of septicemia caused by contaminated infusion solutions. This septicemia has led to hypotension and death in some cases.

A. The infusion may be contaminated within the hospital, during the addition of drugs, electrolytes, or nutrients to the IV infusion. One potential source of spread is drug solutions from which small doses are extracted on multiple occasions. Each usage adds to the risk of introducing contamination. For this reason it is advisable to use single-dose vials.

B. Contaminated IV infusion fluid and irrigation solutions have been traced to the manufacturing process. In the most famous epidemic an unusual pathogen, *Enterobacter agglomerans,* which most likely has its reservoir in soil, was introduced through a elastomer-lined, screw-cap closure.

The microorganisms that have been isolated from IV infusions are somewhat different from those associated with catheter-site infections:

Gram-negative bacilli
Klebsiella pneumoniae
Enterobacter cloacae
Enterobacter agglomerans
Serratia marcescens
Ps. thomasii
Citrobacter freundii
Flavobacterium

Fungi
Penicillium
Trichoderma

Some unusual organisms in this list have caused common-source epidemics. Curiously, some of the usual pathogens are absent from the list. The likely explanation is that certain microorganisms do not grow well or in fact perish when exposed to 5% dextrose in water. These poor survivors include

Staph. aureus
Ps. aeruginosa
Proteus
E. coli
Herellea
Candida albicans

V. Contaminated arterial lines. Infections may be introduced through arterial lines, now being used with increased frequency in cardiovascular and pulmonary surgery. The sources of risk are as follows:

A. The intraarterial catheter may be contaminated in the same manner as the intravenous lines.

B. Small-dose heparin administration, used to maintain clear flow through the line, may introduce infection. The multiple-use heparin bottle, and even the syringes storing heparin, can be contaminated with gram-negative bacilli.

C. Blood gas determinations through an arterial line can be the site of contamination. In one outbreak, the syringes used for obtaining intraarterial blood were cooled in ice that was contaminated by a *Flavobacterium* species. This organism was introduced into the arterial line and caused septicemia.

VI. Antibiotic

A. There is no evidence that systemic antibiotics reduce or in any way alter the incidence of catheter-associated infections.

B. Topical antibiotics, such as an ointment containing bacitracin, neomycin, and polymyxin, often are used at the infusion site. Some studies have shown a reduction in skin colonization by normal flora, and perhaps a lower rate of septicemia. These benefits have been partially counterbalanced by an increase in the recovery of *Candida* and resistant gram-negative bacilli from the infusion site. The only strong indication for using topical antiseptic ointments (e.g., povidone-iodine ointment) is a cutdown.

VII. Recommendations for prevention of intravascular infections*

Category I† = Strongly recommended for adoption
Category II = Moderately recommended for adoption
Category III = Weakly recommended for adoption

A. Indications for use. IV therapy should be used only when there are definite therapeutic or diagnostic indications for it. **Category I.**

B. Choice of cannulas for peripheral infusions

1. Plastic cannulas are acceptable for routine peripheral IV infusions if and only if the hospital can be sure that cannulas are replaced every 48–72 hours, such as can be done by an IV team. **Category II.**
2. Otherwise, stainless steel cannulas should be used for routine peripheral IV infusions, and plastic cannulas should be reserved for those clinical settings in which a secure route for vascular access is imperative. **Category II.**

C. Handwashing

1. Hospital personnel should wash their hands before inserting an IV cannula. **Category I.**

*U.S. Department of Health and Human Services, Centers for Disease Control, Center for Infectious Diseases, Atlanta Georgia, *Guidelines for Intravenous Catheter*. October 1981, pp. 1–5.
†See pages 306–307 for complete explanation of ranking system.

2. Soap and water is adequate for handwashing for most insertions, but an antiseptic should be used before insertion of central canulas and cannulas requiring a cutdown. **Category II.**
3. Sterile gloves should be worn for insertion of central cannulas and cannulas requiring a cutdown. **Category I.**

D. Choice of site. In adults, the upper extremity (or, if necessary, subclavian and jugular sites) should be used in preference to lower extremity sites for IV cannulation. All cannulas inserted into a lower extremity should be changed as soon as a satisfactory site can be established elsewhere. **Category I.**

E. Site preparation

1. The IV site should be scrubbed with an antiseptic prior to venipuncture. **Category I.**
2. Tincture of iodine, 1–2%, is preferred, but chlorhexidine, iodophors, or 70% alcohol can be used. The antiseptic should be applied liberally and allowed to remain in contact for at least 30 seconds prior to venipuncture. **Category II.**
3. Neither aqueous benzalkonium-like compounds nor hexachlorophene should be used to scrub the IV site. **Category I.**

F. Procedures accompanying insertion

1. A topical antibiotic or antiseptic ointment should be applied at the IV site immediately after cannula insertion, especially for insertions by cutdown. **Category II.**
2. The cannula should be secured to stabilize it at the insertion site. **Category I.**
3. A sterile dressing should be applied to cover the insertion site. The dressing, not the tape, should cover the wound, unless the tape is sterile. **Category I.**
4. The date of insertion should be recorded in a place where it can be easily found. **Category I.** (The date may be recorded in the medical record and, if feasible, also on the dressing or tape.)

G. Maintenance of IV site

1. Patients with intravenous devices should be evaluated at least daily for evidence of cannula-related complications. This evaluation should include gentle palpation of the insertion site through the intact dressing. If the patient has an unexplained fever, or if there is pain or tenderness at the insertion site, the dressing should be removed and the IV site inspected. **Category I.**
2. For peripheral cannulas that must remain in place for prolonged periods, the IV site should be inspected and dressed with a new sterile dressing at 48–72 hours. Thereafter, the site should be inspected and dressed regularly (the optimal frequency of dressing cannula sites in this situation is not known). **Category II.**
3. Antibiotic or antiseptic ointment, if used, should be reapplied with each dressing change. **Category II.**

H. Replacement of peripheral cannula. If prolonged IV therapy with a peripheral cannula (including heparin-lock devices and peripheral cannulas inserted by a cutdown) is indicated, the cannula should be changed and a new cannula inserted every 48–72 hours, provided that no IV-related complications requiring cannula removal are encountered before this. Cannulas inserted without proper asepsis—for example, those inserted in an emergency—should be replaced at the earliest opportunity. **Category I.** (Peripheral cannulas may occasionally have to be used for longer than 48–72 hours if another peripheral site cannot be found.)

I. Special procedures for central cannulas (those whose tips lie in the large central vessels)

1. Central cannulas should be inserted with aseptic technique and sterile equipment. Gloves and drapes are usually required to achieve this objective. **Category I.**
2. All central cannulas should be removed when they are no longer medically indicated or if they are strongly suspected of causing sepsis. **Category I.**
3. Central cannulas that are inserted by a subclavian or jugular approach, except those used for pressure monitoring, need not be changed routinely. **Category I.** (The proper frequency for changing cannulas that are used for

pressure monitoring—for example, those used to measure pulmonary artery or central venous pressure—is not known.)

4. Central cannulas that are inserted through a peripheral vein should be treated as peripheral cannulas (see appropriate recommendations above). **Category I.**
5. In the case of central cannulas that must remain in place for prolonged periods, the insertion site should be inspected and dressed with a new sterile dressing every 48–72 hours. **Category II.**

J. Maintenance of administration sets

1. IV administration tubing, including "piggy-back" tubing, should be routinely changed every 48 hours. **Category I.**
2. Tubing used for hyperalimentation should be routinely changed every 24–48 hours. **Category II.**
3. Tubing should also be changed after the administration of blood, blood products, or lipid emulsions. **Category III.**
4. Between changes of components, the IV system should be maintained as a closed system as much as possible. All entries into the tubing, as for administration of medications, should be made through injection ports that are disinfected just before entry. **Category I.**
5. Flushing or irrigation of the system to improve flow should be avoided. **Category II.**
6. Blood specimens should not be withdrawn through IV tubing except in an emergency or when immediate discontinuation of the cannula and tubing is planned. **Category II.**

K. Changing parts of the IV system for infection or phlebitis

1. The entire IV system (cannula, administration set, and fluid) should be changed immediately if purulent thrombophlebitis, cellulitis, or IV-related bacteremia is noted or strongly suspected. **Category I.**
2. For phlebitis without signs of infection, the cannula should be changed. **Category I.**

L. Culturing for suspected IV-related infections

1. If an IV system is to be discontinued because of suspected IV-related infection, such as purulent thrombophlebitis or bacteremia, the skin at the skin-cannula junction should be cleaned with alcohol and the alcohol allowed to dry before cannula removal, and the cannula should be cultured by a semi-quantitative technique. **Category II.**
   - **a.** If an IV system is discontinued because of suspected fluid contamination, the fluid should be cultured and the implicated bottle saved. **Category I.**
   - **b.** If an IV system is discontinued because of suspected IV-related bacteremia, the fluid should be cultured. **Category III.**
   - **c.** If contamination of fluid is confirmed, the implicated bottle and the remaining units of the implicated lot should be saved, and the lot numbers of fluid and additives should be recorded. **Category I.**
   - **d.** If intrinsic contamination (contamination during manufacturing) is suspected, the local health authorities, CDC, and United States Food and Drug Administration should be notified immediately. **Category I.**

M. Quality control during and after admixture

1. Parenteral and hyperalimentation fluids should be admixed (compounded) in the pharmacy, unless clinical urgency requires admixture in patient-care areas. **Category II.**
2. Personnel should wash their hands before admixing parenterals. **Category I.**
3. All containers of parenteral fluid should be checked for visible turbidity, leaks, cracks, and particulate matter and for the manufacturer's expiration date before admixing and before use. If a problem is found, the fluids should not be used and should be sent to (or remain in) the pharmacy. **Category I.**
4. In the pharmacy, a laminar flow hood should be used for admixing parenteral fluid. **Category II.**
5. Single-use (single-dose) containers (vials) should be used for admixture whenever possible. When multiple-use containers intended for intravenous

use are opened, they should be marked with the date and time that the container is entered. The product label or package insert should be consulted to determine whether refrigeration of the container is necessary. **Category II.** (The proper storage temperature is product-specific and is determined by many factors, such as stability of ingredients and optimal activity of antibacterial preservatives; bacterial survival in some containers may be enhanced by refrigeration. Unless an expiration date is stated on the product label or package insert, it is not known whether multiple-use containers, once entered, should be discarded after a specific or arbitrary length of time.)

6. A distinctive supplementary label should be attached to each admixed parenteral stating, as a minimum, the additives and their dosage, the date and time of compounding, the expiration time, and the person who did the compounding. **Category I.**
7. All admixed fluid should be refrigerated or started within 6 hours of admixing.
8. If necessary, admixed parenterals may be stored in the refrigerator for up to a week before use, provided that refrigeration is continuous and begins immediately after admixing. Other factors, such as stability of ingredients, may dictate a shorter storage time. **Category II.** (This recommendation is intended to prevent waste of parenterals that are admixed for immediate use but, unexpectedly, cannot be used.)
9. Once started, all parenterals should be completely used or discarded within 24 hours. **Category I.**
10. Infusions of lipid emulsions should be completed within 12 hours of starting. **Category I.**

N. IV Filters. Usage of IV in-line filters is not recommended as a routine infection control measure. **Category II.**

O. IV Teams

Using professional, specially trained IV teams that insert and maintain IV cannulas may decrease the risk of IV-related infections. **Category III.**

Total Parenteral Nutrition (TPN)

TPN has brought great benefit to many surgical patients, but the procedure is also fraught with difficulty, especially in the area of sepsis. When total parenteral nutrition was first introduced, septicemia was encountered in 10–30% of TPN administrations. This figure was obviously unacceptable if the technique was to continue being used, so radical changes, including the establishment of "TPN teams," have been instituted at most hospitals. The result has been a reduction in sepsis to < 5%—in some institutions, to < 1%.

I. Microbiology. The microbiology of TPN-associated sepsis is somewhat different from that associated with conventional IV cannulas.

A. *Candida* accounts for 50% of TPN sepsis.

B. The remaining cases are divided between gram-negative bacilli, especially *Klebsiella,* and *Staph. aureus.*

C. Most cases of fungemia at present can be traced to TPN administration. While many episodes are self-limited, a small percentage of patients will develop disseminated candidiasis, *Candida* endocarditis, and *Candida* endophthalmitis. *Candida* emerges as the leading pathogen in patients receiving TPN, for three reasons:

1. The patients are extremely ill, often immunosuppressed, owing either to their severe illness or as a result of drugs such as steroids and chemotherapy.
2. Most are receiving antibiotics. In those receiving systemic therapy, there is suppression of the normal flora with overgrowth of fungi. Even the use of topical antibiotics favors the overgrowth of *Candida* at the infusion site, offering an easy portal of entry into the TPN line.
3. *Candida* can proliferate with great ease in TPN fluid, in contrast to many other organisms that grow poorly or not at all.

II. Recommendations for TPN control

A. Insertion of the catheter.

1. The catheter should be inserted under conditions of operating room sterility. If the placement is done in a treatment room, the operator and his assistants should each wear a cap, mask, gown, and gloves.
2. The area for insertion should be suitably shaved and prepared as for a surgical procedure.
3. The patient should be placed head down to minimize the possibility of air embolism.
4. The subclavian vein is used most often in adults, the internal or external jugular in infants. Other sites can be used, but catheters placed in the extremities are particularly vulnerable to infection and thrombosis, so this is not recommended. Because of risk of infection, the cervical route should not be used if there is a tracheostomy.
5. **X-ray confirmation of the position of the catheter is mandatory.** A surprisingly high number pass to the opposite side or even an opposite jugular vein. The correct position is the tip of the catheter in the superior vena cava just above the right atrium.
6. The use of povidone-iodine ointment at the site of insertion of the catheter is recommended, together with an occlusive dressing with tape securing the catheter to prevent accidental dislodgment.

B. Precautions.

1. All solutions should be mixed in the pharmacy, preferably under laminar flow conditions with maximum aseptic technique. If additional electrolytes are needed, they should be given by separate IV infusion. Certain alterations in the standard formula may increase the risk of infection; for example, adding bicarbonate facilitates the growth of staphylococci in the solution.
2. **Absolutely nothing** should be added to the solution once it leaves the pharmacy. Strict adherence to this rule is necessary in order to prevent infection. When insulin is needed (quite rare), it should be given separately. When antibiotics or electrolyte supplements are needed, they should be given by separate IV infusion.
3. The solution is administered through an 0.45-μ Millipore filter, the last item in the line. An intravenous pump is recommended.
4. The line and catheter must not be used for drawing blood samples, central venous pressure measurement, or other purposes (except for periodic blood cultures).
5. Certain infusion pumps, such as the Harvard pump, drive fluids into the tissue at increased pressure, producing infiltration and eventual skin sloughs. This presents a serious hazard of sepsis, not to mention the severe pain and discomfort accompanying the mishap. Gravity feed can be used in many situations; if a pump is to be used, the choice should be one that shuts off or sounds an alarm when the infusion pressure is excessive.

C. Line care

1. A special TPN team, which may be the same as the IV team, should be trained for care of this important device.
2. The entire intravenous administration set, including the Millipore filter and the occlusive dressing about the catheter site, is changed three times per week (Monday, Wednesday, Friday) using aseptic technique (mask and gloves). This also should be done by the TPN nurse.
3. Solutions are provided by the pharmacy in amounts to last no more than 8 hours. The bottles should be kept refrigerated until 1 hour before they are hung for use, when they are allowed to warm to room temperatures.
4. Some institutions prefer to draw a blood sample through the catheter for a culture at the change of line. The value of this culture has not been established, and in our view it is not necessary. However, a culture of the skin site at the time of dressing change is useful in predicting infection. A positive culture has a 60% predictive value of infection, whereas a negative culture has a 98% predictive value for absence of infection.

D. Indications for removing catheter because of sepsis

1. Two consecutive "routine" blood cultures, drawn from different IV sites, which are positive for the same pathogen in an asymptomatic patient.
2. One positive blood culture in a patient who has otherwise unexplained fever.
3. Strong clinical evidence of local infection, even if blood cultures are negative.
4. Evidence of local complications about the catheter site: inflammation, pus, thrombosis, or extravasation.
5. An otherwise unexplained fever. In this setting it may be necessary to stop TPN and withdraw the IV line. The catheter line segment, any local discharge, and a sample of the TPN fluid should be sent for culture and Gram's stain. Report of a positive Gram's stain may be sufficient indication to initiate treatment in the case of a patient with fever. The guidelines given later (pp. 329–330) for catheter-induced infection are to be followed. In the case of TPN, however, greater consideration should be given to the possibility of *Candida* infection, and a decision to start therapy with amphotericin B must be weighed.

Intravascular Pressure Monitoring Systems

Transducers used for monitoring arterial pressures have been the source of contamination with gram-negative organisms such as *Serratia* and *Klebsiella*.

I. Problems with transducers

A. There are various manufacturing companies with different levels of quality control.

B. Certain companies use disposable domes for the supposed reason that the instrument can be used without lengthy sterilization. However, these disposable domes have been the source of contamination in certain epidemics.

C. Many intensive care units within the same hospital are using transducers, often without a standardized program for sterilization. Because these instruments are in frequent use, sterilization is often reduced to a substandard minimum, setting the stage for an epidemic.

D. Contamination has occurred in the interspace between the transducer and the protective dome membrane, in the stopcocks and sampling ports, and in the exterior ports, perhaps at the assembly. Bacteremia can arise from contamination of the flush fluid and from infection at the skin site of insertion, especially if the transducer is left for more than 4 days.

II. Recommendations for prevention of infections in intravascular pressure monitoring systems*

Category I† = Strongly recommended for adoption.
Category II = Moderately recommended for adoption.
Category III = Weakly recommended for adoption.

A. Use

Invasive pressure monitoring should be used only in clinical situations in which information gathered by this technique can clearly influence decisions in patient management. **Category I.**

B. Assembly

1. Disposable components that are preassembled and sterile-packaged by the manufacturer should be used when possible. **Category II.**
2. Pressure-monitoring systems should be assembled in the simplest arrangement possible. Sterile items, including disposable domes and lines, should be

*U.S. Department of Health and Human Services, Centers for Disease Control, Center for Infectious Diseases, Atlanta Georgia, *Guidelines for Prevention of Infection Related to Intravascular Pressure Monitoring Systems*. October 1981, pp. 1–5.
†See pages 306–307 for complete explanation of ranking scheme.

kept in their sterile wrapping until needed. These items and the transducer should not be assembled hours or days before the time of actual need, even to prepare for a possible emergency. Most important, systems should never be filled with flush solution and stored (since even a few microorganisms inadvertently introduced into the solution at the time of assembly can rapidly multiply during storage). **Category I.**

3. In disposable domes and transducers, the space between the transducer head and dome membrane should be left dry or, if fluid is required, the space should be filled with normal saline, bacteriostatic water, or 70% alcohol (if the manufacturer states that it will not damage the dome or transducer); glucose-containing solutions should not be used, since they are known to support the growth of microorganisms. **Category I.**

C. Flushing lines

1. Patency of pressure-monitoring cannulas should be maintained by a closed flush system rather than an open system that requires use of a syringe and stopcock. **Category II.**
2. Flush solutions, i.e., those whose main purpose is to maintain patency of the cannula and that are infused very slowly or are given as intermittent boluses, should not contain glucose for the reasons stated in sec. **B.3. Category I.**

D. Handwashing

1. Hospital personnel should wash their hands before inserting a pressure-monitoring cannula or manipulating a pressure-monitoring system, such as to draw a blood specimen. **Category I.**
2. An antiseptic handwashing agent is preferred, but soap and water can be used. **Category II.**
3. **a.** Sterile gloves should be worn for insertion of central cannulas for pressure monitoring (for example, pulmonary artery and central venous cannulas) and for peripheral cannulas requiring a cutdown. **Category I.**
   b. Sterile gloves should be worn for insertion of other intravascular cannulas used for pressure monitoring. **Category III.**

E. Insertion and maintenance. Recommendations for insertion and maintenance of intravenous pressure-monitoring systems are similar to those recommended for intravenous cannulas.

1. The site chosen for cannula insertion should be scrubbed with an antiseptic prior to insertion of the cannula. **Category I.**
2. Tincture of iodine (1–2%) is preferred for the insertion site, but chlorhexidine, iodophors, or 70% alcohol can be used. The antiseptic should be applied liberally and allowed to remain in contact for at least 30 seconds before insertion. **Category II.**
3. Neither aqueous benzalkonium-like compounds nor hexachlorophene should be used to scrub the insertion site. **Category I.**
4. A topical antibiotic or antiseptic ointment should be applied at the site immediately after cannula insertion, especially for insertions by cutdown. **Category II.**
5. Central and cutdown cannulas should be inserted with aseptic technique and sterile equipment. Gloves and drapes are usually required to achieve this objective. **Category I.**
6. The cannula should be secured to stabilize it at the insertion site. **Category I.**
7. A sterile dressing should be applied to cover the insertion site. The dressing, and not tape, should cover the wound, unless the tape is sterile. **Category I.**
8. The date of insertion should be recorded in a place where it can be found easily. **Category I.** (The date may be recorded in the medical record and, if feasible, on the dressing or tape.)
9. Patients with intravascular devices should be evaluated at least daily for evidence of cannula-related complications. This evaluation should include gentle palpation of the insertion site through the intact dressing. If the patient has an unexplained fever or there is pain or tenderness at the insertion site, the dressing should be removed and the site inspected. **Category I.**

10. In the case of peripheral cannulas that must remain in place for prolonged periods, the insertion site should be inspected and dressed with a new sterile dressing at 48–72 hours. The site should be inspected and dressed regularly thereafter. (The optimal frequency for dressing cannula sites in this situation is not known.) **Category II.**
11. In the case of central cannulas that must remain in place for prolonged periods, the insertion site should be inspected and dressed with a new sterile dressing every 48–72 hours. **Category II.**
12. Antibiotic or antiseptic ointment, if used, should be reapplied with each dressing change. **Category II.**

F. Calibration. During calibration of a pressure-monitoring system, contact should not occur between the sterile fluid column in the cannula and tubing and non-sterile solutions or equipment. **Category I.**

G. Obtaining specimens

1. Ideally, pressure-monitoring systems should be maintained as closed systems. Stopcocks, if used, should be covered. **Category I.**
2. Arterial pressure-monitoring systems should be used primarily to monitor blood pressure and to obtain specimens for arterial blood-gas analysis. Routine blood specimens, if they are to be drawn from the arterial line, should be drawn at the same time as those for blood-gas analysis, if possible, to keep the number of manipulations to a minimum. **Category I.**
3. Care should be taken to ensure that all specimens be obtained aseptically; for example, syringes chilled in ice should not be allowed to contaminate the stopcocks or sampling ports. **Category I.**

H. Replacement of intravascular monitoring systems in patients requiring prolonged monitoring

1. The container of flush solution should be changed every 24 hours. **Category I.**
2. The chamber dome, administration tubing, and continuous flow device (if used) should be replaced at 48-hour intervals. **Category II.** (It is not known whether the transducer needs periodic disinfection or sterilization during prolonged use on a single patient.)
3. Under special circumstances, such as following the reflux of blood into the tubing or domes or following countershock (which could damage the protective membrane of some disposable domes), replacement of the tubing and dome is desirable. **Category III.**
4. Peripheral arterial cannulas should be left in place no longer than 4 days if other sites for cannula insertion are available. **Category II.**
5. Central cannulas for pressure monitoring that are inserted through a peripheral vein should be removed in 48–72 hours. **Category I.** (These cannulas may occasionally have to be used for longer than 48–72 hours if another insertion site cannot be found. The proper frequency for changing pressure-monitoring cannulas inserted through a subclavian or jugular approach is not known.)
6. Cannulas for pressure monitoring should not be replaced over a guide wire if this is done solely for infection control. **Category II.**
7. Intravascular pressure-monitoring systems should be removed when they are no longer medically indicated and promptly discontinued or placed at another site if the initial site becomes infected or if the monitoring system is suspected as the source of clinical sepsis or bacteremia. **Category I.**

I. Processing transducers before reuse

1. Disposable components of the pressure-monitoring system should not be resterilized and reused. **Category I.**
2. **a.** After use, transducers (including transducer heads and reusable domes) should be cleaned, disinfected (high-level) with a chemical agent or sterilized with ethylene oxide, and stored in a manner to prevent recontamination before use on the next patient. **Category I.** (The manufacturers of the transducer and reusable dome should be asked for recommenda-

tions about classes of disinfectants that will not injure the equipment and about proper methods of cleaning, sterilizing, and storing components.)

b. Sterilization with ethylene oxide is recommended, unless the manufacturer states that this method is not satisfactory. **Category II.**

Contaminated Blood Products

I. Approximately 1–6% of blood products administered to patients are found to be contaminated. Despite these alarming figures, clinical infection is rare, probably because the inoculum size is relatively low and the organisms often are of low virulence.

II. The product of greatest risk is **platelets,** since they are pooled from several donors and stored at 25°C, which ensures not only the survival of platelets, but also of microorganisms.

III. Other microorganisms besides bacteria and fungi that are transmitted by blood products are as follows:

A. Hepatitis virus
B. Epstein-Barr virus
C. Cytomegalovirus
D. *Toxoplasma*
E. Malaria

IV. Recommendations for control of sepsis from blood products

A. Once delivered from the blood bank, the blood products should be administered without delay.

B. After infusion, the entire administration line, down to the cannula insert, should be replaced.

C. When sepsis is suspected from the onset of chills and fever (which, of course, may be due to a hypersensitivity reaction), the infusion is stopped, and appropriate cultures are obtained from the apparatus and the remaining blood products.

D. Most contamination is owing to gram-negative bacilli. Initial decisions are guided by Gram's stain of the infused product. If this fluid is unavailable or the stain results are inconclusive, the recommendations for catheter-associated infections (see below) should be followed.

Catheter-Associated Infections

I. Diagnosis. Catheter-related sepsis should be suspected in any patient with an indwelling plastic catheter, especially with the risk factors already mentioned (pp. 318–319). The presence of phlebitis or a discharge from the skin site adds further credibility to this diagnosis. Procedures to be followed are:

A. Blood cultures should be obtained from two different intravenous sites, while the catheter is in place.

B. If the IV fluid is thought to be contaminated, an aliquot of 20 ml should be saved for bacteriologic culture. This volume is required to recover organisms present in small numbers.

C. The catheter should be removed under aseptic conditions. The intravascular segment is deposited carefully into a sterile container and delivered to the bacteriology lab for culture. A semiquantitative technique for culture is the preferred method. High-density growth correlates with IV-related bacteremia and local inflammation. If there is a discharge from the local area, it should be cultured and used for Gram's staining. The skin should be cleaned and dressed. When phlebitis is present, a warm pack and elevation are useful measures.

II. Treatment

A. The majority of patients can be cured by simple **removal** of the catheter. Indications for systemic antibiotics are

1. Severe sepsis with fever, chills, or hypotension.

2. Persistent fever, along with signs of phlebitis, for more than 8 hours after removal of the catheter. Even though the patient is not severely ill, it has become obvious that the infection is not resolving.
3. Severe local signs of inflammation and phlebitis, even in the absence of fever.

B. If **systemic antibiotics** are required, the following guidelines should be used, based on the Gram's stain of the exudate from the infusion site or from the catheter tip:
1. **If gram-positive cocci are seen,** they are probably *Staph. aureus* or *Staph. epidermidis*. The treatment is a semisynthetic penicillin such as oxacillin or nafcillin, 2 gm IV q6h.
2. **If gram-negative bacilli are seen,** an aminoglycoside, such as gentamicin, tobramycin, or amikacin, should be started in the appropriate dosage (see p. 254); plus carbenicillin, 5 gm IV q4–6h, or ticarcillin, 3 gm q4–6h.
3. If **yeasts** are seen, a careful decision is required whether to initiate amphotericin B treatment. Most patients do not require such therapy and can be cured by removing the catheter. Again, the clinical condition of the patient is the best guide. The eye grounds should be examined for the presence of fluffy, white exudates, which are the characteristic lesions of *Candida* endophthalmitis. In an extreme situation such as this, the amphotericin B dose should be accelerated. After a test dose of 1 mg, the 1st day's dose can then be given to a total of 5 mg; 2nd day's dose, to 10 mg; and the dosage increased sequentially (see pp. 281–282).
4. If the **Gram's stain fails to reveal organisms,** or if **no material is available for study,** start a cephalosporin, such as cefazolin or cephalothin, and an aminoglycoside (gentamicin, tobramycin, or amikacin).

C. Whether or not antibiotics have been started, repeat blood cultures, at different sites, should be obtained on the 2 subsequent days in order to determine the presence of continued bacteremia. This finding suggests suppurative thrombophlebitis.

D. The usual duration of therapy for this infection is 7–10 days, allowing ample opportunity for the local site to heal.

III. A special problem is that of the patient with catheter-based **Staph. aureus bacteremia** who has a **heart murmur.** This pathogen may implant on a previously damaged cardiac valve, producing endocarditis. In this setting the following steps should be taken:

A. Any patient with either Gram's stain or blood culture evidence of *Staph. aureus*, in the presence of a cardiac murmur, should receive antistaphylococcal medication (either a penicillinase-resistant penicillin, such as oxacillin or nafcillin, or a cephalosporin).

B. There should be a scrupulous examination for other signs of endocarditis, such as Osler's nodes, hematuria, and petechial hemorrhages in the conjunctivae, skin, or beneath the nails (see Chap. 7).

C. There should be daily inspection for changing heart murmur, new murmurs, and cardiac failure, along with examination for the signs of endocarditis.

D. Blood cultures should be obtained every 2–3 days during therapy.

E. If the patient has become afebrile, and there are no changes in the cardiac status, no signs of persistent bacteremia, and no physical findings of endocarditis, antibiotic treatment can be stopped at 7–10 days. The patient should remain in the hospital for an additional 48 hours, during which time new sets of blood cultures are obtained and the patient is observed for fever or changing status.

F. If, after 48 hours, the patient remains well and blood cultures are negative, he or she can be discharged, with careful instructions that, should any fever or skin lesions develop, the doctor be contacted immediately.

Suppurative Thrombophlebitis

I. The main difficulty is making the diagnosis, since approximately 50% of patients lack local findings of phlebitis. The clinical setting is continuous bacteremia with fever and chills, leading eventually to septic shock and death. The therapeutic approach is as follows:

A. Appropriate antibiotics, based on the sensitivity of the organism isolated from the bloodstream, should be started. Since 80% of cases are associated with gram-negative organisms, especially *Klebsiella,* the treatment should include an aminoglycoside, such as gentamicin, tobramycin, or amikacin, plus a second drug—a cephalosporin such as cephalothin or cefazolin (in the case of *Klebsiella*), or carbenicillin or ticarcillin (in the case of *Enterobacter* and other resistant organisms).

B. If phlebitis is recognized, warm, moist packs and elevation have an ameliorating effect.

C. Anticoagulation by heparin or coumadin has no demonstrable benefit in this disease.

D. If the patient fails to respond to these measures a surgical approach is indicated, as follows (it should be noted that the vast majority of patients will improve with conservative management):

When local findings of inflammation, erythema, swelling, or discharge are present, an incision is made over the venotomy site, and the underlying vein is milked down to demonstrate whether pus extrudes from the distal end. Further exploratory incisions may be required more proximally, since the area of phlebitis can be rather localized. When the thrombotic site is found, the full extent of the involved vessel is identified, and a ligature is placed at the most proximal area. An excision of the entire length of the involved vein and its tributaries is undertaken. The wound is packed open, and systemic antibiotics are continued.

II. The most difficult problem is the patient with continuous, gram-negative bacteremia without a source, who lacks local findings of phlebitis. If the patient has failed to respond to antibiotics, and the clinical condition is worsening, it may be necessary to make exploratory incisions over the previous catheter sites to search for suppurative phlebitis. In our experience, this situation arises very rarely, and usually there are alternative explanations for gram-negative sepsis.

15 Specimen Collection for Microbiology

Blood Cultures

I. General principles. Blood cultures should be obtained from any septic patient. The total number of cultures and the interval between samplings are dictated by the clinical setting. If the patient is acutely ill, at least two cultures should be obtained from separate venipuncture sites prior to initiation of antibiotics. In cases of suspected endocarditis, five blood cultures should be obtained. When the patient is less severely ill, it is often possible to delay treatment and collect blood cultures over several hours or days. If antimicrobials have already been given, it may be desirable in certain settings to suspend treatment and obtain cultures 24–48 hours later; suspected intravascular infections, such as infected graft and endocarditis, are examples.

II. Forms of bacteremia

A. Intermittent bacteremia represents periodic hematogenous seeding associated with **extravascular** infections such as abscess, pyelonephritis, pneumonia, and intraabdominal sepsis. The fever pattern usually is characterized by intermittent spikes; blood cultures are most likely to be positive just prior to or during the chill or on the ascending limb of the temperature spike.

B. Continuous bacteremia is noted with **intravascular** infections such as endocarditis, infected vascular graft, suppurative thrombophlebitis, and arteritis; and occasionally with overwhelming extravascular infections such as typhoid fever and brucellosis. Blood cultures are positive on repeated occasions, so the timing of samples is less critical.

C. Transient bacteremia commonly occurs with trauma of mucosal surfaces that harbor an indigenous microflora, as with dental procedures or urinary tract manipulation. The bacteremia is self-limited, and there are either no symptoms or only a transient, self-limited temperature elevation. In the setting of a dental procedure, the organisms isolated from the bloodstream are streptococci, especially the *viridans* group, diphtheroids, and microaerophilic or anaerobic streptococci. Enterococci or even coliforms may be found in patients undergoing procedures on the GI or GU tract. The major concern is with patients who have underlying cardiac lesions that predispose to endocarditis, since these organisms may colonize heart valves and roughened endocardial surfaces. (For recommendations concerning antibiotic prophylaxis, see pp. 295–296.)

III. Culture technique

A. The skin is vigorously cleaned with 70% alcohol followed by 2% tincture of iodine. Povidone-iodine (Betadine) is an alternative agent for skin decontamination. In patients with hypersensitivity to iodine, only 70% alcohol should be used.

B. Once the skin is prepared, the vein should not be palpated, unless the finger is prepared in a similar fashion or covered with a sterile glove.

C. The diaphragm tops of culture bottles, which are potentially contaminated, should be swabbed with 70% alcohol.

D. The volume of blood delivered to culture bottles should result in a blood-broth ratio of 1:10–1:20, in order to dilute the antibacterial properties of serum. In most instances 5–10 ml is drawn from adults and 1–5 ml from children. The practice of collecting larger volumes in a single syringe for inoculation of several culture sets is deplored; the results are often misleading, since the same contaminants may be present in all bottles. Therefore, specimens from one venipuncture should constitute a single culture. Additional cultures should be drawn with a new needle from a different site.

IV. Laboratory procedures

A. Media. All-purpose blood culture media include trypticase soy broth, brain-heart infusion broth, thioglycollate broth, and Columbia broth. Media should be supplemented with sodium polyanetholsulfonate (SPS), bottled under a vacuum with CO_2, and capped with a rubber diaphragm top. All these media are considered equally efficacious, although the yield of positive cultures is increased when two bottles are used rather than one. Many hospital laboratories routinely employ a two-bottle system—one bottle for anaerobes and a second (which is vented in the laboratory) for aerobes. The optimal medium for recovering fungi in blood cultures is vented diphasic brain-heart infusion media. Additional blood culture media that are occasionally advocated include:

1. Hypertonic broth (for cell wall–defective bacteria, i.e., L-forms).
2. Supplemented peptone broth (Vacutainer)
3. Prereduced anaerobically sterilized brain-heart infusion broth (for anaerobes)
4. Radiometric broth (for early detection of bacteremia)

These media have not proved superior to conventional media for routine use.

B. Processing of cultures: Blood cultures should be observed daily for evidence of growth. Gram's stain of broth will sometimes reveal bacteria before growth is grossly visible. Any suspected positive culture should be immediately Gram's-stained, subcultured, and reported. Before the culture is discarded at the end of 3 weeks, the broth should be Gram's-stained to search for indolent growth.

C. Buffy-coat examination. A smear of leukocytes from the buffy coat of peripheral blood can demonstrate bacteria in 5–10% of positive blood cultures. This provides immediate information concerning the morphotype of the organism responsible. **Technique:** Unclotted, anticoagulated blood is pipetted into two sterile Wintrobe hematocrit tubes. These are centrifuged for 10 min at 300 g. All but approximately 1 ml of plasma is removed. The remaining plasma and buffy coat are pipetted, spread evenly on a clean slide, Gram's-stained, and examined microscopically.

V. Interpretation. *Staph. epidermidis,* diphtheroids, *Bacillus,* and *Propionibacterium* usually represent blood culture contaminants. These organisms normally colonize the skin, and they may be inadvertently introduced during venipuncture or with subsequent laboratory manipulation. When the patient has a prosthetic device, however, these "contaminants" are given more respect, since they may be pathogens. Repeat blood cultures are indicated to resolve their status.

Urinary Tract Specimens

I. General principles. Few infections more readily yield to accurate bacteriologic analysis than those involving the urinary tract. Quantitative culture of a properly collected, voided specimen of urine is adequate to establish the diagnosis in most cases. In occasional cases specialized sampling techniques are required in order to avoid contaminants or to localize the site of infection.

II. Voided urine specimens

A. Female

1. Spread the labia and wash the vulva with several soaped 4 × 4 sponges, using a slow front-to-back motion.
2. Use a final rinse of sterile water to remove the soap.
3. Collect urine in a sterile container during the middle of an uninterrupted stream.

4. The reliability of the urine specimen is improved if the patient is in the lithotomy position, the perineum is adequately cleaned, and the midstream sample is collected by a trained person.

B. Male

1. Retract the foreskin and wash the glans with several soaped 4 × 4 sponges, followed by a final rinse with sterile water to remove soap.
2. Circumcised males require no local preparation.
3. Collect urine in a sterile container during the middle of an uninterrupted stream.

C. Processing. Since the doubling time of bacteria in urine is 30–45 minutes, an excessive delay in culture leads to spurious results. Specimens should either be processed within 30 minutes of collection or refrigerated.

D. Interpretation of culture results

1. Quantitative urine cultures show 95% of patients with untreated urinary tract infections have $\geqslant 10^5$ bacteria/ml urine. These high counts are most readily found in morning specimens, when the bacteria have had sufficient time to multiply in the bladder, since bladder urine serves as an excellent growth medium. Lower concentrations are noted in "spot" urines and in patients who void frequently.
2. Contaminants are usually present in counts of $< 10^3$/ml.
3. Counts of 10^3–10^4/ml are of uncertain significance, and the culture should be repeated. These low counts can be found in patients with urethritis (both male and female) and prostatitis.
4. Because of the high incidence of perineal and urethral contamination in females, a single, early-morning, clean-catch specimen of urine with 10^5 bacteria/ml indicates true bacteriuria in only 80% of cases; with two specimens yielding the same type and concentration of bacteria, the accuracy is 95%. Asymptomatic female patients with significant bacteriuria should be asked to produce a 2nd specimen for confirmation. In the case of symptomatic women, a single specimen is sufficient. Reliability of a single, properly collected specimen in males is virtually 100%.
5. Urinary tract infections usually involve a single bacterial species. Two or more types of bacteria are most likely to appear in a single specimen of urine with infections complicating an anatomic defect, Foley catheter, stone, or foreign body; otherwise, polymicrobic bacteriuria indicates contamination, and the culture should be repeated.
6. Urinary tract infections usually are caused by enteric bacteria, such as *E. coli, Klebsiella, Proteus, Enterobacter, Pseudomonas,* or enterococci. *Staphylococcus saprophyticus* is found in 5% of patients with urinary tract infection. Other staphylococci, such as *Staph. aureus* and *Staph. epidermidis,* are either contaminants (usually) or have seeded the kidney via bacteremia. Diphtheroids, lactobacilli, and micrococci generally represent urethral contaminants.
7. False-negative cultures result from previous antibiotic therapy, vigorous hydration, infection behind a stone or proximal to an obstructed ureter, contamination of the specimen with cleansing solution, or infection with a fastidious or slow-growing organism.

E. Direct microscopic examination of properly collected fresh urine provides immediate diagnostic information and serves as a quality control of culture results. One drop of **uncentrifuged** urine is placed on a clean slide and allowed to dry without spreading. The slide may be examined without staining under reduced light, or it may be stained with methylene blue or by Gram's stain. One or more bacteria per oil immersion field indicates a count of 10^5/ml. (Correlation with quantitative urine culture is 80–90%.)

F. Urinalysis. All changes are nonspecific for infection. Pyuria (>5 WBC/high power field [HPF]) depends to some extent on urine flow rates and pH. Pyuria is present in 50% of patients with asymptomatic bacteriuria and in most patients with symptomatic urinary tract infection. Pyuria may also occur with vaginal infections as well as with many noninfectious diseases of the GU system, such as interstitial nephritis and lupus nephritis.

III. Urethral catheterization. This procedure is seldom required for bacteriologic studies per se. The risk of introducing bacteria into the bladder, particularly in elderly and bedridden patients, interdicts this procedure when alternative methods are available.

Technique

1. Preparation is the same as described for clean-catch urine specimens.
2. A #12 French catheter is passed, using aseptic technique.
3. Initial urine is allowed to wash through the catheter, and only the later portion is collected for culture.
4. Quantitative counts may be lower than with voided specimens: 10^3/ml is regarded as significant, if techniques are optimal.

IV. Indwelling catheters. Freshly passed urine is collected with a a 26-gauge needle passed into the proximal portion of the catheter tubing after it has been cleaned with 70% alcohol. Urine drainage bags should not be sampled, since bacterial multiplication may have occurred in the stagnant collection. Catheter tips should not be cultured, since the tip becomes contaminated during passage through the urethra.

V. Condom (external) drainage system. These systems allow large concentrations of contaminants to proliferate in the stagnant urine at the attachment site. Despite obvious difficulties, an attempt should be made to obtain freshly passed urine by means of needle aspiration of the tubing after preparation with 70% alcohol.

VI. Cystoscopy procedures, ureteral catheters, cystostomies, and nephrostomies. Urine collected from these systems is a reliable culture source. Lower concentrations of bacteria are considered significant, since these specimens are less likely to be contaminated.

VII. Suprapubic bladder aspiration. This is a safe, rapid, bedside method of obtaining urine that is free of urethral and perineal contaminants.

A. Indications

1. Patients who, owing either to age or to underlying disease, are unable to provide a voided specimen. It is the preferred specimen source in infants with suspected urinary tract infections.
2. Situations in which voided urine specimens are likely to yield contaminants, as in the case of male patients with condom drainage and female patients with marked obesity or redundant labia.
3. Situations in which bacteriologic results of voided urine specimens are difficult to interpret i.e., the recovery of an unlikely pathogen, polymicrobic bacteriuria, or conflicting results with repeated samplings.
4. When an anaerobic organism is suspected to be the urinary pathogen. (Because it is so rare, the result has to be confirmed.)

B. Technique (adult patient)

1. The bladder should be full as determined by palpation, by the urge to void, or by the urge to void with suprapubic pressure. A gentle penile clamp for several hours may be required for incontinent male patients.
2. Cleanse the suprapubic skin area with antiseptic solution, but do not shave. The application of local skin anesthesia is optimal.
3. Aspirate bladder urine with a 3½-inch 22-gauge needle 2 cm above the symphysis pubis in the midline. The needle should be advanced rapidly and straight back, i.e., perpendicular to the bed with the patient in the supine position.
4. Urine cannot be aspirated in 5–10 percent of cases, because the bladder either is in the retropubic area or is inadequately filled.

C. Complications are rare but may include perforation of the bowel, prostatitis, bacteremia, hematuria, and induction of premature labor or abortion in pregnant females.

VIII. Transvaginal bladder aspiration. This is an alternative to suprapubic aspiration for women undergoing gynecologic examination. The patient is placed in the lithotomy position, a speculum is inserted, and the anterior blade is removed, leaving the posterior blade as a perineal retractor. The needle puncture site is the anterior vaginal wall just proximal to the urethrovesical junction. This is prepared with antiseptic and punctured with a 22-gauge spinal needle attached to a syringe. The forward part of the speculum blade is pushed down as the needle is advanced straight forward (parallel to the floor), while slight suction pressure is maintained on the syringe. Urine should be collected after the needle is advanced approximately 2–3 cm. Discomfort with this procedure is minimal; slight vaginal bleeding is common, but hematuria is rare.

IX. Localization of lower urinary tract infection in male patients. Quantitative cultures of fractionated urine and prostatic secretions are useful for diagnosing prostatitis, urethritis, and cystitis.

A. Indications. This procedure is particularly helpful in identifying the prostate as a residual focus of infection in males with recurrent urinary tract infections in the absence of an anatomic abnormality of the genitourinary tract. The principal disadvantage is the **cost** of processing four bacteriologic specimens. It may be justified, however, by the benefits derived from optimal treatment, made possible by accurate diagnosis.

B. Technique

1. **First voided bladder urine (VB_1).** The clean-catch method (see sec. **II.B**) is used for collecting the 1st 10 ml of voided urine.
2. **VB_2.** After approximately 200 cc has been voided, a 2nd or midstream sample is collected.
3. **Expressed prostatic secretions (EPS).** The patient is instructed to stop voiding and, during prostatic massage, urethral discharge is collected. This specimen cannot be obtained in 10–20% of cases.
4. **VB_3.** Immediately after massage, the patient voids again, and the 1st 10 ml is collected.
5. The procedure should not be performed when significant bacteriuria is present on routine urine culture. Sampling during antimicrobial administration is acceptable, since an infected prostate continues to shed bacteria in expressed secretions.

C. Interpretation of results is based on relative counts in the four specimens:

Condition	**VB_1**	**VB_2**	**EPS**	**VB_3**
Urethritis	+ + (VB_3)	+	—	+
Prostatitis	±	±	+ + (VB_3)	+ (VB_1)
Bladder bacteriuria	+ +	+ +	—	+ +

Quantitative counts are often less than 10^5/ml, but they should be considered significant in relation to the other specimens. Therefore the microbiologist should be instructed to use a larger quantitative loop (i.e., 0.01 ml) than usually employed for routine urine culture.

X. Methods of differentiating upper and lower urinary tract infections. These studies are of limited value in the routine assessment of urinary tract infections, since the usual goal of treatment is elimination of bacteria from all portions of the genitourinary system. Differentiation of upper and lower tract bacteriuria may be important in cases of recurrent infection without apparent anatomic abnormality.

A. Urethral catheterization. Paired samples from each ureter are obtained for quantitative culture after the bladder has been carefully washed out to avoid contamination by bladder urine. The assumption that bacteriuria in the ureter or renal pelvis indicates renal parenchymal involvement is usually, but not invariably, correct. False positives may occur due to ureterovesical reflux or pyelitis (as opposed to pyelonephritis). The technique is excessively invasive for routine use but can be employed when the patient is undergoing cystoscopy for other indications.

Technique

1. The patient must be well hydrated.
2. The cystoscope is passed into the bladder, and urine is collected.
3. The bladder is washed with 1–2 liters of sterile irrigating solution and emptied.
4. A #5 French ureteral catheter is introduced into the bladder, the inflow

stopcocks are closed, and the irrigating solution is collected via the ureteral catheters. Growth in these specimens represents the maximal concentration of bacteria that could contaminate the ureteral specimens.

5. Ureteral catheters are quickly passed to the mid points of the ureters bilaterally. The cystoscope stopcocks are opened to ensure an empty bladder and prevent ureteral reflux.
6. Simultaneous paired urine samples are collected from each ureter for quantitative culture after the first 5–10 ml is discarded.

B. Fairley technique. The assumption is that a bladder rinse with antibiotics eliminates bacteria localized in the bladder, while those bacteria originating from the upper tract persist. There are, however, many false positives and equivocal results. On the other hand, the procedure is relatively benign and involves only a Foley catheter.

Technique

1. A Foley catheter is inserted.
2. The bladder is emptied and there is instilled into it a solution containing 50 ml of 0.1% neomycin (to sterilize the bladder) and two ampules of Elase or Varidase (to remove fibrinous exudate from the bladder wall).
3. The solution remains in the bladder for 30 minutes, and then the bladder is rinsed with 2–3 liters of sterile water.
4. The final bladder washout and three sequential 10-minute specimens are cultured quantitatively.
5. The criterion for upper tract infection is $> 10^3$ bacteria/ml in each postwashout sample. **Note:** Infection restricted to the bladder often is cured by this washout procedure.

C. Renal biopsy. This procedure is never indicated for the purpose of localizing urinary tract infections. Cultures may be performed when the biopsy is obtained for other reasons, and positive results are considered diagnostic. Negative cultures are meaningless, since the usual needle biopsy specimen consists of only about 10 mg of cortical tissue, and pyelonephritis usually is a focal disease involving primarily the medulla and calyxes.

D. Urine concentrating ability. Patients with bilateral upper tract infections generally are unable to concentrate their urine to > 800 mOsm/kg following fluid restriction and administration of antidiuretic hormone. The test is of limited use in routine practice, because of false negatives with unilateral upper tract disease and false positives with nonbacterial renal disease.

E. Serologic studies. These studies are available only in research laboratories.

1. **Circulating antibody.** A significant elevation in circulating antibody to the urinary pathogen is found in most cases of pyelonephritis but not with infections confined to the bladder. Most studies involve hemagglutination titers to somatic or K antigens of *E. coli*.
2. **Immunofluorescence of bacterial antigen in renal tissue.** The test uses antiserum against a common antigen in *E. coli* 014 that is shared by most Enterobacteriaceae. Specimens should consist of at least 250 mg of tissue obtained during a surgical procedure and should include medulla and calyxes. This procedure has proved useful in identifying infections as a cause of renal disease, even when urine and renal tissue cultures are negative.
3. **Indirect immunofluorescence test for antibody-coated bacteria in urine.** This method is used to distinguish pyelonephritis and cystitis, since secretion of antibody is supposed to be confined to the kidney. There may be an antibody coating of bacteria in the prostate, however, so the test may be subject to some inaccuracies in localizing the site of infection in males. For unknown reasons the test has also proved disappointing in females.

Respiratory Tract

I. General principles. Infections of the lung and pleural space represent the **lower respiratory tract,** and the pathogens may not be found necessarily in sputum and other secretions from the upper respiratory tract. A specimen's reliability in accurately reflecting the bacteriology of the lower respiratory tract is largely determined by the amount of oropharyngeal contamination during collection. A complex aerobic and anaerobic flora colonizes the upper airways, with concentrations of bacteria in oropharyngeal secretions in the range of 10^7–10^{10}/ml. The respiratory tract below the larynx is sterile in healthy individuals. The trachea and bronchi may become colonized with bacteria due to loss of normal clearing mechanisms in persons with chronic pulmonary disease, especially those with chronic bronchitis. On the basis of these observations, specimens for the diagnosis of pleuropulmonary infections can be divided into reliable and unreliable according to the absence or presence of microbial contaminants from the upper airways:

Reliable specimens (unlikely to be contaminated)
Transtracheal aspirate
Transthoracic lung aspiration
Empyema fluid
Bronchial brushing (transcricothyroid entry)
Blood culture

Unreliable specimens (likely to be contaminated)
Expectorated sputum
Nasopharyngeal aspirate
Bronchoscopy aspirate using the usual collection methods (see Sec. **IV**)
Endotracheal tube aspirates
Tracheostomy aspirates

The preferred specimens for implicating a specific pathogen depend on the biology of the organism, the ease of identifying it by conventional or special stains, and its ability to grow in the laboratory (Table 15-1). Another important consideration is whether antimicrobial treatment has been initiated, since antibiotics rapidly alter the cultivable flora of the lower respiratory tract. Thus, the optimal specimen is one from the reliable list, collected prior to antimicrobial treatment.

II. Expectorated sputum. A portion of purulent material is teased away from salivary secretions for Gram's stain and culture.

A. Gram's stain, to be considered significant, should show

1. Large numbers of polymorphonuclear leukocytes (PMNs).
2. A dominant bacterial morphotype with the likely pulmonary pathogen present in large numbers (10–100/HPF). The Gram's stain is often more reliable than the culture in establishing the pathogen, since the organism may be fastidious and may not survive transport and delayed processing.
3. Absence or paucity of large squamous epithelial cells. These cells are from the upper airway and indicate that saliva, and not sputum, is being examined.

B. Culture—processing and results:

1. Only specimens that are grossly purulent and show the absence or paucity of squamous epithelial cells on microscopic examination are suitable for culture.
2. Immediate processing of specimens increases the likelihood of reliable results.
3. Common lower respiratory tract pathogens (*Strep. pneumoniae* and *Hemophilus influenzae*) are relatively fastidious and easily overgrown by oropharyngeal contaminants.
4. Aerobic gram-negative bacilli and *Staph. aureus* are easily cultivated from sputum. Their absence in deep-coughed specimens generally excludes them as the pathogen in a pulmonary infection. However, these organisms often colonize the upper airways in hospitalized patients, so their presence in sputum does not necessarily indicate an etiologic role in infection.
5. Guidelines for interpretation of culture results are summarized in Table 15-2.

III. Nasopharyngeal aspiration. This is an alternative way to obtain sputum from patients unable to provide an adequate expectorated specimen. It should be appreciated that the catheter is contaminated by the nasopharyngeal flora during passage through the upper airways. Thus, interpretations of Gram's stain and culture have the same limitations as those for expectorated sputum.

Table 15-1. Preferred specimens for implicating specific agents of pulmonary infections

Agent	Specimens	Microscopy	Culture	Serology
Bacteria				
Aerobes	Expectorated sputum, uncontaminated specimens	Gram's stain	X	
Anaerobes	Uncontaminated specimens	Gram's stain	X[a]	
Legionella	Uncontaminated specimens	IFA, Dieterle	X[b]	micro IFA
Nocardia	Expectorated sputum, uncontaminated sputum	Gram's stain	X[a]	
Chlamydia	Nasopharyngeal swab, uncontaminated specimen	—	X[b]	CF, micro IFA
Mycoplasma	Expectorated sputum	—	X[b]	CF, IFA
Mycobacterium	Expectorated sputum, bronchoscopy aspirate, uncontaminated specimens	Carbolfuchsin Fluorochrome	X[a]	
Fungi				
Pathogenic	Expectorated sputum, uncontaminated specimen	KOH with phase contrast, GMS stain		
Blastomyces			X[a]	
Coccidoides			X[a]	CF, ID, LA
Histoplasma			X[a]	CF, ID
Opportunistic organisms				
Cryptococcus	Expectorated sputum	H&E, GMS	X[a]	LA
Phycomyces	Expectorated sputum, lung biopsy	H&E, GMS	X[a]	
Candida	Lung biopsy	H&E, GMS	X	
Aspergillus	Expectorated sputum, lung biopsy	H&E, GMS	X	ID
Viruses	Nasal washings, nasopharyngeal swab	—	X[b]	CF
Pneumocystis	Transthoracic aspirate and lung biopsy	H&E, GMS		

KOH = potassium hydroxide; GMS = Gomori methenamine silver; H&E = hematoxylin and eosin; IFA = immunofluorescent antibody; CF = complement fixation; ID = immunodiffusion; LA = latex agglutination.

[a] Indicates requirement for specialized media; the organism suspected should be indicated on the culture request.

[b] Most clinical microbiology laboratories do not culture viruses, *Legionella*, *Chlamydia*, or *Mycoplasma*.

Table 15-2. Interpretation of cultures in expectorated sputum

Organisms	Comment
Normal flora (colonizes upper airways of nearly all persons)	
α-Hemolytic *Streptococcus*	
Neisseria	
Hemophilus parainfluenzae	
Anaerobic streptococci	
Fusobacterium	
Actinomyces	
Bacteroides	Other than *B. fragilis*
Colonizers	Transient colonization in some persons
Streptococcus pneumoniae	Colonization rate of 10–40%, especially in winter, children, and patients with chronic lung disease
H. influenzae	Colonization rate of 20–60%
Neisseria meningitidis	Colonization rate of 5–15%
Staphylococcus aureus	Most frequently colonizes nasal mucosa
Coliforms, *Pseudomonas*	Colonization rate of 3–15% in healthy persons, 15–60% in patients, depending on severity of illness
Candida	Colonization rate of 20–50%, especially high in patients receiving antibiotics
Intruders	Presence implies active or potential disease
Mycobacterium tuberculosis	
Nocardia	
Legionella	
Blastomyces	
Coccidioides	
Histoplasma	
Cryptococcus	
Aspergillus	Although part of the normal flora, its isolation in a **susceptible** host usually indicative of infection

IV. Bronchoscopy aspirates. These specimens often are unreliable for microbiologic study for the following reasons:

A. Topical anesthetics, such as lidocaine (Xylocaine) solution, dilute the specimen and also are toxic to many bacteria, including *Mycobacterium tuberculosis*. The antibacterial effect can be minimized by using small amounts of the least toxic agent—lidocaine without preservatives. Specimens should be collected and processed rapidly to reduce the duration of contact between anesthetic and bacteria.

B. Bronchoscopes are invariably contaminated during passage through the upper airways, so specimens obtained from the instrument tip contain bacteria from the oropharynx. This contamination can be partially or completely avoided by using a commercially available double-lumen catheter with a protected plug at the distal end of the outer cannula. Topical anesthesia is achieved with nebulized Xylocaine or lidocaine. The catheter is passed into the lower airways, and the inner cannula is advanced to dislodge the protecting plug. The brush, on a retractable wire, is advanced to obtain the specimen, than retracted into the inner cannula, and the entire unit is removed. The brush is then severed from the wire and placed into 1 ml of diluent, and this is submitted for direct or quantitative bacteriologic analysis, using a 0.001-ml inoculating loop. Specimens obtained with the brush average 0.01 gm, so any growth generally reflects bacteria in concentrations exceeding 10^5/ml.

Two admonitions to remember with this technique are

1. Avoid injecting anesthetic solutions through the tube. This contaminates the lower airways with bacteria in oral secretions that collect during instrument passage.
2. Quantitative cultures are useful in distinguishing contaminants from true pathogens. Direct culture can be used, however, with caution in interpretation.

V. Tracheostomy and endotracheal tube aspirates. The lower respiratory tract rapidly becomes colonized following endotracheal intubation or tracheostomy. Endotracheal aspirates commonly yield multiple bacterial species, including *Staph. aureus,* coliforms, *Pseudomonas aeruginosa,* and *Candida.* The diagnosis of infection should be based primarily on **clinical grounds** (fever, dyspnea, purulent secretions, x-ray changes); the bacteriologic results are used as a guide to the likely pathogen.

VI. Transtracheal aspiration (TTA). This technique is a rapid and effective way to obtain bronchial secretions devoid of oropharyngeal contaminants. The procedure is safe, provided that the patient has no contraindications and the operator is experienced in the technique. TTA should be performed before treatment with antimicrobial drugs to ensure accurate results.

A. Indications. TTA should be performed when the etiology of a pulmonary infection is difficult to predict and the expected morbidity and mortality of the infection itself are relatively high. Examples are **hospital-acquired pneumonia, pneumonia in the compromised host,** and **necrotizing pneumonia.** Additionally, this procedure is useful for excluding bacterial infection in patients with pulmonary lesions of unknown etiology. A transtracheal aspirate that yields no pulmonary pathogens from a patient who has not received prior antimicrobial treatment virtually excludes bacterial infection.

B. Contraindications

1. Moderate or severe hemoptysis
2. Bleeding diathesis
3. Uncooperative patient
4. Severe dyspnea and uncorrected hypoxemia ($PO_2 < 50$ mm)
5. Pediatric patients (< 15 years)

C. Technique

1. The patient is placed in the supine position with the neck hyperextended. Patients receiving oxygen should have it continued during the procedure.
2. The notch between the lower border of the thyroid cartilage and the cricoid cartilage is prepared, draped, and infiltrated with 1–2% lidocaine containing epinephrine. (The epinephrine facilitates hemostasis.)
3. An intermediate-sized Intracath (14-gauge needle) is inserted through the cricothyroid membrane; it is angulated with the needle tip directed caudad, so that the catheter is passed into the trachea rather than the oropharynx.
4. The catheter is advanced quickly to its full extent into the lower trachea, almost invariably stimulating a vigorous cough reflex.
5. The needle is withdrawn, leaving the catheter in place.
6. Aspiration is performed with a tight-fitting 30-cc Luer-Lok syringe or, preferably, by suction into a Luken's trap. The Luken's trap is fitted with a Y connector to permit thumb control of suction.
7. Saline (without a bacteriostatic additive) may be injected into the catheter to facilitate aspiration. This should be avoided, however, because saline is toxic to some bacteria, and dilution of the specimen makes semiquantitative bacteriologic analysis impossible.
8. As soon as a few drops of secretion are obtained, the catheter should be rapidly withdrawn. Firm pressure is applied to the needle puncture site for several minutes.
9. Subsequent expectorations induced by the procedure can be collected for tuberculous and fungal cultures and for cytology.

D. Complications

1. Subcutaneous emphysema at the needle puncture site. This affects 10% of patients but is seldom severe and does not produce tracheal compression.

Occasional patients have soft-tissue emphysema involving the mediastinum, chest wall, or face.

2. Abscess at needle puncture site.
3. Vasovagal reaction with arrhythmias (atropine should be readily available).
4. Bleeding from a pulmonary lesion or at the needle puncture site (rare when patients with contraindications are avoided).
5. Severe dyspnea and hypoxemia during coughing paroxysm.

VII. Transthoracic lung puncture aspiration

A. Indications

Similar to those for TTA, although TTA is generally preferred because of fewer complications. Principal indications for transthoracic aspiration are as follows:

1. Patients with certain contraindications to TTA, especially those in the pediatric age group.
2. When TTA is negative or inconclusive, especially in the compromised host. Transthoracic aspiration is more likely to reveal the pathogen in cases of nocardiosis and aspergillosis.

B. Contraindications

1. Bullous pulmonary disease
2. Bleeding diathesis (platelet transfusions may correct this defect in thrombocytopenic patients)
3. Severe lung disease in which a pneumothorax could not be tolerated
4. Pleural effusion or empyema overlying the parenchymal lesion
5. Lesions localized to areas adjacent to the heart or major vessels

C. Technique

1. The area of involvement is determined by posteroanterior and lateral chest x-rays.
2. An appropriate location along a superior rib margin is prepared; local anesthesia is optional.
3. The midaxillary line is the preferred site of aspiration in patients with diffuse pulmonary involvement. Small or deep lesions require localization under fluoroscopy.
4. Aspiration is performed with a 20- or 22-gauge needle, 1½ inches or longer, depending on the thickness of the chest wall and the depth of the infiltrate. The needle is rapidly inserted and withdrawn slowly under constant suction. When possible, the patient should be instructed to hold his breath or to take shallow respirations.
5. The specimen is stained and cultured for bacteria, fungi, and mycobacteria. Suggested stains are Gram's, acid-fast bacteria, and methenamine silver (for fungi and *Pneumocystis carinii*).

D. Complications

1. Pneumothorax: 20% of patients develop a small pneumothorax; about 1% will require a chest tube.
2. Intrapulmonary hemorrhage
3. Empyema

VIII. Thoracentesis

A. Indications. All patients with undiagnosed pleural effusions should have a thoracentesis. The only contraindication is a severe bleeding diathesis.

B. Method

1. The site of needle penetration is determined by auscultation and upright x-rays of the chest.
2. The skin is prepared and infiltrated with lidocaine at a point low in an intercostal space to avoid injury to intercostal vessels and nerves.
3. An intracatheter, attached to a three-way stopcock and syringe, is inserted until fluid is encountered. The syringe and stopcock are then disconnected, and the needle is occluded with a gloved finger to avoid air entry. A straight needle, without intracatheter, can also be used, by attaching it directly to the three-way stopcock.
4. The intracatheter is inserted through the needle and directed downward. The needle is then withdrawn, leaving the catheter in proper position and

taped to the chest wall. (The needle is withdrawn to prevent trauma to the lung surface during aspiration.)

5. The syringe and stopcock are attached to the catheter, and fluid is aspirated.
6. When larger needles are used, the puncture site should be packed with petroleum jelly gauze.

C. Complications

1. Pneumothorax (from external air entry or lung surface trauma)
2. Intrapleural hemorrhage (rare, except in patients with bleeding diathesis or improper needle placement through intercostal vessels)
3. Pulmonary edema due to rapid removal of excessive quantities of fluid

D. Fluid analysis

1. Cell count—red and white blood cells, with differential
2. Cytology
3. Gram's stain and acid-fast stain
4. Glucose, total protein, LDH, amylase, and pH
5. Culture—aerobic, anaerobic, fungal, and mycobacterial
6. Rheumatoid factor and complement level (if indicated)

Soft-Tissue Infections

I. Wound cultures

A. Wound preparation. Extensive surface contamination is to be anticipated with open wounds such as burns, decubitus ulcers, and traumatic injuries. The area should be carefully debrided prior to culture. Surface preparation is accomplished by cleansing from the center of the wound outward in a concentric fashion, using 70% isopropyl alcohol and povidone-iodine (Betadine) or similar agents. The antiseptic should be air-dried or wiped dry with sterile pads prior to specimen collection.

B. Specimen collection

1. **Aspirates** of exudate should be collected from the depths of the wound, preferably with a large-bore needle or polyethylene catheter attached to a syringe. If no exudate is obtained, an adequate liquid specimen can usually be produced by massaging the wound edge.
2. **Tissue** specimens can be obtained by excision from the wound edge with a scalpel or punch biopsy.
3. **Swabs are considered inferior culture sources compared to liquid or tissue specimens.** When necessary, the swab specimens should be obtained from the depths of the wound.

II. Quantitative tissue cultures. Quantitative culture of wound tissue has proved useful in predicting wound sepsis and delayed healing. This approach is predicated on the hypothesis that bacteria within the tissue are more important than those on the surface, and that bacteria reach a critical concentration prior to overt infection.

A. Applications. Significant tissue concentrations of bacteria ($>10^5$–10^6 bacteria/gm) herald septic wound complications. This type of analysis has proved to be a useful predictor in the following clinical settings: **skin graft survival, burn wound sepsis, healing of decubitus ulcers,** and **successful secondary closure of granulating wounds.**

B. Technique

1. Cleanse the open wound with 70% isopropyl alcohol.
2. Obtain a tissue biopsy with a 3–4-mm dermal punch or scalpel. Weigh the specimen aseptically.
3. Dip the specimen in isopropyl alcohol, flame it briefly to remove surface contamination, and place it in a measured volume of thioglycollate broth to achieve a 1:10 dilution (1 gm tissue/10 ml broth).
4. Following homogenization, perform four serial 10-fold dilutions (1:10–1:100,000) in saline and plate an aliquot (0.1 ml) onto appropriate media for aerobic and anaerobic incubation.

C. **Interpretation.** Conceptions of 10^5–10^6 bacteria/gm tissue are considered significant. *Strep. pyogenes* (group A β-hemolytic *Streptococcus*) is an exception, since this organism can cause infection even when initially present in low concentrations.

D. **Gram's stain.** The same approach can be used to obtain a specimen for Gram's stain in order to provide immediate information. The method described in **B** is followed to obtain a 1:10 thioglycollate dilution. Exactly 0.02 ml of this suspension is spread on a glass slide with a 20-lambda Sahli pipette. The slide is oven-dried (15 minutes at 75°C) and Gram's stained. If any bacteria are observed in the entire specimen the count is considered to be $\geq 10^5$/gm.

III. **Soft-tissue abscess**

A. **Undrained lesion.** The surface is prepared with antiseptic, and exudate is collected by needle aspirate or surgical incision.

B. **Previously drained lesions** (either spontaneously or surgically). Exudate is obtained either by (1) needle aspiration at an area away from the drainage site or (2) through the drainage site after careful surface preparation to remove superficial exudate.

IV. **Cellulitis.** Needle aspiration is performed at the advancing edge of inflammation, usually with a 22–26-gauge needle. It may be necessary to inject lactated Ringer's solution or saline (without preservative) to obtain a specimen. **Note:** Pathogens cannot be recovered by this method in many cases of active infection.

V. **Intravenous catheter sites**

A. The optimal specimen is exudate from the needle site, obtained after surface preparation and milking of the involved vein.

B. Polyethylene catheter tips can be withdrawn after surface preparation, cut with sterile scissors, and deposited in fluid culture medium.

C. **Note:** Care must be taken to interpret clinical and bacteriologic observations properly. Many intravenous infusions (especially those containing cephalosporins, tetracyclines, erythromycin or amphotericin B) cause a chemical phlebitis that may be difficult to distinguish from infection. The isolation of *Staph. epidermidis,* diphtheroids, and *Propionibacterium* usually is of little concern, since they are skin flora and generally represent colonization or contamination. Blood cultures from another vein should be obtained from any patient who is septic.

VI. **Bullae, blebs, and vesicles.** Intact lesions are preferred; these should be aspirated after careful surface preparation.

VII. **Fistulae and sinus tracts.** Adjacent skin surfaces are prepared, and exudate is aspirated with a needle or polyethylene cannula inserted to the depths of the lesion. If no fluid is available, and none can be expressed, a swab is inserted.

Body Fluids

I. Pericardial, pleural, peritoneal, synovial, or cerebrospinal fluid is collected after appropriate skin surface preparation.

II. These fluids may require the addition of sterile anticoagulant (heparin or sodium oxalate) to prevent clotting.

III. Thick, purulent specimens should be examined with direct Gram's stain. Thin (watery) specimens can be centrifuged for Gram's stain.

Biopsy Material

I. Biopsy material should be divided, one portion for histologic study and the other for culture.

II. The portion for culture is placed in a sterile tube or Petri dish **without fixative** for immediate transfer to the laboratory.

III. If any delay in processing is anticipated, the specimen should be placed in a sterile liquid broth to avoid drying.

Stool

I. **Cultures.** Routine stool cultures are generally examined for *Salmonella, Shigella* and *Campylobacter* only. *Campylobacter* is the most important of this list; at present, it is being isolated in 5–15% of cases of diarrhea, even outnumbering *Salmonella* and *Shigella* in many communities. It is our view that serotyping for enteropathogenic *E. coli* should not be performed for sporadic cases of diarrhea, but rather reserved for epidemic situations, especially in the newborn nursery. *Yersinia,* enterotoxigenic and invasive *E. coli,* and vibrios require specialized techniques that may not be available in all microbiology laboratories.

II. **Methylene blue stool examination for fecal leukocytes.** A fleck of mucus or stool is mixed with two drops of methylene blue, and a coverslip is put on it. The specimen is examined under low power for cells and under high power for a differential count. Less than 10 WBC/HPF is noted in normal conditions and in most diarrheal illnesses, including those caused by enterotoxin-producing organisms such as *Vibrio cholerae,* enterotoxigenic *E. coli,* and food-poisoning strains of *Staph. aureus* and *Clostridium perfringens,* viral gastroenteritis, and most antibiotic-induced diarrheas. The presence of over 10 WBC/HPF suggests bacillary dysentery caused by *Shigella* or invasive *E. coli; Campylobacter; Yersinia;* inflammatory bowel disease; antibiotic-associated colitis; or *Salmonella.*

Index

The Little, Brown SPIRAL® Manual Series

Little, Brown, SPIRAL® manuals are available at all medical bookstores. You may also order copies from Little, Brown by filling in and mailing this postage-paid card.

☐ MANUAL OF **MEDICAL THERAPEUTICS,** 24th Edition — Washington University Department of Medicine: Frietag & Miller, Editors (#923958) **U.S. $16.95**/Can. $21.95*

☐ MANUAL OF **CLINICAL PROBLEMS IN INTERNAL MEDICINE:** ANNOTATED WITH KEY REFERENCES, 3rd Edition — Spivak & Barnes (#807168) **U.S. $17.95**/Can. $22.95*

☐ PROBLEM-ORIENTED **MEDICAL DIAGNOSIS,** 3rd Edition — Friedman, Editor (#293598) **U.S. $16.95**/Can. $21.95*

☐ MANUAL OF **CLINICAL PROBLEMS IN INFECTIOUS DISEASE:** WITH ANNOTATED KEY REFERENCES — Gantz & Gleckman (#303518) **U.S. $16.95**/Can. $21.95*

☐ MANUAL OF **ACUTE BACTERIAL INFECTIONS** — Gardner & Provine (#303275) **U.S. $16.95**/Can. $21.95*

☐ MANUAL OF **CORONARY CARE,** 3nd Edition — Alpert & Francis (#035084) **U.S. $16.95**/Can. $21.95*

☐ MANUAL OF **CARDIOVASCULAR DIAGNOSIS AND THERAPY** — Alpert & Rippe (#035025) **U.S. $16.95**/Can. $21.95*

☐ MANUAL OF **CLINICAL PROBLEMS IN CARDIOLOGY:** WITH ANNOTATED KEY REFERENCES, 2nd Ed. — Hillis, Firth, & Willerson (#364010) **U.S. $16.95**/Can. $21.95*

☐ MANUAL OF **ELECTROCARDIOGRAPHY** — Mudge (#589179) **U.S. $14.95**/Can. $18.95*

☐ MANUAL OF **CLINICAL PROBLEMS IN PULMONARY MEDICINE:** WITH ANNOTATED KEY REFERENCES — Bordow, Stool & Moser (#102644) **U.S. $16.95**/Can. $21.95*

☐ MANUAL OF **SURGICAL THERAPEUTICS,** 5th Edition — Condon & Nyhus, Editors (#152692) **U.S. $16.95**/Can. $21.95*

☐ MANUAL OF **MEDICAL CARE OF THE SURGICAL PATIENT,** 2nd Edition — Papper & Williams (#690481) **U.S. $15.95**/Can. $19.95*

☐ MANUAL OF **EMERGENCY AND OUTPATIENT TECHNIQUES** — Klippel & Anderson, Editors (#498688) **U.S. $16.95**/Can. $21.95*

☐ MANUAL OF **ACUTE ORTHOPAEDIC THERAPEUTICS,** 2nd Edition — Iversen & Clawson (#434310) **U.S. $15.95**/Can. $19.95*

☐ MANUAL OF **PEDIATRIC THERAPEUTICS,** 2nd Edition — Children's Hospital Medical Center, Boston; Graef & Cone, Editors (#139114) **U.S. $17.95**/Can. $22.95*

☐ MANUAL OF **PATIENT CARE IN VASCULAR SURGERY** — Hallett, Brewster & Darling (#340502) **U.S. $16.95**/Can. $21.95*

☐ MANUAL OF **CANCER CHEMOTHERAPY** — Skeel (#795720) **U.S. $15.95**/Can. $19.95*

☐ MANUAL OF **INTRODUCTORY CLINICAL MEDICINE:** A STUDENT-TO-STUDENT GUIDE — Macklis, Mendelsohn & Mudge (#542466) **U.S. $14.95**/Can. $18.95*

☐ MANUAL OF **CLINICAL PROBLEMS IN SURGERY:** WITH ANNOTATED KEY REFERENCES — Cutler, Dodson, Silva & Vander Salm (#165751) **U.S. $18.95**/Can. $24.95*

☐ MANUAL OF **CLINICAL PROBLEMS IN PEDIATRICS:** WITH ANNOTATED KEY REFERENCES — Roberts, Editor (#749842) **U.S. $16.95**/Can. $21.95*

☐ MANUAL OF **NEONATAL CARE** — Cloherty & Stark (#147494) **U.S. $16.95**/Can. $21.95*

☐ MANUAL OF **OBSTETRICS,** 2nd Edition — Niswander (#611417) **U.S. $16.95**/Can. $21.95*

☐ MANUAL OF **ANESTHESIA,** 2nd Edition — Snow (#802220) **U.S. $16.95**/Can. $21.95*

☐ MANUAL OF **NEUROLOGIC THERAPEUTICS,** 2nd Edition — Samuels, Editor (#769916) **U.S. $16.95**/Can. $21.95*

☐ MANUAL OF **PSYCHIATRIC THERAPEUTICS** — Shader, Editor (#782203) **U.S. $15.95**/Can. $19.95*

☐ MANUAL OF PATIENT CARE IN **NEUROSURGERY,** 2nd Edition — Howe (#375756) **U.S. $16.95**/Can. $21.95*

☐ MANUAL OF **RHEUMATOLOGY AND OUTPATIENT ORTHOPEDIC DISORDERS** — Beary, Christian, & Sculco (#085758) **U.S. $15.95**/Can. $19.95*

☐ MANUAL OF **ALLERGY AND IMMUNOLOGY** — Lawlor & Fischer (#516651) **U.S. $17.95**/Can. $22.95*

☐ MANUAL OF **DERMATOLOGIC THERAPEUTICS,** 3rd Edition — Arndt (#051810) **U.S. $15.95**/Can. $19.95*

☐ MANUAL OF **OCULAR DIAGNOSIS AND THERAPY** — Pavan-Langston (#695378) **U.S. $16.95**/Can. $21.95*

☐ MANUAL OF **CLINICAL PROBLEMS IN ONCOLOGY:** WITH ANNOTATED KEY REFERENCES — Portlock & Goffinet (#714240) **U.S. $16.95**/Can. $21.95*

☐ MANUAL OF **NEPHROLOGY** — Schrier (#774774) **U.S. $15.95**/Can. $19.95*

☐ MANUAL OF **CARDIAC SURGERY,** 3rd Edition — Behrendt & Austen (#087564) **U.S. $16.95**/Can. $21.95*

☐ MANUAL OF **ACUTE RESPIRATORY CARE** — Zagelbaum & Pare, Editors (#984671) **U.S. $15.95**/Can. $19.95*

☐ MANUAL OF **CLINICAL PROBLEMS IN OBSTETRICS AND GYNECOLOGY:** WITH ANNOTATED KEY REFERENCES — Rivlin, Morrison & Bates (#747645) **U.S. $16.95**/Can. $21.95*

☐ MANUAL OF **PATIENT CARE IN PLASTIC SURGERY** — Barrett (#082171) **U.S. $18.95**/Can. $24.95*

☐ MANUAL OF **BURN THERAPEUTICS** — Salisbury, Newman & Dingeldein (#769584) **U.S. $15.95**/Can. $19.95*

☐ MANUAL OF **BEDSIDE ONCOLOGY** — Casciato & Lowitz (#130680) **U.S. $17.95**/Can. $22.95*

☐ MANUAL OF **NUTRITIONAL THERAPEUTICS** — Alpers, Clouse & Stenson (#035092) **U.S. $16.95**/Can. $21.95*

☐ MANUAL OF **INTENSIVE CARE MEDICINE** — Rippe & Csete (#747084) **U.S. $16.95**/Can. $21.95

☐ MANUAL OF **CLINICAL PROBLEMS IN NEUROLOGY:** WITH ANNOTATED KEY REFERENCES — Mohr (#577472) **U.S. $18.95**/Can. $24.95*

☐ MANUAL OF **CLINICAL PROBLEMS IN ASTHMA, ALLERGY** AND RELATED DISORDERS: WITH ANNOTATED KEY REFERENCES — Bukstein & Strunk (#114731) **U.S. $18.95**/Can. $24.95*

NAME ______________________________

ADDRESS ______________________________

CITY ______________________________

STATE & ZIP ______________________________

☐ **My check for $**__________ **is enclosed.** Publisher pays postage and handling. MA, CA, NY residents please add state sales tax.

☐ **Please bill me for book(s) plus postage and handling.** (Outside continental U.S.A., payment *must* accompany order.)

HANDLING CHARGE: 50¢ per book, not to exceed $2.50 per total order.

T denotes a tentative price. Prices listed are Little, Brown prices, current as of May 31, 1984, and do not reflect the prices at which books will be sold to you by suppliers other than Little, Brown. All prices subject to change without notice.

***CANADA:** Order directly from Little, Brown (Canada) Ltd., Medical Division, 25 Hollinger Rd., Toronto, Ontario M4B 3G2. Note special Canadian prices in Canadian dollars.